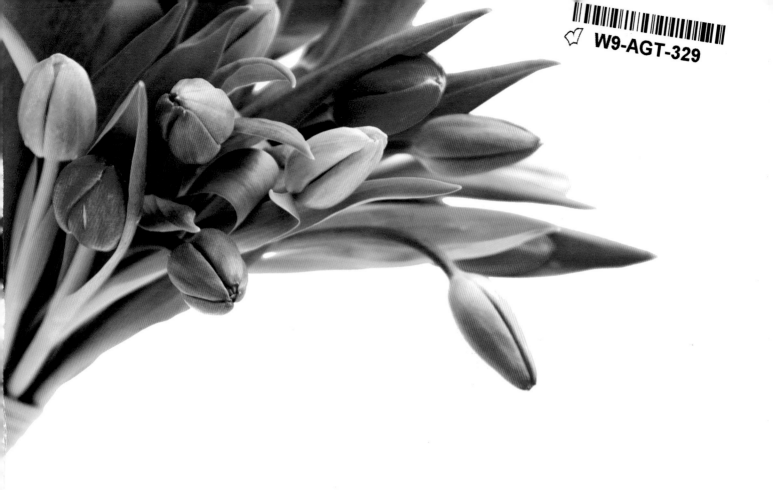

W9-AGT-329

Breast cancer has invaded my body,
but it need not invade my spirit.

There may be scars on my chest,
but there need not be scars on my heart.

—Judy Kneece

Breast Cancer
Treatment Handbook

Understanding the Disease, Treatments, Emotions and Recovery from Breast Cancer

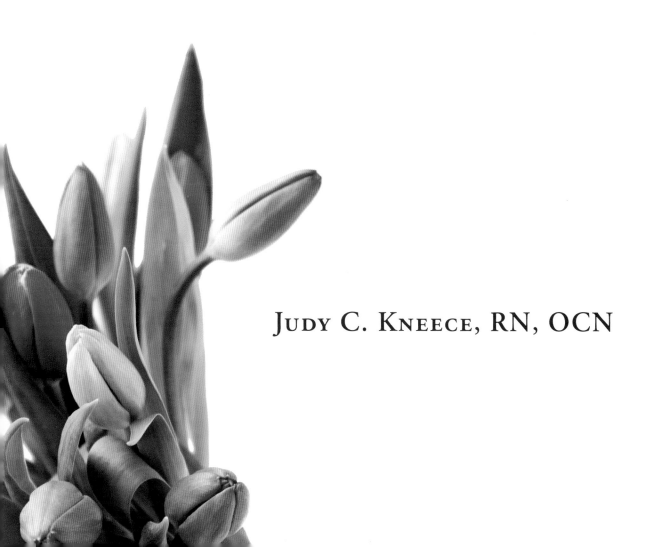

Judy C. Kneece, RN, OCN

Copyright © 2009 Judy C. Kneece, RN, OCN

All rights reserved. Reproduction or use of editorial or pictorial content in any manner is prohibited without written permission, except in the case of brief quotations embodied in articles or reviews. Readers accessing an on-line version of this work in an authorized manner are permitted to download or print one copy for personal viewing. Other reproduction, distribution or use of copyrightable content without the express written consent of the copyright owner is prohibited. Permission can be requested by contacting the author at: 3294 Ashley Phosphate Rd., Ste. 1-A, North Charleston, SC 29418.

No patent liability is assumed with respect to the use of the information contained herein. While every precaution has been taken in the preparation of this book, the publisher and author assume no responsibility for errors or omissions. Neither is any liability assumed for damages resulting from the use of the information contained herein. This book has been written to enlighten patients and motivate them to discuss the issues with their healthcare team. Each patient should determine the best treatment protocol based on physicians' recommendations and her own needs, assessments and desires.

All trademarks used in this book are the property of their respective owners.

2011: 7th Revised Edition; 2009: 7th Edition; 2005: 6th Edition; 2003: 5th Edition; 2001: 4th Edition; 1998: 3rd Edition; 1997: 2nd Edition; 1995: 1st Edition
ISBN: 978-1-886665-23-1
Library of Congress Card Number: 2009931734
Printed in the United States of America
Published by EduCareInc.com

To order:

EduCare
3294 Ashley Phosphate Road, Suite 1-A
North Charleston, SC 29418
1-800-849-9271 or Fax: 843-760-6988
www.educareinc.com or www.breasthealthcare.com

Illustrations: Debra Strange, Setsuko Lawson

Publisher's Cataloging-In-Publication Data
(Prepared by The Donohue Group, Inc.)

Kneece, Judy C.
    Breast cancer treatment handbook : understanding the disease, treatments, emotions and recovery from breast cancer / Judy C. Kneece.—7th ed.

        p. : ill. ; cm.

    Originally published as: Your breast cancer treatment handbook : a patient's guide to understanding the disease, treatment options, and the physical and emotional recovery from breast cancer.
    Includes bibliographical references and index.
    ISBN: 978-1-886665-23-1

1. Breast--Cancer--Patients. 2. Cancer--Treatment. I. Title.

RC280.B8 K54 2009
616.99/44906   2009931734

Dedication

This book is dedicated to all of the brave women and their families who have faced the pain of diagnosis and the challenge of emotional recovery from breast cancer and now serve as an inspiration for this handbook.

My appreciation is extended to the hundreds of women and families who shared openly and honestly as I served as their Breast Health Navigator. I am also grateful for the hundreds of breast cancer survivors who participated in national focus groups and shared their cancer experiences so that others could learn from their struggles and victories. Their openness about their fears, questions, challenges and hopes during their breast cancer journey made this book possible. From the privilege of being there with them, I learned the basic education and recovery needs of women diagnosed with breast cancer. They shared their struggles and how they learned to cope so that other patients could benefit from their journey.

This is also dedicated to the nurses and physicians with whom I have worked and learned. I am especially grateful to Henry Patrick Leis, Jr., M.D., F.A.C.S., a dedicated breast surgeon and one of the pioneers in breast care. He served as my first tutor in the medical management of breast disease.

To the two thousand Nurse Navigators I have trained to work with patients during the past fifteen years, I pass the torch of caring. Their encouragement to continue writing educational support materials has kept me motivated.

My gratefulness is extended to my support staff that made this Seventh Edition a reality: Heather Bennett for editorial guidance; Jerri White and Saralyn White for editorial assistance; Bianca Schumacher for graphic design and layout; Nicole Cendrowski for cover concept; Debra Strange and Setsuko Lawson for medical illustrations; and to Mindy Wilson for her support in all aspects of the project. Their dedication to serve breast cancer patients unselfishly brought this project to fruition.

Finally, to my husband, Dr. Robert Karl Hetz, who served as my cheerleader and surprisingly had to learn to be a "nurse" after I broke all of the bones in my ankle during the writing of this edition. His unceasing support made it possible for me to keep writing against all odds.

Someone once asked, "Have you had breast cancer?" My reply was, "No, my body has not, but my heart has been diagnosed hundreds of times as I shared the pain my patients and family members were feeling as they walked through their unexpected journey with cancer." It is to those of you who now face the same experience that I make this final dedication. You are the reason for this book!

Acknowledgements

A special word of appreciation to the following people for their contributions to this work:

Peg Baim, MS, NP, Associate in Medicine, Harvard Medical School; Clinical Director, Center for Training, Benson Henry Institute of Mind/Body Medicine at Massachusetts General Hospital

Susan Casella, RN, OCN, Breast Health Coordinator, Northside Hospital, Atlanta, Georgia

Calvin Chao, MD, Director, Medical Affairs, Genomic Health, Inc.

Anna Cluxton, MBA, Survivor; President, Young Survival Coalition, Columbus, Ohio

Edward P. Dalton, MD, FACS, Elliot Hospital Breast Center, Manchester, New Hampshire; Past President, National Consortium of Breast Centers

Carla J. Daniels, MSN, AOCNP, Springfield Clinic, Oncology Department, Springfield, Illinois

Jennifer L. Harper, MD, Assistant Professor of Radiation Oncology, Medical University of South Carolina

Robert Karl Hetz, MD, Family Practice, Charleston, South Carolina

Kevin Hughes, MD, FACS, Surgical Director, Avon Foundation Comprehensive Breast Evaluation Center, Massachusetts General; Co-Director, Breast and Ovarian Cancer Genetics and Risk Assessment Program; Assistant Professor of Surgery, Harvard Medical School

George P. Keogh, MD, Medical Oncologist, Charleston Hematology Oncology Associates, Charleston, South Carolina

Karl Kibler, DC, East Cooper Rehabilitation and Pilates, Charleston, South Carolina

Rosemary Lambert-Falls, MD, Medical Oncologist, Columbia, South Carolina

Lisa Martinez, RN, BSNM, JD, Survivor, Founder and Executive Director of The Women's Sexual Health Foundation, Cleveland, Ohio

Maurice Nahabedian, MD, FACS, Associate Professor of Plastic Surgery, Georgetown University, Washington, DC

Stephanie D. Page, MSPT, MBA, Premier Physical Therapy, North Charleston, South Carolina

John S. Ravita, MD, FACRO, Medical Director, Georgia Center for Total Cancer Care at Cowles Clinic, Greensboro, Georgia

Ervin Shaw, MD, Chief of Pathology, Lexington Medical Center, West Columbia, South Carolina

Harriett Barrineau, Earnestine Brown and *Anna Cluxton,* The Voices of Experience, Breast Cancer Survivors

Debbie Metts, Breast Cancer Survivor

Bianca Schumacher, Graphic Design and Layout

Jerri White, Graphic Design Production

Nicole Cendrowski, Cover Concept

Debra Strange and *Setsuko Lawson,* Medical Illustrators

About the Author

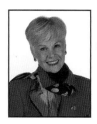

Judy C. Kneece, RN, OCN, is a certified oncology nurse with a specialty in breast cancer. She began her career as a Breast Health Navigator in a hospital where she developed her concept of nursing patient navigation in 1991. She started EduCare Inc. to train other nurses as Breast Health Navigators and to write educational information for breast cancer patients in 1994.

During the past seventeen years, EduCare has been a leader in developing educational materials and in training nurses to support breast cancer patients. Judy has trained over 2,000 registered nurses to fill the Breast Health Navigator role in hospitals, breast centers and physicians' offices. Her forty-hour training program focuses on patient education, support and bridging the gaps between specialties. In 1998, she began holding Comprehensive Strategic Planning trainings for breast centers and hospital administrators. Over 500 hospitals and breast centers have used her principles to implement breast care programs that emphasize pre-treatment interdisciplinary care conferences and the role of the Nurse Navigator.

The first edition of the *Breast Cancer Treatment Handbook* was published in 1995. This patient handbook has been in continuous publication and is now in its seventh edition. A companion book for the support person, the *Breast Cancer Support Partner Handbook* was also published in 1995 and is being released in its seventh edition. Judy has authored three other books and created the COPE Library, a collection of 427 topics designed to help nurses and doctors support and educate their patients.

Her background working in a hospital as a Breast Health Navigator gave her new insights into the needs of women and their families going through breast cancer. Judy has also done extensive research on the experiences of breast cancer patients by holding national focus groups on the struggle with breast cancer, recurrent breast cancer and sexuality issues after chemotherapy treatments. Her research serves as a basis for understanding the breast cancer experience and the needs of patients and their families.

Judy presently serves as a national consultant for breast centers and hospitals in the area of developing and implementing a comprehensive educational and support program for breast cancer patients. She has served as a contributing editor for numerous national women's magazines on the issues of breast health and cancer and speaks widely to patients on triumphant survivorship.

Quoted in *Cope* Magazine, Judy says, "Empowering patients with an understanding of their disease, treatment options and providing tools for recovery management are essential for complete recovery. Breast cancer is more than scars on the breast; it can also scar the heart. We must address the psychological and social issues breast cancer brings if a woman is to successfully manage her disease. Getting well is more than surgery and treatments; it is a woman understanding the vital role she can play in managing her own recovery."

You Are Not Alone...

Unwanted as the diagnosis must be, you have joined a host of other women who have experienced the overwhelming anxiety of hearing the words, "You have breast cancer," and are now living examples of survivorship. Among those survivors are:

Christina Applegate	Rue McClanahan
Shirley Temple Black	Martina Navratilova
Diahann Carroll	Olivia Newton-John
Sheryl Crow	Cynthia Nixon
Jill Eikenberry	Justice Sandra Day O'Connor
Linda Ellerbee	Nancy Reagan
Melissa Etheridge	Cokie Roberts
Edie Falco	Robin Roberts
Peggy Flemming	Happy Rockefeller
Betty Ford	Betty Rollin
Laura Ingraham	Carly Simon
Kate Jackson	Jaclyn Smith
Ann Jillian	Suzanne Somers
Hoda Kotb	René Syler
Evelyn Lauder	Marcia Wallace

As you can see from this list, although breast cancer is an unwelcome experience, it is one that can add depth and influence to your life. These well-known women are now advocates in education and support for other women living with cancer. As you begin your journey to understand and recover from breast cancer, be assured that you, too, can master the experience. You can learn, as they learned, how to take the crisis of breast cancer and transform it into an opportunity for personal growth. You can become a triumphant survivor.

"Seeds of faith are always within us; sometimes it takes a crisis to nourish and encourage their growth."

—Susan Taylor

Dear Survivor

I almost began this letter "Dear Patient," but then I changed my mind. I do not want you to see yourself or think of yourself as only a patient. You will be a patient for a short time. You will be a survivor for the rest of your life. I want you to know that you are, from the innermost parts of your being, a breast cancer survivor.

"You have breast cancer" are four words that have changed your life. A cancer diagnosis is most often an unexpected journey—a journey that you did not choose. Cancer has not only invaded your body, but your life. It has interrupted all of your plans and probably left you feeling unprepared to face this new challenge. If you feel this way, you are sharing the feelings of thousands of other women after their diagnoses. Diane Rice said shortly after her diagnosis, "The first 24 hours were dreadful for me because I didn't have any answers and didn't know who would help me find them. For me, losing control over what was happening in my life was the most difficult part."

Like Diane, most women find that not knowing what to do and what is ahead—the loss of personal control over their bodies and their lives—is the hardest part to deal with. Most likely, this may be your feeling. How do you regain your control? This is my job. From my personal experience, first as a Breast Health Navigator working directly with patients and then in seventeen years of training other Breast Health Navigators to educate and support patients, I write this book as your guide. In the following chapters of this book, I will lead you through the process of regaining your control. We will go step-by-step through breast cancer treatment and recovery, but this book is about more than breast cancer treatment. It is about you regaining your control and planning to emerge stronger, emotionally and physically.

Your goal is to convert your emotional distress and helplessness into a plan for action. The challenge is to take this time to make positive changes and emerge with a new and improved life. At this time in your diagnosis, this statement may seem trite. The truth is that no one likes the process, but people most often emerge stronger from their personal struggles with cancer. Now is the time to re-examine your life and plan how you want to redefine your life's goals.

Cancer is certainly not a good thing, but good things can come from the cancer experience. Let's get started on our journey to making cancer a positive change. By learning about your disease, you are beginning your journey to survivorship like millions of other women.

It is my privilege to share this journey with you,

Judy

The Voices of Experience

As I worked with newly diagnosed breast cancer patients, I quickly learned the value of their early interaction with other women who had experienced breast cancer. They needed to talk to a peer who had survived all of the decisions that they were going to have to make over the next weeks and months. While writing this guide for you, I immediately decided to include other women's experiences with breast cancer so that you, too, could benefit from what they have learned. To serve as your peers throughout this book, three women from very different situations share their experiences, fears and thoughts on their journeys with breast cancer. Let me introduce you to Harriett Barrineau, Anna Cluxton and Earnestine Brown.

Harriett's Story

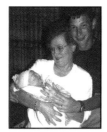

Harriett was diagnosed with breast cancer in 1991 at the age of 44. At the time of diagnosis, she was married and had four sons. Today she also has four daughters-in-law and eight grandchildren. Harriett says, "This is what survival means."

Because of the characteristics of her tumor, she had a modified radical mastectomy and followed her surgery with chemotherapy. Over a year later, the resulting posture shift caused back pain and spurred Harriet's decision to have a prophylactic second mastectomy and immediate bilateral reconstruction.

As a Breast Health Navigator, I had the opportunity to work with Harriett. She often shared her fears, feelings, failures and triumphs during her breast cancer experience. Her honest and insightful reflections during her diagnosis, treatment and recovery are a source of comfort to other women who are just beginning their journeys. Harriett openly shares with other women what she has experienced. She tells them that they will not always feel hopeless and that there are going to be problems, but that with determination, they, too, can make it. She is the epitome of survivorship—the quality of using present coping skills and learning new skills to triumph over a seemingly insurmountable task.

Today, Harriett works full-time in her husband's accounting firm and has served as a Reach to Recovery volunteer. Harriett remembers how after her diagnosis, she searched for people who would share with her the ins and outs of the experience.

Harriett's quotes in this book serve as the voice of one who personally knows the perils of the journey you are undertaking; she is a woman who has been where you are and where you are going—a woman who has survived! Al, her husband, provides the same type of commentary in the *Breast Cancer Support Partner Handbook*.

Anna's Story

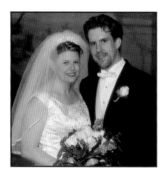

*A*nna was 32 years old and single when she noticed a flattened area below her left nipple. She performed monthly breast self-exams, but she had never felt anything different in this area. Gradually, she noticed that the area would flatten out more when she raised her arm. Anna mentally dismissed it as hormonal changes or recent weight loss, but continued to keep her eye on it. She had other important things to do—she was planning her wedding.

The wedding went as planned without any problems. She and her new husband, Brian, went to Jamaica for their honeymoon. During the trip, she noticed that she could now feel a lump under the flattened area of her breast. When they arrived home, she called her OB/GYN, who performed an ultrasound. The doctor immediately decided a mammogram was needed. Anna saw a surgeon and had a fine needle biopsy seven days after she had been sitting on the beach in Jamaica. Twenty minutes after the biopsy, she was told that it looked positive for cancer. "Brian and I were completely shocked," Anna told me. "I can't even remember what else the doctor said to us after those words."

One month after the wedding, Anna underwent seven hours of surgery for a mastectomy with an immediate TRAM flap reconstruction. All 16 lymph nodes removed during the surgery came back negative. Anna had chemotherapy. The day of her first chemo treatment, Brian shaved his head to show his support. "When other couples are supposed to be starting their new life together, Brian was sitting on the bathroom floor holding me as I was throwing up."

Anna recalls the experience: "Cancer changed our lives as individuals and as a couple. I was young—too young for breast cancer, some would think. But I learned from experience that breast cancer does happen to young women. I also learned that having cancer at an early age brings different types of problems to a woman and her spouse. Because of this I became involved in the Young Survival Coalition, an organization focused on supporting young women with breast cancer. I went on to get my MBA in healthcare administration and work in breast health. I am presently serving as President of the Young Survival Coalition. I feel like I am making a difference every day so that no one, in particular a young woman, has to feel alone when she is diagnosed with cancer."

Anna and Brian's life changed quickly. They were a very young couple facing a breast cancer diagnosis, but they allowed an unexpected visitor to turn their lives into a mission to help others. I asked Anna to share how a young woman thinks and responds to the different decisions that have to be made. Throughout this book, you will read Anna's response to her cancer diagnosis as a young woman. Brian provides the same type of commentary in the companion book, *Breast Cancer Support Partner Handbook.*

Earnestine's Story

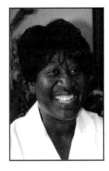

*E*arnestine was in her late forties in June of 2007 when she was diagnosed with infiltrating ductal carcinoma. She had seen cancer in her extended family, so she says that her diagnosis didn't come as a complete surprise. She was, though, concerned about how her family would cope with the changes cancer would bring. Her three children, Shannon, Krystle and Amber, needed her. Her aging mother needed her. She was the head of her household and, at the time of her diagnosis, held two jobs to pay the bills.

She didn't have time for cancer, but once she was diagnosed, she was anxious to learn what could be done. She underwent lumpectomy with lymph node dissection, chemotherapy and radiation therapy. She is currently being treated with Herceptin® and close follow-up care.

Her commentary throughout the book explains how she learned to slow down and take care of her health. During her treatment, she also learned to depend on her family for support. Her children provide commentary in the companion volume to this book, the *Breast Cancer Support Partner Handbook*.

Now, two years out from treatment, the side effects are mostly gone, and Earnestine has a new focus on taking care of herself and enjoying her children and grandson. She demonstrates the best of survivorship when she says, "For me, cancer had its ups and downs—but I'm still here."

As Survivors, we learn that survivorship is an attitude we adopt. It is the one component of recovery that no one else can do for us. We have to decide for ourselves how we intend to respond to our illness and how we will approach our recovery. We, alone, decide to become Survivors.

—Judy Kneece

Table of Contents

TEAR-OUT WORKSHEETS

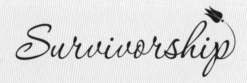

Take Life With Cancer One Day at a Time

As you begin your journey with breast cancer,

Remember to take life with cancer one day at a time.

Don't spend too much time looking at the past and wondering, "Why?"

Or spend too much time looking into the future asking, "What's next?"

Know that life can only be lived today; concentrate on today's problems.

Cancer is a new experience, and there is so much to learn.

If you take one day at a time, and one problem at a time,

You can overcome your fears, self-doubt and pain.

Surrounded by your family, friends, humor, prayers and faith,

You can, as you have in the past, move through this season with courage.

Just take life with breast cancer one day at a time.

—*Judy Kneece*

xiv

CHAPTER 1

The Emotional Impact of Breast Cancer

"My emotions were on a constant roller coaster ride. One minute I was so grateful I had a good prognosis. Then anger, fear and depression took over. I realized I was going to need help working through my emotions."

—Harriett Barrineau

"I made peace with death—and then I asked for strength ... I had a child who was in college. It was important for me to be there for my child's graduation."

—Earnestine Brown

Understanding Your Emotions

Shocked. Scared. Angry. Disappointed. Numb. Irate. Crushed. Disarmed. Brokenhearted. Furious. Speechless. Overwhelmed. A complete loss of control over my life. These are all terms women have used to describe their emotions upon hearing the words, "You have breast cancer." Most women report that they heard or remembered little after hearing the diagnosis. Their fears took control as they recalled all that they knew in the past about breast cancer. Most thought, "Will I die?" Often, they remembered someone who had gone through a similar diagnosis, and they mentally substituted themselves into the role. In the midst of this mind-boggling experience, the physician informed them of surgery options and possible treatments. "Overwhelmed" is usually an inadequate word for the experience. How do you begin to work through this complicated maze of emotions and unexpected decisions you have to make?

Foremost, you must realize that breast cancer is usually a very treatable disease. Survival rates are at an all-time high. Strong emotions are normal for all women at this time. Fears are natural. Most importantly, you need to know that breast cancer is usually not a medical emergency. You can take several weeks to sort through your emotions and seek answers to your questions without endangering your health. Your physician will discuss the

"I didn't process everything for a few days after hearing I had breast cancer. Then several days later, at six o'clock in the morning, I had an emotional meltdown. Having my husband there to comfort me helped. But I also needed time by myself to reflect on what was happening to me. I had an unplanned future to consider."

—Anna Cluxton

1

appropriate time frame with you. Use this time to understand the treatment options you have and the advantages and disadvantages of each. It will be best for you, both emotionally and physically, to take the time to make informed, rational decisions about your treatments.

What Is a Normal Response?

Women experience an array of emotions and respond to the diagnosis according to their basic personalities and previous life experiences. The only thing that everyone has in common is that this is a new experience, one that demands a great deal of physical and emotional energy. Most women cry and face depression as they sort through their potential losses. Remember, tears are okay. They confirm that you are dealing with reality and are using a very natural and appropriate response to deal with loss. Do not deny yourself the right to grieve. Grieving and tears are signs that your emotional healing has begun.

Some women experience great anger. They may direct this anger against themselves for not taking steps toward an earlier diagnosis, toward a physician or even a family member. Anger is an emotion people use to try to regain control over a situation in which control has been lost. Usually, it is not a productive way to solve problems; however, it is a natural response. A sense of control will return as you begin to understand and learn about the disease and how you can participate in your recovery. Loss has to be acknowledged before steps to recovery can be effective.

Communicating With Family

Eventually, your thoughts will turn from yourself to your family and friends and the effect your diagnosis will have on them. They, too, are in emotional pain over your news. The diagnosis is also a shock to them. Like you, they have a need to express their sad feelings, usually by crying, feeling down and questioning what is ahead as they grieve with you over your news. This is also a necessary and natural part of the family's emotional adjustment to your diagnosis.

You can play a vital part in facilitating their recovery by talking openly of your feelings and allowing them to ask questions and express their thoughts. This is probably one of the hardest parts of the breast cancer experience—open, honest communication. If honest communication begins at the time of diagnosis, it will help both you and your family. Often, we think that if we say nothing or do not let anyone see us crying or feeling depressed, we are making it easier for other people. The opposite is true. Hiding and not talking about feelings creates an atmosphere of uncertainty. People don't know what to say or do, and this uncertainty results in increased anxiety among family members.

Positive attitudes are needed. However, attitudes that seem overly optimistic may block communication in families because they set the stage for everyone to be in denial and mask their feelings. Your family needs to see you express a full range of emotions and be able to do so themselves. Begin to share as soon as you can, and ask them to share with you. They may need your permission before they talk because they don't want to "upset" you. They want to help you through this time. When you talk openly, they can find how to best help you. Let them to be a part of your recovery by allowing them to do things for you. For example, when they offer to do a chore, accompany you to the doctor or do something special for you, accept the offer. Feeling useful helps facilitate their emotional healing.

Communicating during times of stress may not be easy. You may find it difficult to open up and talk. The ones closest to you may not respond if you open up and share. Breast cancer doesn't change your basic personality or emotional responses to life. If you, your partner or other family members found it difficult to talk before the diagnosis, it may still be difficult to share during this time. However, you need someone with whom you can openly share your thoughts and fears in an understanding, nonjudgmental atmosphere.

Since you can't force people to participate in communication, it may be necessary for you to look outside the family unit for someone who can best respond to your needs. Consider your friends, a professional counselor or a support group. It is necessary and helpful for you to locate a support system in which you will be free to communicate and share your feelings, whatever they may be. You need a safe place to talk where your feelings, thoughts and fears will not be criticized or condemned but will be listened to instead.

Studies have shown that women who have good support systems adjust and respond to treatment more effectively. Ask your physician, Breast Health Navigator or clinic nurses for names of counselors or support groups for breast cancer patients in your area. Breast cancer support groups provide a safe and helpful environment where you can share, learn and receive support from women who know exactly how you feel and what you are facing. The American Cancer Society or Susan G. Komen for the Cure will also have a list of groups that meet in your area. The goal is to find somewhere to communicate your feelings! Acknowledging your emotional responses as normal and communicating openly will set the stage for a successful emotional recovery.

Communicating With Friends

After a diagnosis of breast cancer, many people are concerned about you and are interested in knowing how you are doing. This is encouraging, but answering numerous phone calls and emails in the midst of making decisions and undergoing treatment can become burdensome. Technology can help ease the burden of keeping friends and family informed. A Web site service called CaringBridge® offers anyone going through a health crisis a free online communication site. Setting up a hub at CaringBridge® allows you to update your health status online and for your friends to access the site at any time to follow your recovery. Friends can communicate by leaving a message that you can access at your convenience.

Setting up your own communication hub at www.caringbridge.org is a simple, three-step process that takes just a few minutes.

Getting the Facts Straight

Often family and friends who are trying to be helpful will offer you information and suggestions concerning your surgery and treatments. They do this because they care. However, it may only serve to confuse you and increase your anxiety. It is best to listen but not let this interrupt your quest to learn specific information concerning your diagnosis from the professionals guiding your treatment. There have been great advancements in the treatment and management of breast cancer. Drugs have been developed that have changed many of the side effects of chemotherapy. Surgical treatment is often less disfiguring because of newer surgical procedures, and survival rates are at an all-time high.

Learning about your disease, surgeries and treatment is important in order to regain a sense of control in your physical recovery. Breast cancer is a disease with many variables. There are approximately 15 types of breast cancer, many that require different surgical management and treatment. For this reason, you cannot compare notes with a friend who had breast cancer or listen to well-meaning family or friends because there are too many differences in treatments. Your information needs to come from someone who knows your exact diagnosis and has up-to-date information on the medical management of your disease. Your physician and healthcare staff will be the best source for accurate information.

Decisions, Decisions, Decisions!

Starting with the day you are diagnosed, the need to make multiple treatment decisions begins. Making treatment decisions can be overwhelming because most women know little about breast cancer options. There is so much to learn about breast cancer, so many decisions to make, and you're often required to make them within a short period of time. This definitely increases your stress.

There seem to be two extremes in making decisions. One is being so fearful that a person refuses to learn about treatment options and the other is a never-enough, never-ending search for information. Either extreme only leads to increased stress. Letting your fear cause you to avoid examining options and wanting to leave decisions completely up to others leaves you feeling powerless. On the other hand, incessant over-analysis in search of the perfect answer is emotionally exhausting. There has to be a balance.

If you lean toward fear-based decision making, thinking, "I'm afraid of what I may find out," I encourage you to face your fears and find out all you can. Remember that knowledge is power. The more you understand about something, the less power it has over you. Most often, you will find that even unpleasant news is better than a lurking fear. When you know the facts, you can take appropriate steps of action. The old saying "forewarned is forearmed" is true because it allows you time to prepare for the experience. In Chapter Four, we will discuss facing your fears in more detail.

If you tend to be a person who can not get enough information to make a decision, this can also hamper your ability to cope. Incessant searches on the Internet or multiple physicians' second, third and fourth opinions can serve as a way of avoiding making a decision altogether. "Paralysis of analysis" is certainly true; it will immobilize you. Have you ever noticed how much better you feel once you make a decision about how you are going to deal with something? You should take the time to carefully study your options—but set a time limit on your search so that you can make a decision and reduce your anxiety.

Managing the Breast Cancer Experience

As you are communicating, actively learning about your disease and making decisions, you will find yourself experiencing mood swings. There will be periods when you feel that you are doing well. Then you may find that you once again feel overwhelmed, asking, "Why?" and "What did I do to deserve this?" or saying, "I don't think I can go through this." These are normal responses while you are working through a crisis. You won't always feel in control. Feelings of depression, with periods of crying, may be dispersed throughout your recovery. When these times occur, don't be too hard on yourself for not being "brave." Acknowledge them as normal and then take steps to restore your positive mood. For some, it helps to get out of the house for a special outing, to spend time with friends or to work on a hobby.

It is also necessary that you monitor your rest during this time. A crisis can drain us of normal energy and require that we get more sleep. Listen to your body and get adequate rest. Most women need seven to eight hours of uninterrupted sleep daily. This may mean that you have to ask family members to assume some of your household duties for a time. Remember to plan some fun events. It is important to do things you enjoy. This will reduce stress as well.

Breast cancer is not an event you would have invited into your life. You will need to learn how to best participate with your healthcare team in your recovery, but don't allow yourself to make a "career" out of cancer. Try to see it as an experience to rekindle your life. Many women believe that the breast cancer experience caused them to grow into happier and healthier women, adding new dimensions to their lives that they had never taken time to enjoy before. Look at this time as an opportunity to grow, learn and make positive changes in your life. Consider an exercise program. Change your nutritional habits, or take time to start a hobby that brings you joy. A crisis can serve as an opportunity to grow into a physically and emotionally stronger and happier individual. Seek to make this a time of personal growth.

Managing the breast cancer experience requires information, support and a plan. This is what this book is all about—helping you master this unexpected challenge.

CHAPTER 2

Relationship With Your Partner

"I needed reassurance from my husband. I needed to hear, 'I love you.' I needed attention from him. His faith had to be strong enough for both of us for a short time. But, later, I realized he also needed support. He, too, was hurting. He found this unique source of understanding in a mates' support group."

—*Harriett Barrineau*

At diagnosis, your partner is confronted with the same surprise and faces the same overwhelming emotions as you. In the midst of all of this, though, they often strive to be strong, understanding and supportive. The way your partner responds to this crisis is determined by their basic personality and previous coping experiences. Behaviors may vary among people, but under it all are the basic emotions of fear, loss and uncertainty. A partner's love for you causes a strong emotional experience and an extreme feeling of helplessness when you are diagnosed with breast cancer. This is one thing they cannot fix. In an interview concerning support partners, Dr. Marilyn T. Oberst stated:

Learning to live with cancer is no easy task. Learning to live with **someone else's** *cancer may be even* **more difficult,** *precisely because no one recognizes just how hard it is to deal with someone else's cancer.*

Communicating With Your Partner

It is difficult to see you, the one they love, suffering emotionally and physically. Some partners may withdraw emotionally as they mentally sort out the situation. They may not say anything. Others may be very verbal. Remember, this is a new experience for them also. They too are hurting emotionally and often feel inadequate in their responses. You can help them by sharing your needs verbally. Do not wait, hoping that they will know what you need them to do or how you wish for them to respond. Most people want to meet their partner's needs and be helpful, but they are not sure how to respond. Recent studies by Dr. Oberst show

"I was so afraid of what having 'damaged goods' for a wife would do to our young marriage. It became very important to both of us to know when to reach out to each other and when to let go."

—*Anna Cluxton*

that during the first six months after a diagnosis, some partners may experience greater degrees of emotional problems than the patient because of personal fears and the anxiety created by not knowing what is expected of them in their new role as a support partner. You can help by encouraging them to talk to others who understand the role of a support partner. Call your cancer treatment center or local American Cancer Society office for the name of support groups for partners or ask for the name of a volunteer. Chaplains working in cancer treatment centers are an excellent source of support because they understand the unique stressors that families face with a cancer diagnosis. Encourage your partner to reach out to others to meet their own personal needs.

Intimate Relationship Changes

"What effect will my diagnosis and surgery have on my intimate relationship?" "Will I still be loved?" "How will my new body image affect our sexual relationship?" These thoughts are in the back of most women's minds. They are valid questions that need to be explored and understood. Intimate relationships are built on mutual love, trust, attraction, shared interests and common experiences in life. Breast cancer will not change these shared feelings.

What may change is how you view your body, and how that can affect your sexual intimacy. The physical aspect of lovemaking may temporarily change because of loss of energy resulting from your treatments. However, you can resume your sexual relationship as soon as you feel able. You are still the same person your partner selected and loves. You can bring a new dimension to this relationship by openly discussing your feelings about the changes in your body image. Try to communicate honestly about these concerns.

Often, you will need to be the one to initiate the discussion of these fears or needs. Your partner may feel these issues are too personal or sensitive. It is helpful if these concerns are addressed as soon

as you are diagnosed. Allowing time to pass only makes the conversations more difficult and walls of silence easier to build.

After surgery, early viewing of your incision area is very helpful in restoring the relationship and preventing distance between you and your partner. You may feel embarrassed or afraid to talk about your changed body image or to be seen nude. These feelings are best confronted and faced early. Viewing the incision is a necessary step. It has been proven that these feelings can be overcome if you share openly. Accepting the changes while reaffirming your love and joy of being alive and together will help you work through these feelings.

Partners often fear that their physical closeness may cause pain or injury to the incision site. It is helpful for you to share your need for physical closeness and what is comfortable or uncomfortable to you. Many times what women mistakenly sense as sexual rejection is really an effort on the part of the partner to protect the one they love. Therefore, state your desire for physical contact and share what is pleasurable. This will reduce the unspoken fear in your partner's mind concerning physical intimacy.

Open communication will decrease anxiety for both you and your partner, enabling your personal and sexual relationship to grow even stronger. There may be a period of adjustment, but most couples put their fears behind them and reestablish a satisfying and loving relationship. By sharing both the troubles and triumphs of cancer openly, you and your partner will have the opportunity to strengthen bonds of affection, trust and commitment.

Changes in the Family

Cancer is a family affair. It emotionally affects every member of the family. A cancer diagnosis is similar to throwing a stone into a body of water. The stone causes ripples that are greatest to those closest to the person diagnosed and diminish in intensity as they reach those further away emotionally. Naturally, the partner and the children feel the greatest impact. However, extended family and friends are also impacted. An essential part of healing and recovery is allowing each person to handle the pressures in a way that matches their basic coping skills. Some will be very talkative and want to come and share this time with you. Others may find themselves without words and withdraw emotionally for fear of not knowing what to say. It is helpful if you remember that this is a new experience and they have to process their responses over time, just as you do. Cancer presents not only a challenge to family unity but also an opportunity to strengthen bonds and increase love, respect and understanding. Studies report that most family relationships improve or become closer after a diagnosis.

Support Partner's Guide Available

A companion to this book, the *Breast Cancer Support Partner Handbook*, is available for your support partner. This book is designed as a guide to help support partners understand how to best help you while understanding their own emotional responses to the diagnosis. It addresses the unique emotional issues that a person faces during a partner's breast cancer diagnosis and explains what they can do. Ask your healthcare provider about this book, or you may order it from www.EduCareInc.com or at the address provided in the front of this book.

Remember

Your partner suffers emotionally from the diagnosis, just as you do.

Most support partners are unsure about how best to help. Helping them adapt to the role of support partner requires open communication. You must let your partner know how to best help during the experience by verbalizing your needs and expressing your desires.

Encourage your support partner to reach out for support from others who understand the unique needs of a support partner.

Intimate relationships are based on love, trust, shared interests and common experiences; breast cancer does not change this.

Sexual intimacy after surgery is dependent upon open communication. Discuss your change in body image, view the incision early and verbalize your need for continued intimacy.

Breast cancer can bring a couple closer and strengthen the bonds of affection, trust and commitment.

The entire family is affected by your diagnosis. All members will respond differently according to their personalities and previous coping skills.

Survivorship

Loss has a way of changing our lives dramatically. We become transformed. However, the idea that learning and personal growth could come from our loss when we are in the middle of our pain is an almost disgusting idea. This is how most people feel the first six months or longer. It takes time and we have to move past our crisis to see the changes that have occurred.

—Anne Kaiser Stearns

As survivors, we take a misfortune in life and change it into something that produces personal growth and somehow benefits others.

As survivors, we choose hope after loss. We choose to look at what we can do now that cancer has invaded our lives. We acknowledge our loss and nurse our pain, but we move on to make the diagnosis a source of motivation for a new direction in our lives.

—Judy Kneece

CHAPTER 3

Telling Your Children

"When I told my children, I found out that they handled it the way I handled it."

—*Earnestine Brown*

"My young cousins asked questions, and we were open and honest with them—after checking with their parents."

—*Anna Cluxton*

Children react to a parent's illness in various ways according to their ages, developmental stages and personalities. As a parent, you want this illness to create as little negative effect as possible on their lives. How do you handle this situation so that it causes the least amount of emotional distress for your children? From the beginning, tell the truth and answer their questions honestly. Often, it may appear that keeping the facts from them would be more helpful, but this is not wise. Children are very perceptive; they instinctively sense when something is wrong in the family. Not knowing what is wrong will often cause them to imagine things, which results in more anxiety than knowing the truth. It is also important that they hear the news first from you or the family, not from strangers. When information is presented truthfully, on their level of understanding, they can interact with you and receive answers to their questions and fears. It may be helpful to ask your medical team if they have information about how to talk with children about cancer.

In the *Journal of Psychosocial Oncology*, Karen Greening, MSW, LCSW, summarizes a child's five basic needs during a parent's diagnosis:

1. A need for clear information on what is happening

2. A need to be involved and to help out

3. A need for realistic reassurance

4. An opportunity to express thoughts and feelings

5. A need to maintain normal interests and activities

"Having always been the caretaker in my family, I found it difficult to let my four sons know I needed anything. I finally told them that I needed to talk about my fears and feelings, even though talking about Mom's breasts was not the most comfortable subject. Our love for one another and deep faith in God brought us closer together during this crisis."

—*Harriett Barrineau*

Impact of Diagnosis on Children

In his book, *How Do We Tell The Children?* David Pertz, M.D., explains:

> *A child's first question about illness and death is an attempt to gain mastery over their frightening images of abandonment, separation, loneliness, pain and bodily damage. If we err on the side of overprotecting them from emotional pain and grief with 'kind lies' we risk weakening their coping capacities.*

Tips for Telling the Children:

- If possible, wait until you and your partner have some control of your emotions. For some, this may take a day or two; others may be able to share the first day.

- Ask your treatment team for information, or call your local American Cancer Society for information written for children.

- With your partner or family member, plan what you will say to the children. Plan a time when both of you can share with them and not be interrupted.

- Turn off the television and hold telephone calls to prevent interruptions.

- Start by sharing something similar to the following: "Mommy has found a lump in her breast. The doctor says that the lump is cancer (call it by the right name). Cancer cells grow too fast. The doctors say that they need to take this lump out because these are not good cells. The doctors and nurses can also help by giving medicine." Continue to share truthfully and simply what the facts are. If you have an example, it will be helpful.

- Young children's greatest concern is often themselves—"Who will take care of me?" "Where will I stay?"

- Assure your children that their thoughts or actions did not cause your cancer and that they cannot catch your cancer.

- If you or your partner begins to cry, assure your children that this is because you are sad and it is okay to be sad and to cry.

- Allow the children to ask questions. Answer to the best of your ability. If you do not know the answers, be honest and say you do not know. Keep your answers age-appropriate.

- Reassure them that you will continue to tell them what is happening.

- Involve them in the process of helping Mom adjust to surgery and possible treatments. Help them feel as if they are part of the solution to the problem by sharing chores that contribute to the well-being of the family.

Teenage children and grown children also need to communicate openly and honestly. However, don't be surprised if they don't seem to be overly concerned and quickly return to their normal duties and interests. Take this as a compliment; your openness has restored their confidence that, as a family, you can cope with your new situation.

Telling the Teachers

Inform your child's teachers or instructors that your child is dealing with a cancer diagnosis (or family crisis) at home. This alerts them and allows them to identify potential changes in a child's behavior as stress reactions to the change in the home environment. They will also be able to recognize if the child is suffering from overwhelming sadness and needs emotional support, or they can offer additional help with schoolwork if stress makes it hard for your child to concentrate.

Older children and teens may feel more comfortable sharing their feelings with adults outside the home rather than with their parents. Knowing that there is a health concern at home allows these trusted adults to offer valuable emotional support to your child.

Teachers are also often in a position to request help and assistance from other school personnel, such as trained professional counselors and school psychologists, in order to offer additional professional emotional support to a child.

Other Parenting Tips:

- Allow your child time for active or aggressive play as an outlet for frustration and anxiety. For a young child, this may include pounding on a hammering toy or drum or playing with fierce toys (sharks, dinosaurs, etc.). Older children may enjoy basketball or video games.

- Try to arrange for a little extra love and attention for your children during this stressful time. Fathers, family members and friends may be willing to devote extra time to the children.

- If possible, plan family time every day. Resume your normal activities together as soon as possible.

- Guard against the tendency to make a teen your only source of emotional support.

- Ask the family to help see that teens maintain their social activities as much as possible.

- Be aware of teens' social concerns and possible embarrassment if you use humor about your breast as a coping mechanism.

When to Seek Professional Help:

- Marked change in school performance

- Poor grades despite trying very hard

- Extreme worry or anxiety manifested by refusing to go to school, go to sleep or take part in age-appropriate activities

- Frequent angry outbursts or anger expressed in destructive ways

- Hyperactive activities, fidgeting, constant movement beyond regular or normal behaviors

- Persistent anxiety or phobias

- Accident proneness, possibly self-punishment or a call for attention

- Persistent nightmares or sleeping difficulties

- Stealing, promiscuity, vandalism, illegal behavior (drug/alcohol use)

- Persistent disobedience or aggression (longer than six months) and violations of the rights of others

- Opposition to authority figures

Families often worry about the effect the illness will have on their children. The most important factor in how children respond is how they see you and your partner respond to the illness. If they see you communicating openly, honestly and sharing with a positive attitude, they will be more likely to respond the same way. The family can value this time as one of growth and maturity in problem solving. If you find it difficult to know what to say or realize problems are developing in the family with your children, contact your cancer treatment center and ask for a counselor trained in dealing with children.

Children's Support Resource

For the cost of postage (approx. $6.95), Kids Konnected will send care packages to families experiencing cancer. Packages are individually tailored to each family, depending on the ages of the children, who has cancer and what stage the cancer is in. Packages contain books, workbooks, brochures and additional information to help the child or teen better cope with what cancer brings. Every package includes a "Hope" teddy bear for each child and a security blanket for children under five.

Kids Konnected
26071 Merit Circle, Suite 103
Laguna Hills, CA 92653
949-582-5443
www.kidskonnected.org

Remember

Children need to be told the truth, at the level of their understanding, by you or a close family member.

Children need all of their questions answered honestly.

Truthfulness, coupled with love, will enable your child to grow stronger through this family crisis.

Children need to feel a part of the family by assisting with household chores.

Teens need to maintain their social life as much as possible and not become the only source of communication or support for the parent.

Breast cancer does not have to be a negative experience for children. It can serve as a time when families grow stronger.

CHAPTER 4

Calming Your Fears

"My husband's first reaction to my diagnosis was that we had been given a death sentence. Mine was just the opposite. I saw death as the easy choice. My greatest fear was having to live with the aftermath of breast cancer."

—Harriett Barrineau

At diagnosis, the struggle with cancer is often more difficult mentally than physically. Most women feel physically well when diagnosed, but they struggle after they hear the word "cancer." Many patients feel paralyzed and isolated by their fear. In support groups, women are often surprised to hear other women express exactly the same fears. In fact, most fears women have are common to everyone coping with a diagnosis. Your personality, previous coping experiences and your present support system may change your fear's intensity, but the underlying concerns are often the same.

The Most Commonly Expressed Fears:
- Will I die?
- How do I need to plan for the future?
- Are they telling me the truth?
- Can I still have children?
- Will I live to see my children grow up?
- How can I protect my loved ones from the pain this causes?
- What will I look like after surgery?
- Can I cope with my new body image?
- Will treatment be painful?
- Will treatment work?
- How will I know if cancer recurs?
- I feel helpless. What can I do about cancer?

"I remember coming across a Web site about a young woman who died from breast cancer and it scared me to death. Until that moment I don't think I had made the actual connection in my mind that I could die from this. Talking to my doctors and getting honest answers helped me put everything into perspective."

—Anna Cluxton

First, know that fear is natural. In fact, women who do not express fear are the most at risk psychologically. Disarming fear begins with recognizing its presence, expressing the fear to the appropriate person and taking steps of action against the fear. Do not hold onto your fears in silence. Identify your fears and express them. Often, when fears are expressed, strategies can be developed to help you deal with your fear.

Where Do You Start?

Continuing to live in a state of fear is like sitting in a dark room, imagining what might be there, while refusing to turn on the lights to see what really surrounds you. The same principle is true with a cancer diagnosis. If you don't take the steps to turn on the light, you will be trapped forever by your uncertainties and will never feel the sense of power that comes from knowing exactly what you are dealing with. Addressing your fears about cancer eliminates the clutter that consumes a lot of mental and physical energy. Decide not to waste your energy on the unknown—identify your fears, get answers to your questions and take appropriate steps of action.

Remember that turning on the light does not mean that you will not feel fearful. You will still feel a sense of fear. That's normal. You have simply ruled out "imagined fears" by knowing what you are dealing with.

It is important to start with understanding the facts about your cancer diagnosis. Ask your physician about your breast cancer's stage. Breast cancer is staged on a scale from 0 through 4. Stage 0 is the least aggressive and stage 4 means that your cancer has spread to other organs in your body and has the greatest potential to be life-threatening. In any stage, breast cancer most often requires learning to live with cancer rather than dying from it.

Learning the facts about your own cancer frees you to make appropriate decisions about living your life with cancer and alleviates many unfounded

fears. If you do not ask questions and understand the facts, your fear will become an inner source of tension that drains your energy—precious energy that could be better used in living life to the fullest.

Plan to Address Fears

Make a list of the fears that are clouding your mind (see example below). Be honest. You do not have to show anyone the list. After you have made your list, in a column beside each fear, list the people or person that the fear involves. If another person is involved, such as your partner or physician, express your fear to that person. Think about the fear and actions that you can take to understand or to change it.

FEARS	PERSON(S) INVOLVED	THINGS I CAN DO
"Will I still be sexually attractive?"	Partner	Express fear Purchase attractive lingerie Express desire for closeness Plan for special times
"Are they telling me the truth?"	Physician/ Nurses	Ask for honesty and all the facts Read about my disease
"What can I do about living with cancer?"	Support Group Professional Counselor	Attend a support group Ask for the name of a counselor

A worksheet for listing your fears and your planned strategies to disarm them is located on page W • 3. When you are ready to express your fears to the appropriate person, state your fear questions using "I" language. Example: "I am very concerned about the effect of my surgery on our sexual relationship. I don't want it to change." You may say to your physician, "I want to know all of the details about my disease and the side effects of treatment."

Fear can be a great impediment to recovery. Expressing the fear, determining your resources and developing a plan of action will cause the fear to be less of a threat. Communicate openly with your healthcare team to clear up any misinformation. Verbalizing your fears to the team allows them to help you seek a strategy to deal with your anxieties. Not all uncertainty will be alleviated, but the fears can certainly be brought to a manageable level.

Support groups, professional counselors and spiritual faith have been proven to assist in the management of fear. These sources offer a wealth of strength for dealing with a cancer diagnosis. As your physician and healthcare team are working to eradicate the cancer from your body, you can help them by keeping your body as free from stress and fear as possible.

Support Groups

Support groups are a "safe" place to express your fears and have your cancer questions answered by those who truly understand. You may have loving support from your family and friends, but often they do not seem quite able to understand what you really feel. In a breast cancer support group, the shared experiences of other women help you adapt and resume your fighting spirit. It is helpful to see those who are months ahead of you living full, productive lives after mastering the crisis of breast cancer. They have many tips and lots of encouragement to share with you. Avail yourself of this source of strength and understanding.

Ask your treatment team for names of groups or call your local American Cancer Society or Susan G. Komen for the Cure. When you have identified a support group or groups, you may wish to call and ask about the organization and goals of the group. Select a group that is affiliated

with a medical facility, if possible. These groups are usually facilitated by professionals who have an understanding of breast cancer and are able to get accurate answers to your questions.

Visit the group at least twice before making a judgment. If you do not feel the group meets your needs, visit another group if possible. Try to avoid any group that is allowed to become a "pity party." Select one which offers education and sharing among participants and promotes an optimistic approach to recovery.

It is also helpful if your partner can attend a support group. Often, partners have very few people with whom they can confide and receive helpful support. Ask about local support groups for your partner. A companion to this book, the *Breast Cancer Support Partner Handbook*, is available from EduCareInc.com and offers tips on becoming an effective support partner.

Some cancer centers also offer educational classes for children. This allows young family members to meet with other children and learn about cancer and cancer treatment on their level of understanding. Ask about children's classes for educational support.

Most patients feel that support groups were helpful to their recovery. Women who participate in groups or seek support from professionals have been proven to adjust more quickly both physically and emotionally than non-participants. Support groups are a way to reduce your fears and get answers to your questions.

Professional Counseling

Support groups are a valuable source of free information and support. However, some women do not feel comfortable in a large group or do not have access to a support group because of time or distance. If you find that a support group cannot meet your needs, ask your healthcare team for the name of a specialized counselor, therapist or psychiatrist. This is not a sign of weakness but of strength. Seeking appropriate support is as necessary as seeking appropriate medical treatment. The difference is that you may have to express your need for this service.

Individual counseling allows you to express your feelings and fears in an atmosphere of trust and support. Your selected counselor helps you plan strategies to make this crisis a manageable event in your life. This is usually short-term crisis counseling.

Spiritual Faith

Inherent in each of us is a deep need for understanding our existence and our future. Cancer causes a real threat to our sense of safety and forces these issues to be foremost in the mind. Answers to your struggles to understand "why," "how" and "what about tomorrow" are found in your faith. It will be helpful if you reach out and seek the help of your spiritual counselor during this time. If you do not have a pastor, priest, rabbi or spiritual leader, ask your hospital for the name and number of their chaplaincy service. Chaplains are trained in dealing with the adjustment to the crisis of cancer. Avail yourself of this valuable service.

In the book *Cancervive*, Susan Nessim shares her feelings as a cancer survivor:

> *Cancer has taken us on an amazing journey. When we look in the mirror we may see our faces as unchanged, but the person they belong to has undergone a spiritual metamorphosis. We have shed our old skins. Now we must assess who we've become and where we're headed. We've gained new insights into the depths of our spiritual strength, physical resiliency and courage.*

Looking at the cancer experience through the eyes of spiritual faith gives the experience meaning and purpose. Susan continues:

> *In the school of life, cancer survivors feel as if they've just completed an accelerated course—not that anyone, given the choice, would sign up for that course again. But for those fortunate enough to have gained a new perspective, the lessons learned are as precious as life itself.*

Why Do I Keep Losing It Emotionally?

Feelings and fears are a lot like holding on to Jell-O®. Just when we think we have them in our hands and under our control, they slip right out of our grasp.

This is the natural course of dealing with a crisis. We are not always in control of our feelings. We may think we are doing well and handling our emotions. Then, seemingly without warning, new problems arise, fears of the future return, tears begin to flow and depression comes to visit. Dealing with a cancer diagnosis is not an easy task. It keeps bringing new problems and fears as you progress through treatment and recovery. If you feel that your emotions slip out from under your control at times, you are normal. Most people dealing with a cancer diagnosis have this happen. When it does, you just have to start all over and look behind the cause of your present fears and see what, if anything, you can do. Don't be too hard on yourself. You don't have to be a superwoman.

Tear-out Worksheet
Managing My Fears - Page W • 3

Facing Fear

"Fear is the thief of progress because it paralyzes its victims, making them captives of the unknown."

—*Author **Unknown***

"Fighting fear is like trying to sack fog; you just can't get a handle on it. Giving your power away to the fear is worse than suffering the consequence that you're afraid of. Choose to give yourself the chance. It's normal to be anxious and afraid, but you can't be dominated by the fear."

—*Dr. **Phil McGraw***

"My best advice to newly-diagnosed women is don't be fearful. Fear can ruin you. Trust your doctors—they're going to do everything they can for you, and if they don't, get someone else. Demand the best out of whoever's taking care of you. Ask hard questions. Never stop learning. This is your life we're talking about."

—*Earnestine **Brown***

Remember

Fear is common to all women diagnosed with breast cancer. If you feel fearful, relax—you are normal.

Fear is not a sign of weakness.

Keep in mind that fears vary in intensity according to an individual's personality, previous coping experiences and support systems.

Fears lose their power when expressed openly and when steps are taken to disarm them.

The first step is to name the fears and questions that cloud your mind. Write them down.

Support groups offer emotional help and answer many fears and questions.

Some women are not comfortable in a large group and can benefit greatly from individual professional counseling.

Spiritual faith is a strong component in giving meaning to fear and providing a sense of strength to surmount the crisis of diagnosis. Reach out for spiritual understanding.

Keeping control of our emotions is often like holding on to Jell-O®. Sometimes they ooze out or slip from our control for a while. This is normal.

Survivorship

You gain strength, courage and confidence by every experience in which you really stop to look your fear in the face. You are able to say to yourself, "I have lived through this horror. I can take the next thing that comes along." You must do the thing you think you cannot do.

—Eleanor Roosevelt

Many of our fears are tissue-paper thin, and a single courageous step would carry us right through them.

—Brendan Francis

Courage is not the lack of fear. It is acting in spite of it.

—Mark Twain

I have a lot of things to prove to myself. One is that I can live life fearlessly.

—Oprah Winfrey

CHAPTER 5

What Is Breast Cancer?

reast cancer is not a sudden occurrence but a process that has been developing for a period of time. Therefore, when a biopsy confirms a cancerous breast tumor, you are most often **not** facing a medical emergency. You have time to get answers to your questions and learn about your particular disease and treatment options. Most physicians recommend surgery within several weeks of biopsy. There are exceptions; for example, inflammatory carcinoma requires immediate treatment with chemotherapy for maximum control. Whereas, women who have a family history of breast cancer may need genetic testing prior to surgery to guide treatment decisions. Ask your physician what recommendations will be made regarding your particular tumor.

Some tumors characteristically spread more rapidly to other parts of the body, while others do not spread as quickly. Breast cancer spreads to other parts of the body through the lymphatic system or the blood system. The spread of cancer can be local (in the area of the breast), regional (in the nodes or area near the breast) or distant (in other organs of the body).

What Causes Breast Cancer?

The female breast is a very complicated glandular organ and is the site of the most common cancer in women—breast cancer. No one knows exactly what causes breast cancer. Genetics (having a family history of breast cancer) increases the risk. Factors that do not cause cancer, but may promote it, include lifestyle factors such as diet and hormonal function.

Cancer begins when the cells of the breast gland undergo changes. The normal cell is damaged and converts into a cell that has an uncontrolled growth pattern. The cancer cells continue to divide and grow and may spread to other parts of the breast and then to other parts of the body if not removed. The cancer cells can invade neighboring tissues and spread throughout the body, establishing new growths at distant sites. This process is called metastasis.

"Breast cancer is not the unconquerable enemy I thought it was."

—*Harriett Barrineau*

" 'Know thy enemy'— what an understatement. I learned so much about cancer in the first few weeks after my diagnosis. And I continue to learn as much as possible, as this is an unending battle!"

—*Anna Cluxton*

"Breast cancer saved my life ... I had spent my whole life taking care of people—my mother for twenty years, getting my kids through college. My husband left me with a mess, and I took care of that. Now, I had to learn to take care of myself."

—*Earnestine Brown*

Internal Structure of the Female Breast

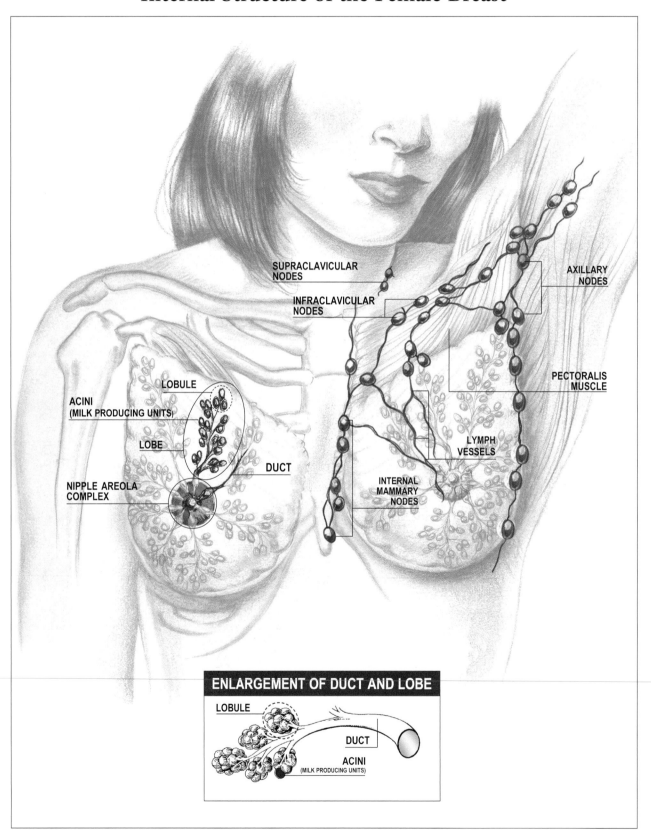

SUPRACLAVICULAR NODES

INFRACLAVICULAR NODES

AXILLARY NODES

LOBULE

ACINI (MILK PRODUCING UNITS)

LOBE

NIPPLE AREOLA COMPLEX

DUCT

PECTORALIS MUSCLE

LYMPH VESSELS

INTERNAL MAMMARY NODES

ENLARGEMENT OF DUCT AND LOBE

LOBULE

DUCT

ACINI (MILK PRODUCING UNITS)

Types of Breast Cancer

Cancers are first classified according to their relationship to the lobule or duct walls where they begin. The two major divisions are in situ and invasive/infiltrating. In situ means still inside; invasive or infiltrating means the cancer is now outside the walls of where it began. Approximately 15 different types of breast cancer have been identified. The term carcinoma is used by physicians to describe a malignant or cancerous growth. Tumors that develop from different types of breast tissue, in different parts of the breast, may have varying characteristics of development.

DUCT WITH NORMAL CELLS

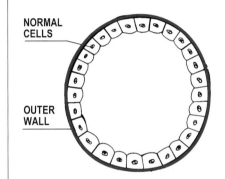

NORMAL
CELLS

OUTER
WALL

Normal ducts and lobules are lined with one or more layers of orderly cells.

IN SITU CANCER CELLS

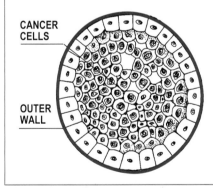

CANCER
CELLS

OUTER
WALL

In situ carcinomas are cancers that are still contained within the walls of the portion of the breast in which they developed. The cancer has not grown through the outer wall and invaded surrounding tissue.

INVASIVE CANCER CELLS

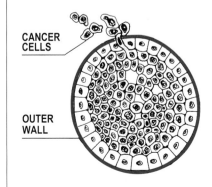

CANCER
CELLS

OUTER
WALL

Infiltrating or invasive carcinomas are cancers that have grown through the duct or lobular walls and into surrounding connective tissues.

Breast Cancer Names Depend on Where the Cancers Develop

DUCTAL CARCINOMA

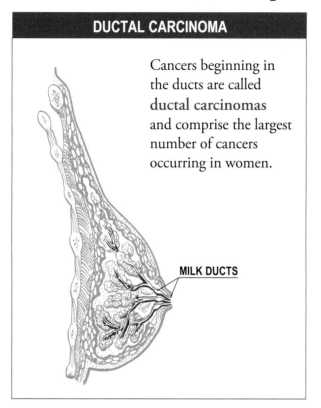

Cancers beginning in the ducts are called **ductal carcinomas** and comprise the largest number of cancers occurring in women.

MILK DUCTS

LOBULAR CARCINOMA

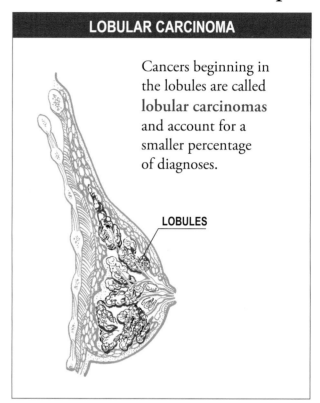

Cancers beginning in the lobules are called **lobular carcinomas** and account for a smaller percentage of diagnoses.

LOBULES

INVASIVE AND IN SITU CANCERS

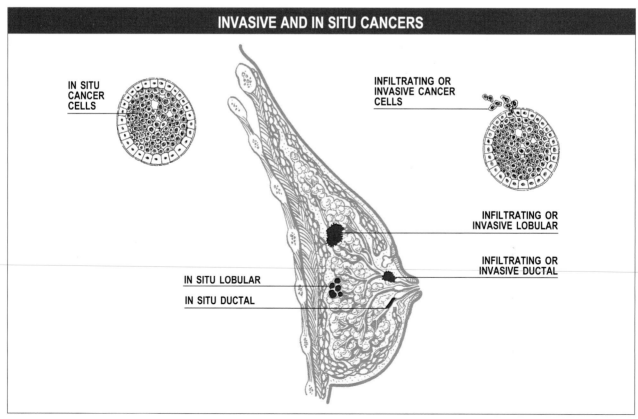

IN SITU CANCER CELLS

INFILTRATING OR INVASIVE CANCER CELLS

INFILTRATING OR INVASIVE LOBULAR

INFILTRATING OR INVASIVE DUCTAL

IN SITU LOBULAR

IN SITU DUCTAL

Cancer Growth Rate

Some cancers grow rapidly, while others grow more slowly. Breast cancers have been shown to double in size every 23 to 209 days. A tumor which doubles every 100 days (the estimated average doubling time) would have been in your body approximately eight to ten years when it reaches about one centimeter in size (⅜ inch)—the size of the tip of your smallest finger. The cancer begins with one damaged cell and doubles until it is detected on mammography or by finding a lump or other symptom. The cancer must be surgically removed from the body, killed with chemotherapy or radiation therapy or controlled with hormonal therapy. Some people believe that cancers may grow in spurts and the doubling time may vary at different times. However, by the time a one centimeter tumor is found, the tumor has already grown from one cell to approximately 100 billion cells.

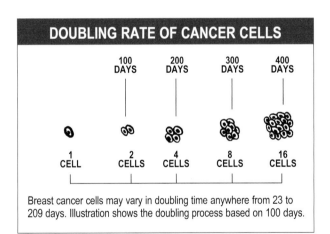

DOUBLING RATE OF CANCER CELLS

| 100 DAYS | 200 DAYS | 300 DAYS | 400 DAYS |

| 1 CELL | 2 CELLS | 4 CELLS | 8 CELLS | 16 CELLS |

Breast cancer cells may vary in doubling time anywhere from 23 to 209 days. Illustration shows the doubling process based on 100 days.

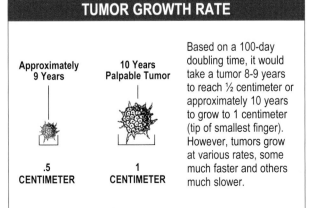

TUMOR GROWTH RATE

Approximately 9 Years

10 Years Palpable Tumor

.5 CENTIMETER

1 CENTIMETER

Based on a 100-day doubling time, it would take a tumor 8-9 years to reach ½ centimeter or approximately 10 years to grow to 1 centimeter (tip of smallest finger). However, tumors grow at various rates, some much faster and others much slower.

Role of the Lymphatic System

Lymph nodes play an important role in the discussion of your treatment decisions. It is helpful if you understand how the lymphatic system functions and affects many treatment decisions.

The lymphatic system is a network of thin, tube-like vessels that carry a clear lymph fluid to all parts of the body to remove cellular waste. The lymph vessels follow closely beside the blood vessels and receive the cells' waste products. Lymphatic fluid picks up the cellular waste from tissues and then flows through rounded areas of the lymph system, referred to as lymph nodes, which act as filters. Nodes look like small, round capsules and vary from pinhead to olive size. Lymphocytes and monocytes (cellular components of fluid which fight infection) are produced in the nodes, and the nodes act as filters to stop bacteria, cellular waste and cancer cells from entering the blood stream.

Because this lymphatic fluid passes through these nodes, the lymphatic system is a major route by which cancer spreads or metastasizes. Cancer cells can reach the lymphatic system, filter through the nodes and begin to multiply quickly. They may also pass through the lymphatic system into the bloodstream. The majority of the lymphatic fluid leaving the breast is drained through the nodes located in the area of the armpit, referred to as the axillary nodes. A small amount is drained through the lymph nodes located at other sites. These include the internal mammary and supraclavicular nodes.

Summary

Surgery and treatment with chemotherapy, radiation therapy or hormonal therapy can all vary because of the differences in types of cancer, the size of the tumor, potential lymph node involvement or documented metastasis, aggressiveness of the tumor and hormonal sensitivity. Therefore, it is necessary for you to communicate with healthcare professionals who have access to your final pathology report when seeking any specific information or advice on your breast cancer treatment.

Remember

No one knows exactly what causes breast cancer.

Breast cancer is not a sudden occurrence; it has been developing for years.

Breast cancer is usually not a medical emergency. Most often you have time to gather information and get answers to your questions before surgery or treatments begin.

Don't compare your breast cancer diagnosis with the diagnoses of others. There are approximately 15 different types of breast cancer. Treatment options will vary.

Tear-out Worksheets
Personal Healthcare Provider Records - Page W • 21
Personal Treatment Record - Page W • 23

Special Note:

Pregnant With Breast Cancer

If you are pregnant and discover that you have breast cancer, it can be emotionally overwhelming. At a time when you were preparing to bring a new life into the world, you now find yourself forced to fight to protect your own life. The good news is that you can receive treatment for your breast cancer while you are pregnant. When comparing women diagnosed in the same stage, treatment during pregnancy produces results similar to the treatment of women who are not pregnant. The additional good news is that treatment can be adapted so that your baby will not suffer ill-effects from your treatments. Breast cancer does not appear to harm a baby.

In the past, women were often advised to end their pregnancies when they were diagnosed, but now this advice is rare. Pregnancy termination is only recommended if your cancer requires that you receive chemotherapy during the first three months of your pregnancy. The National Cancer Institute states, "Ending the pregnancy does not seem to improve the mother's chance of survival and is not usually a treatment option." Most treatment options can be adapted to allow you to continue with your pregnancy.

Surgery and Radiation Therapy During Pregnancy

Surgery during pregnancy may require that you have a mastectomy, unless your surgery can be scheduled within six weeks of delivery. Radiation therapy is not considered safe during pregnancy, and surgical breast conservation (lumpectomy) usually requires postoperative radiation therapy as a part of treatment. After mastectomy, you're less likely to need radiation therapy.

Chemotherapy and Pregnancy

Chemotherapy can cause birth defects if given during the first three months (first trimester) of your pregnancy when the embryo's vital organs are forming. If you are diagnosed in the first few weeks of pregnancy and your stage of disease requires immediate chemotherapy (for example, you are diagnosed with inflammatory breast cancer), your doctor may recommend that you end the pregnancy. However, if the stage of your cancer is favorable and you are further along in your first trimester, your doctors will likely delay any recommended chemotherapy until the start of the second trimester (starting the fourth month of pregnancy). Each woman has to be individually evaluated as to the best treatment option for her diagnosis.

Special Note:

Male Breast Cancer

Breast cancer may also occur in men at any age, but it occurs most often between 60 and 70 years of age. Male breast cancer accounts for about one percent of breast cancers diagnosed yearly.

Male breast cancer is usually discovered when the patient notices a change in his breast because there is no routine screening for men. The cancer presents with the same symptoms as in a woman—most often a hard lump or a bloody nipple discharge. Diagnostic and biopsy procedures are the same. Surgery and treatment are also very similar to female breast cancer.

Most Common Types of Cancer Diagnosed in Men:

- Infiltrating or invasive ductal carcinoma (also most common female breast cancer)
- Inflammatory breast cancer
- Paget's disease of the nipple

Survival rates when compared to women diagnosed at the same stage are very similar. However, because of the higher incidence of BRCA2 mutations, men diagnosed with breast cancer are recommended to undergo genetic testing so that the information can be passed on to female relatives. (Refer to Breast Cancer Genetic Testing in Appendix A, page 184.)

Comprehensive information on male breast cancer can be located online (www.cancer.gov/cancertopics/pdq/treatment/malebreast).

CHAPTER 6

Surgical
Treatment Decisions

"I had a limited amount of time to make my surgical decisions. I had to push to meet with a plastic surgeon to fully explore my options. I made my decisions after talking with my healthcare team and based my decision on what I felt was the best choice for me. I couldn't look back or have regrets."

—*Anna Cluxton*

When your acute emotional stress is diminished, you may have many concerns about your diagnosis that need to be clarified. Many women say they were not prepared to hear the diagnosis and that everything the doctor said after the word "cancer" was hazy in their minds. You may want to list your questions and call the physician's office to schedule an appointment to receive accurate answers to your questions. Make this list with the person who accompanied you to the initial appointment.

Before your visit, it will be helpful to begin reading and acquiring a basic understanding of the medical terms used and some of the treatment options that may be offered. This book contains this basic information. Fill out the Patient Treatment Barriers Assessment (page W • 31) and take it to your healthcare provider on your next visit.

Today, women have the opportunity to participate in their care and decide with their physicians which type of treatment will best meet their personal needs and give the best chance for disease-free survival. It is important for you to understand why you are, or are not, offered certain treatment modalities. As an informed patient, you can become an active partner with your physician by understanding the treatments being discussed. It is also helpful if you can select one support person to accompany you to your appointments and participate in this process. This person will be a shoulder you can lean on and can help you remember and evaluate the information that is presented.

"I was frightened by how fast things were happening. I felt totally ignorant about breast cancer and had no idea where to turn for information or education."

—*Harriett Barrineau*

"At diagnosis, I asked my doctor, 'Why can't we just cut my breast off?' He replied, 'If I thought your treatment would be a little better if we took the breast, then I would do it. But it's not going to work like that.' I said, 'Okay, if we're not going to take my breast off, what are we going to do?'"

—*Earnestine Brown*

Obtaining accurate information about your particular disease is very important. Ask your physician for recommended reading material. Women's magazines contain information that is interesting, but it may not apply to the type of cancer you have and may confuse you. Medical terms sometimes have unusual meanings. Using a glossary to clarify the definitions of words will be helpful. As you read and learn, a sense of understanding will replace much of your fear about breast cancer. Sources of free medical information that offer up-to-date material on breast cancer are listed at the end of this book. (Also listed are suggested reading materials, resource lists to assist you in other areas and a glossary of breast cancer terms.)

Treatments for breast cancer are local (breast only) and systemic (pertaining to the entire body). Local treatments include surgery and radiation therapy. Systemic treatments are chemotherapy and hormonal therapy; these treatments travel to all parts of the body. Each type of treatment will be discussed in following chapters.

During your evaluation for breast cancer treatment, you may have a variety of physicians involved in evaluation of your cancer. Each has a special expertise in treating breast cancer. Refer to tear-out worksheets located in the back of the book for a list of questions to ask each physician.

- **Radiologist**—physician who uses diagnostic techniques such as mammography, ultrasound, breast MRI and minimally invasive biopsy to diagnose cancer.

- **Pathologist**—physician who analyzes cells or the characteristics of the tumor removed from your body to determine if disease is present.

- **Surgeon**—physician who removes identified area of suspicion from the body by using surgery.

- **Reconstructive (Plastic) Surgeon**—physician who reconstructs altered or removed breast using body tissues or implants.

- **Medical Oncologist**—physician who specializes in internal medicine and in the treatment of cancer using a variety of methods including chemotherapy, immunotherapy and hormonal therapy. Your surgeon may have an oncologist evaluate you for cancer treatment before or after your surgery. It is very important that you have a good relationship with your oncologist if you are to receive other treatments in addition to your surgery. There will need to be a great deal of interaction between you and the oncologist during the time you are receiving treatments. You should feel comfortable asking questions and participating in treatment decisions. Refer to Chapter 10 for a complete discussion of the role of the oncologist, chemotherapy and hormonal therapy.

- **Radiation Oncologist**—physician who specializes in using radiation (X-ray) therapy to treat local areas of disease. If your physician feels that radiation therapy could kill any remaining cancer cells in an area of your body, you will be referred to a radiation oncologist. Most breast-conserving surgeries are followed by radiation therapy. If you are having radiation therapy, it is helpful to have a consultation with the radiation oncologist before your surgery. Refer to Chapter 11 for a full discussion of radiation therapy and the questions you may wish to ask during your consultation.

Lymph Node Removal

Lymph nodes are removed to determine whether your cancer has spread from the breast into the node area. Whether or not cancer is found in your lymph nodes is one of the most important prognostic factors in breast cancer. Evaluation of your nodes for cancer cells is performed by a surgeon during breast surgery. Nodes may be evaluated by several methods: axillary sampling, complete axillary dissection or a procedure called sentinel lymph node mapping (if your tumor meets certain criteria). For identification purposes, nodes are divided into three levels in the underarm and chest area. (See graphic on next page.) The number of nodes in each level varies from person to person.

LYMPH NODES OF THE BREAST

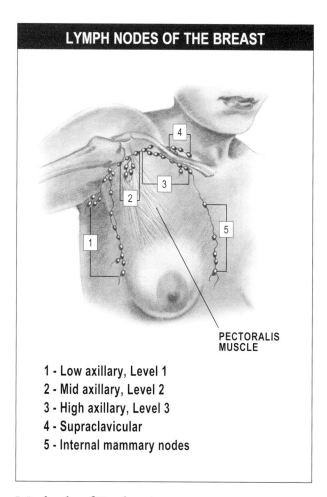

PECTORALIS MUSCLE

1 - Low axillary, Level 1
2 - Mid axillary, Level 2
3 - High axillary, Level 3
4 - Supraclavicular
5 - Internal mammary nodes

Methods of Evaluation:

- **Axillary sampling** is a process in which selected nodes are taken from under your arm.

- **Axillary dissection** is a procedure in which all the nodes under the arm are removed, usually from levels one and two.

- **Sentinel lymph node mapping**—removes the first (sentinel) node(s) that drains the tumor for initial evaluation to see if additional nodes need to be removed.

Node Evaluation Results:

- **Negative nodes** means that your lymph nodes did not have any evidence of cancer.

- **Positive nodes** indicate that the cancer was found in the lymph nodes.

Your surgeon will tell you how many nodes were removed during your surgery and how many

were found to have cancer cells present. Treatment decisions are often based on the number of nodes in which cancer cells are found and the size of your tumor.

Sentinel Lymph Node Mapping

Sentinel lymph node mapping is a procedure that identifies the first node or nodes (sentinel) that receive lymphatic fluid from a cancerous tumor, thus identifying the lymphatic drainage pattern and the node(s) most likely to be cancerous. The sentinel nodes are like the gatekeepers to the rest of the lymph nodes.

Tumors may drain to different node chains, according to the position of the tumor in the breast. The procedure identifies the lymphatic chain and the nodes most likely to indicate whether cancer has metastasized to the regional lymph node area. This identification gives the surgeon and pathologist a reliable guide for more accurate node evaluation without removing a large number of nodes. Not all patients are candidates for a sentinel lymph node procedure.

Factors That May Disqualify You for Sentinel Lymph Node Procedure:

- Pregnancy
- Previous breast surgery in affected breast
- Known or suspicious positive lymph nodes
- More than one tumor in the breast
- History of breast radiation in affected breast
- Certain size tumors
- Ductal carcinoma in situ (surgeon's decision)

TUMOR AND LYMPH NODES

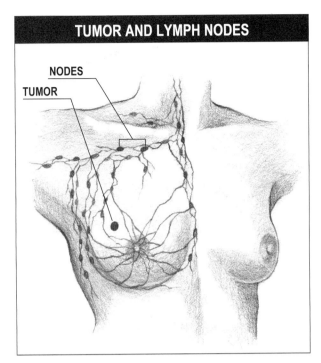

NODES
TUMOR

RADIOACTIVE SUBSTANCE INJECTION

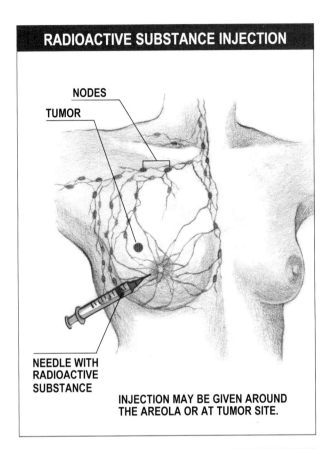

NODES
TUMOR

NEEDLE WITH
RADIOACTIVE
SUBSTANCE

**INJECTION MAY BE GIVEN AROUND
THE AREOLA OR AT TUMOR SITE.**

GAMMA–DETECTION PROBE

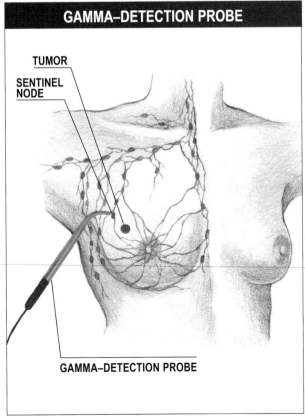

TUMOR
SENTINEL
NODE

GAMMA–DETECTION PROBE

Sentinel Lymph Node Procedure

This procedure begins with an injection of a radioactive substance before you go into surgery. Before surgery begins, the surgeon may also inject a blue dye around the tumor site or areola. The radioactive substance or dye is carried by the lymph fluid to the first node(s) (sentinel) that drains the tumor. During surgery, a hand-held gamma-detection probe first identifies where the radioactive material has concentrated, showing the area for the surgeon to make the incision. The blue dye helps the surgeon visually identify the node (there may be one or several) for removal. Some surgeons may only use the radioactive substance and gamma-detection probe, while others use only the blue dye. After surgery, the pathologist examines these nodes for cancerous cells.

If the sentinel node biopsy shows that there is no cancer, no additional nodes will be removed. If cancer is found in the biopsied node(s), additional node removal is necessary to determine how many nodes are positive. Additional node removal may be performed during your initial surgery or at a later time. Some surgeons prefer to have the biopsy specimen evaluated during surgery, followed by additional node removal.

Others prefer to have the biopsy specimen evaluated later and, if the node(s) is positive, have you return for additional node removal. Ask your physician about your planned procedure and if there is a need for additional node removal.

Side Effects of Sentinel Lymph Node Biopsy:

- Pain during injection or bruising at the injection site.

- Possible allergic reaction to the blue dye.

- Bluish tint of the breast area or of urine may occur if blue dye is used. The discoloration is temporary and is not harmful.

Sentinel node mapping improves the accuracy of selecting nodes to be removed surgically to check for the spread of the cancer. It may also prevent unnecessary removal of nodes not in the lymphatic drainage field of the tumor. Reducing the number of nodes removed can greatly decrease the potential for future lymphedema (a swelling from lymphatic fluid accumulation in the arm, which can cause discomfort and is a lifetime risk) and the likelihood of an infection in the arm if any type of injury should occur.

Determining Factors for Surgery

Surgery is the first line of defense against most breast cancers. Your surgeon will discuss with you the best surgical options for your diagnosis. Your surgeon will consider the following facts when determining which surgery best suits your needs.

- **Type of Tumor**—The type was diagnosed by biopsy and confirmed by the pathology report. There are approximately 15 cell types of breast cancer that vary in tumor growth rate (how aggressively the tumor may spread to other organs and its potential for occurring in the other breast).

- **Size of the Tumor**—Sizes are given in centimeters (cm) and millimeters (mm). (10 mm equal 1 cm; 1 cm equals ⅜ inch; 1 inch equals 2.5 cm)

- **Lymph Nodes**—Possible cancer involvement in lymph nodes.

- **Size of Your Breast**—Some breasts may be too small in comparison to the size of the lump to give good cosmetic appearance when the lump is removed.

- **Location in Your Breast**—Tumors under the nipple sometimes will not give a suitable cosmetic look when the lump is removed. Two tumors in the same breast not located close to each other will not give good cosmetic results.

- **Mammogram**—Determines if your tumor may be multifocal (occurring within one quadrant in the breast) or multicentric (occurring in more than one quadrant in the breast). (Refer to graphic on page 71.) This is sometimes evidenced by microcalcifications (small calcium deposits) or mammographic abnormalities.

- **Involvement of Other Structures**—Skin, muscle, chest wall, bone or other organs.

- **Reconstruction**—Your desire for reconstruction now or later and the desired outcome for the reconstructive surgery (breast enlargement, reduction or matching present size).

- **Health**—Your general health and any treatment limitations due to your present health.

- **Disease Control**—Which surgery will give you the best chance for disease control.

- **Cosmetic Results**—Which surgery will give you the best cosmetic results.

- **Range of Motion**—Which surgery will give you the best functional results for your arm and shoulder.

- **Complications**—Which surgery is associated with the fewest short-term and long-term complications.

- **Personal Desire**—Your priorities regarding the surgery.

Treatment must be evaluated in terms of each tumor's unique and specific features and which surgery will be best for you. Some types of breast cancer may require chemotherapy treatments before surgery, called neoadjuvant chemotherapy.

Discuss the above considerations with your surgeon and ask any questions that will help you make the decision best suited to your needs.

Types of Surgery

Surgery for breast cancer includes several types of surgical procedures. Some types remove the breast (mastectomy), and others remove the tumor and varying degrees of the remaining breast tissue (lumpectomy). These common terms may describe various amounts of tissue removal. You will need to clarify with your surgeon which of the exact procedures will be used. Following are the basic types of surgical procedures and descriptions of the tissues usually removed. After each description, one drawing illustrates the amount of tissue removed, and another drawing illustrates how your body will appear after the surgery. Surgical incisions can vary among different surgeons. A graphic is provided at the back of this book (page W • 8) for your surgeon to draw the procedure that will be used for your surgical treatment and how your scar should appear afterwards.

Breast Conservation Surgery

Breast conservation surgery saves the majority of the breast tissue, including the nipple and the areola. However, there are some reasons that breast conserving surgery may not be the best surgical option.

Factors That May Disqualify You for Breast Conservation Surgery:

- Pregnancy (if radiation therapy will be required before delivery; breast conserving surgery is possible in the third trimester as long as radiation can be postponed until after delivery)

- More than one primary tumor in the breast

- Mammogram with evidence of suspicious scattered microcalcifications

- Location of the tumor in the breast where there may be poor cosmetic results (example: when the tumor is located under the nipple)

- Size of tumor (if the tumor is too large or the breast is too small in relation to the size of the tumor, then there will be poor cosmetic results)

- Prior radiation therapy to breast or chest area

- Collagen vascular disease (lupus, scleroderma, etc.)

- Severe chronic lung disease (because you may not be a candidate for radiation therapy)

- Very large, pendulous breast (may indicate you may not be a good candidate for radiation therapy; you need to have a radiation oncologist's evaluation)

- Evidence of remaining cancer in ducts surrounding tumor after surgical removal (indicating there may be a high risk for recurrence)

- Inability of surgeon to obtain margins with no evidence of cancer after re-excision (second surgery)

- Possibly a positive carrier of a BRCA1 or BRCA2 mutated gene

- Restrictions on travel or transportation to clinic for daily radiation for six to seven weeks

Breast Conservation Procedures

Breast-conserving surgeries do not remove the breast and are commonly called lumpectomies. However, the term lumpectomy may be used inappropriately for other types of surgeries. These surgeries also conserve and do not remove the breast, but the cosmetic results and the amount of tissue removed can vary from procedure to procedure. These variations in the amount of tissue removed have different names which we will discuss below.

Lumpectomy

Lumpectomy removes **only** the tumor and a **small** margin of surrounding tissue. Lumpectomy preserves the basic appearance of your breast, including the nipple and areola. Lymph nodes may or may not be removed by a separate incision under your arm.

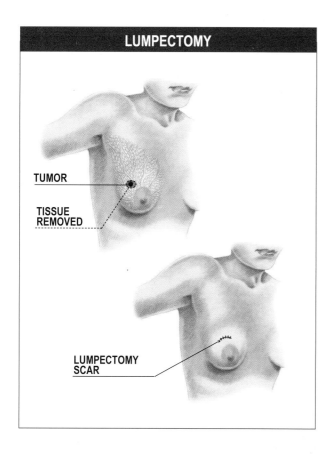

LUMPECTOMY

TUMOR

TISSUE REMOVED

LUMPECTOMY SCAR

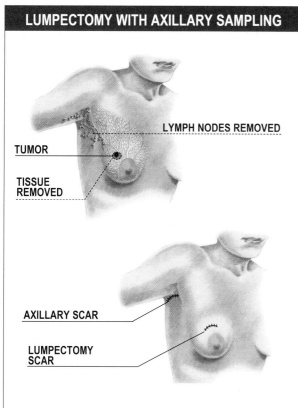

LUMPECTOMY WITH AXILLARY SAMPLING

LYMPH NODES REMOVED

TUMOR

TISSUE REMOVED

AXILLARY SCAR

LUMPECTOMY SCAR

Wide Excision
Breast Conserving Surgeries

A surgery that removes **more** than just the tumor and a small amount of surrounding tissue may be called a partial mastectomy, quadrantectomy, segmental excision, wide excision or tylectomy. In these procedures, the tumor and an area of tissue around the tumor are removed. The overlying skin and a portion of the lining of the chest muscle under the tumor may also be removed.

These are all breast-conserving surgeries, but some may remove up to as much as 25 percent of your breast tissues. If it is necessary to remove a lot of tissue because of the characteristics of your tumor, you may not be as pleased with the cosmetic results of your surgical procedure. Some of these surgeries may require some type of reconstruction using an implant or your own body tissues to restore your breast size. This is the reason you need to inquire how much tissue will be removed. Ask your surgeon to show you how much tissue will be removed and how your incision will appear by filling in the information on page W • 8. This will help you make an informed decision with your physician.

Lymph Node Removal With Breast Conservation

Lymph nodes may or may not be removed from a separate incision, approximately two inches in length, under the arm. Lymph node removal during breast conserving surgery also varies.

You Could Have One of the Following:

- No node removal

- Sentinel node biopsy

- Axillary sampling

- Axillary dissection

Ask your physician what type of lymph node evaluation procedure is recommended for your breast conserving surgery.

33

Mastectomy Procedures

There are several types of mastectomies. Ask your surgeon which of the procedures will be performed and the extent of tissue and lymph node removal you will need to have. The different mastectomies are defined below:

1. Full or Complete Radical Mastectomy

A complete radical mastectomy removes the breast, nipple, areola, all three levels of lymph nodes, small chest muscle, the pectoralis minor, medial pectoral nerve and the lining over the chest wall muscles.

2. Modified Radical Mastectomy

A modified radical mastectomy removes the breast, nipple, areola, underarm lymph nodes and the lining over the chest wall muscles. The procedure may be referred to as a "total mastectomy with axillary dissection," which means that the entire breast and some or all of the level one and two lymph nodes are removed. Sentinel node mapping may also be used. This is the most common mastectomy.

MODIFIED RADICAL MASTECTOMY

TISSUE REMOVED

SKIN REMOVED

MASTECTOMY SCAR

3. Total or Simple Mastectomy

This procedure removes the breast tissue, nipple, areola, and possibly some of the underarm lymph nodes that are closest to the breast. Nodes may also be removed with a sentinel node biopsy.

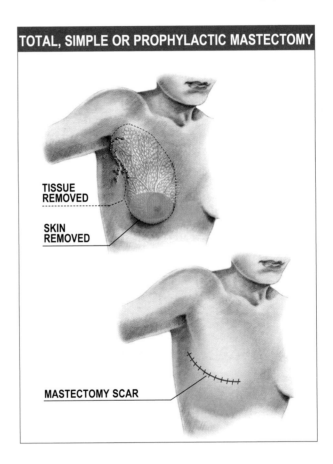

TOTAL, SIMPLE OR PROPHYLACTIC MASTECTOMY

TISSUE REMOVED

SKIN REMOVED

MASTECTOMY SCAR

There is a separate page (page W • 8) in the back of this workbook that your surgeon may fill in for you, showing where your incision will be and how it will look after surgery.

4. Skin-Sparing Mastectomy

Skin-sparing mastectomy is a procedure used when performing a simple or total mastectomy. The method removes the breast tissues from a circular incision around the areola (dark colored circle). The nipple, areola, breast tissues, nodes located near the breast tissues and additional lymph nodes are removed according to the discretion of the surgeon. The procedure is often selected when reconstructive surgery is performed. The sparing of the skin allows reconstructive surgery to be performed with little need for a period of stretching the skin. Sensitivity of the skin over the reconstructed breast remains intact. The reconstructive incision is made using the normal curve of the breast. This incision is not visible because it is usually hidden under the fold of the breast and is concealed by the bra. The incision used to remove the breast is concealed by the reconstruction of a nipple and areola. This is the recommended surgery for women having mastectomy for intraductal disease and desiring reconstruction or for a small peripheral tumor.

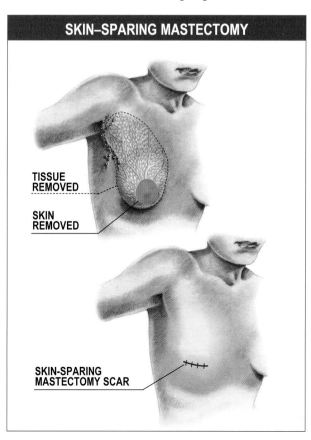

SKIN–SPARING MASTECTOMY

TISSUE REMOVED

SKIN REMOVED

SKIN-SPARING MASTECTOMY SCAR

5. Prophylactic Mastectomy

A prophylactic mastectomy is a total or simple mastectomy performed before cancer has been found. This elective surgery is a decision made collaboratively between the patient, surgeon and oncologist. A second opinion may be required to ensure that this is a physically and psychologically sound decision.

Prophylactic Mastectomy Reasons:
- Desire for bilateral reconstruction with an increase or decrease in the reconstructed breast size
- Family history of breast cancer, including first degree relatives who died of the disease
- Identified positive carrier of BRCA1 or BRCA2 genes
- Repeated breast biopsies for suspicious findings
- Mammograms that show findings which are increasingly difficult to interpret
- Diagnosis of a cancer type that has a high rate of occurrence in both breasts
- When the weight of a very large remaining breast (after mastectomy) creates imbalance, posture changes and back pain
- Overwhelming psychological fear of occurrence in remaining breast

Lumpectomy Versus Mastectomy

If your breast and tumor are within certain size limits, your surgeon may offer you the option of a lumpectomy (breast conservation) versus a mastectomy. If you are in the category that allows you to choose between a lumpectomy and a mastectomy, the decision may be difficult. This needs to be a decision you make in consultation with your physician after a careful review of the advantages and disadvantages of both. Remember, the option to choose is not available for some types of cancer.

It is imperative that you feel comfortable with the decision. Studies document that a lumpectomy, in an appropriate candidate, even if there is local recurrence, does not affect survival rate.

However, it may be inconvenient if a second surgery becomes necessary. Ask your surgeon if there are any additional variables in your surgical decision that may be added to this list.

A self-evaluation for helping you determine which procedure may be more appropriate for you is located in the tear-out worksheet section of the book. (Refer to Decision-Making Sheet on page W • 9.)

Advantages of Lumpectomy:
- Saves a large portion of the breast, usually the nipple and areola
- Preserves body image
- Allows you to wear your own bras
- Rarely requires reconstruction or the wearing of a prosthesis unless a wide-excision lumpectomy was performed
- Recovery time from surgery is usually several weeks shorter than recovery from mastectomy
- Slightly shorter hospitalization time or may be performed as outpatient surgery
- May be psychologically easier to accept, unless monitoring remaining breast tissue for recurrence is too frightening

Disadvantages of Lumpectomy:
- Risk of recurrence of cancer in remaining breast tissue (low risk)
- Several weeks, usually six to seven, of radiation therapy to the remaining breast tissue with external beam radiation or up to five days with brachytherapy
- Changes in texture (lumpiness), color (suntanned appearance) and decreased sensation of feeling in the breast after radiation therapy
- Decrease in size of the remaining breast tissues after swelling decreases following radiation treatments
- Monthly breast self-exam on remaining breast tissue (to monitor for recurrence) becomes more difficult because of increased nodularity (lumpiness) from radiation therapy
- Potential for chronic swelling or accumulation of fluid in the breast (breast lymphedema)
- Possibility of future second lumpectomy or mastectomy if there is a recurrence

Advantages of Mastectomy:
- Removes approximately 95 percent of the breast gland, including the nipple and areola, thus reducing local recurrence to the lowest degree
- Reconstruction of breast is available using your own body tissue or synthetic implants

Disadvantages of Mastectomy:
- Body image changed because of the removal of a breast
- Need for prosthesis or reconstruction to restore body image
- Recovery time is usually several weeks longer than for lumpectomy patients

If you are having problems making your decision, you may wish to speak with a patient who has already made the choice and had one of the procedures. Ask your physician if there is someone who will be willing to talk to you. Your local American Cancer Society's Reach to Recovery program coordinator can provide you with the name of a volunteer who will be willing to share her lumpectomy/mastectomy experience.

If you are considering a lumpectomy, you may wish to have a consultation with a radiation oncologist to discuss radiation treatments. Often this consultation will give you additional insight that may help you make a more informed decision. (See Chapter 11 for more information on radiation therapy.)

Second Opinions
When a medical diagnosis is serious and the suggested therapy hard to accept, some women feel the need for additional information or a second opinion. Surgery, chemotherapy and radiation therapy deserve serious consideration, and you need all of the information necessary to make an informed decision. A second opinion is obtained from another physician

practicing in the same area of medicine. He reviews your records and offers treatment advice. This opinion may help you feel sure about your treatment decision. However, for some women, a second opinion may cause anxiety and increased confusion.

Some insurance providers may require a second opinion before treatment. You will need to check with your insurance provider on this point. Physicians may refer patients for second opinions in order to validate treatment decisions. It is necessary for you to evaluate your needs and decide if a second opinion would be of assistance to you.

Reasons You May Need a Second Opinion:

- You feel insecure or unsure about what you have been told about surgery or treatments.

- Your insurance provider requires a second opinion.

- There has been disagreement or confusion within your family or with your support partner about the right course of action.

- You want information about newer therapies not offered by your treatment team.

How to Obtain a Second Opinion

If you feel a second opinion would help you resolve your indecisiveness, ask your treatment team for the names of several physicians qualified in this area. Ask the treatment team to list the pros and cons of each one in order to help you determine who will best suit your needs. You may also call a major cancer treatment center for a self-referral. Some of the national cancer organizations listed in the reference section of this book will give you the names of the major cancer treatment centers located in your area and the services they provide.

Second opinions are often received through the pretreatment multidisciplinary conferences held at some centers. Physicians from all areas of breast care (radiology, pathology, surgery, medical oncology, radiation oncology, reconstructive surgery) look at your records as a group, discuss your individual case, share their opinions with the group and make treatment recommendations as a team. All of this is done before any of your final treatment decisions are made. These conference recommendations serve as a guide for your own physicians to consider. If you have access to this type of conference, or a group of physicians practicing as a team, it serves as an excellent way not only to get a second opinion, but several expert opinions.

Preparing for the Second Opinion Visit

When seeking a second opinion, you should clarify any questions you have. Make a list of your questions and concerns before the visit and take the list with you. Also, be sure that all requested lab and diagnostic test results are sent to the physician before your visit to ensure that the needed information is available before the consultation. Call several days prior to your appointment and check to see if your records have arrived. The consulting physician will share his or her opinion with you and send recommendations to your physician, who can then take full advantage of the second opinion.

The most common benefit of a second opinion is having peace of mind in knowing that you have gathered all the information that you need to make an informed decision. An informed decision allows you to go through your treatments knowing that this was the best treatment choice for you. Some women feel comfortable with their initial treatment options, feel their questions are answered sufficiently and feel no need for a second opinion. This is acceptable for them. Seeking a second opinion is an individual decision and one that needs to be made according to your needs.

Treatment guidelines for breast cancer
can be requested from:
National Comprehensive Cancer Network
www.nccn.org

Refer to Tear-out Worksheets
Questions About Surgery - Page W • 5
Surgical Decision Evaluation - Page W • 9

Remember

Surgical decisions are the first and often the most challenging for women to make.

Breast cancer is not usually a medical emergency. Take the time to study your options.

If you have an option of mastectomy or lumpectomy, consider all the advantages and disadvantages. Remember that survival rates are equal.

Learn about reconstructive surgery options to help make your decisions.

Ask yourself, "How will I want my body to look a year from now?"

A second opinion is your opportunity to gather all of the information you may need to experience peace of mind about your surgical and treatment decisions.

If the thought of a second opinion creates anxiety for you, it is not a good idea.

CHAPTER 7

Reconstructive Surgery

Even though you are losing a breast or a part of a breast to surgery, you have the option to have your body image restored through plastic surgery. Breast reconstruction has made a big difference, both physically and emotionally, for many women who have undergone surgery for breast cancer. Some have immediate reconstruction at the time of their initial breast surgery. They feel that reconstruction will help bring back their feminine silhouette and alleviate the necessity of wearing a prosthesis. Others wait until their treatments for breast cancer have been completed. Some women choose never to have reconstruction.

If you feel that you would like to have your breast reconstructed, talk to your surgeon prior to your surgery. You may also want to consult a reconstructive surgeon prior to your surgery, even if you plan to have the procedure performed after your treatments. Your surgeon or clinic can provide you with names of reconstructive surgeons who have experience in this field.

A decision to have reconstruction requires a lot of research and discussion. Remember, part of gaining control over your cancer is knowing all the options that are available to you and choosing those that best meet your needs. As you research your choices, keep asking yourself, "How would I like to look a year from now?"

Advantages of Breast Reconstruction:
- Restores feminine body image
- No prosthesis or special bras have to be purchased and worn
- Can wear any clothing, including swimsuits and low-neck attire
- Can go braless for short periods of time, if needed
- Does not have the daily reminder of breast surgery (in the form of a prosthesis)
- Psychologically beneficial in allowing most women to adjust better to the disease

"I had delayed reconstruction about a year after my mastectomy. I chose to have a prophylactic mastectomy on the opposite breast followed by tissue expanders and saline breast implants."

—Harriett Barrineau

"I had immediate reconstruction—a TRAM (used my stomach muscle, skin and fatty tissue to construct a new breast). When I woke up, even though I was bandaged up, I really almost couldn't believe they had removed the breast because the TRAM turned out so well."

—Anna Cluxton

Disadvantages of Breast Reconstruction:

- Physical recovery from surgery will require more time, and you will experience a greater amount of pain

- Increased potential for infection or surgical complications due to the more complex surgery

What May Disqualify You?

Only your reconstruction surgeon can evaluate your past and current physical condition to determine if you are a candidate for breast reconstruction and which surgery best suits your present health condition.

Potential Limiting Factors Are:

- Obesity (especially more than 25 – 35% over ideal body weight)

- History of radiation therapy to the chest wall

- Smoker or recent history of smoking

- Autoimmune disease (lupus, multiple sclerosis, insulin dependent diabetes mellitus, scleroderma, Hashimoto's thyroiditis, fibromyalgia)

- Current or previous history of chronic lung disease

- Psychiatric disorder

- Substance abuse

- Patient compliance (ability to understand procedures and options and the ability to tolerate pain from procedure)

- Abdominal scarring from previous surgery, including liposuction, if choosing a TRAM procedure (may prohibit use of abdominal muscle tissue in breast reconstruction)

The Good News

A woman is never too old for reconstructive surgery if she is in good health. Ask your physician, Breast Health Navigator or nurse for reconstruction information and names of reconstructive surgeons in your facility. The American Cancer Society's Reach to Recovery coordinator can give you names of women who have had reconstructive surgery who may be available to discuss their experiences with you.

Often, women fear that reconstruction may hide or prevent the detection of cancer recurrence in the breast area. There is no evidence of any kind that breast reconstruction, with your own body tissues or with an implant, causes cancer to grow or recur. There is little difficulty in detecting an early local recurrence after reconstruction. This should not be a concern in making your decision.

Reconstruction Reimbursement

In 1998, The Women's Health and Cancer Rights Act (WHCRA) was signed into law, providing coverage of the cost of reconstruction for women who elect to have a mastectomy. This law requires insurance providers to cover not only reconstruction of the surgical breast but also surgery, if needed, to the opposite breast to achieve symmetry (similar shape) between them. It also includes coverage for prostheses and any complications resulting from a mastectomy (including lymphedema, a swelling of the surgical arm). This law allows women to choose a mastectomy knowing that their reconstruction costs will be covered.

Immediate or Delayed Reconstruction

Reconstruction can be done immediately following your cancer surgery or it can be performed at a later time. There is no time limit after cancer surgery for reconstruction being an option to restore your physical image. The decision of when is the best time for you can be made by reviewing the advantages and disadvantages of immediate versus delayed reconstruction. Ask your surgeon for additional comments.

Advantages of Immediate Reconstruction:

- One surgery experience, requiring anesthesia (being put to sleep) only once

- Lower cost than two separate surgeries

- Reduced recovery time in comparison to two separate surgeries

- Body image does not suffer as great a change as has been associated with mastectomy alone

- Psychologically, there may be better adaptation

Disadvantages of Immediate Reconstruction:

- More physical discomfort and longer recovery time following surgery, when anxiety levels are at their highest

- Surgery using body tissues requires a much longer surgery and recovery time

- Surgery using implants requires only slightly longer surgery and recovery time

- Increased potential for infection or surgical complications which could delay treatments for your cancer

Advantages of Delayed Reconstruction:

- Time to carefully study reconstruction methods and talk to patients who have experienced varying procedures

- Time to carefully select reconstructive surgeon and seek several consultations if needed

- Less psychological anxiety over cancer experience at time of reconstructive surgery

- No delay in treatments (chemotherapy or radiation) because of infection or complications from surgery

- Women who choose delayed reconstruction may be happier with their new breast than women who have immediate reconstruction because they have experienced the inconvenience of having to wear a prosthesis and the inability to go braless (thus their expectations were not as great)

Disadvantages of Delayed Reconstruction:

- Need for a second major surgery

- Higher cost because of second major surgery (anesthesia, surgery room, etc.)

- Cost of purchasing a prosthesis and special bras

- Inconvenience of having to wear a prosthesis until reconstructive surgery

- Temporarily unable to go braless or wear some low-cut clothing

- Procedure may fall into another deductible calendar year, requiring deductibles to be met for a second time (Some insurance providers may not pay for both a prosthesis and reconstruction. Only one option for restoring body image may be covered in a policy.)

- Psychological distress from having to deal with an altered body image while waiting on reconstructive surgery

Types of Reconstruction

If you are considering reconstruction, make an appointment for a consultation with a plastic surgeon and openly discuss your options and the different procedures that may be used. After looking closely at your history, recommended surgical procedure (mastectomy or lumpectomy) and treatment recommendations (chemotherapy or radiation therapy), the surgeon will take into account your desired reconstructive surgery outcome and make a recommendation for you.

There are many types of procedures available today which use implants or your own body tissue to reconstruct your breast. Implants may be filled with saline water, silicone or with combinations of both. Implants are placed under your chest muscle. Procedures called autologous reconstructions use body fat, with or without muscle, from your abdomen, back or buttocks to reconstruct your breast.

Surgical Procedure Decisions Depend On:

- Your physical makeup (size of your breast, degree of sagging)

- Your physical health and history

- Your preference for enlargement or reduction of the other breast during surgery

Breast Reconstruction Procedures

Breast Implants

Breast implants are the most common type of reconstructive breast surgery. The procedure may be done immediately after breast cancer surgery or later as outpatient or inpatient surgery. General anesthesia is usually used, and the surgery takes approximately one hour.

Indications for Implant Reconstruction:

- Women with small to medium-sized breasts, with little or no drooping (ptosis)

- Women with a small of amount of abdominal body fat

- Women desiring bilateral (both breasts) reconstruction

- Women not wanting additional scars

- Women who do not want longer, more complicated surgery

- Women in poorer general health or advanced age

- Women with large, drooping breasts who desire implant reconstruction usually require a surgical procerdure on the opposite breast to match the size and contour of the implanted breast.

Implant Procedures

There are two variations in implant procedures: (1) breast implant using an expander before final fixed-volume implant placement and (2) initial placement of a fixed-volume implant.

1. Breast Implants With Expander

Most women need to have their chest muscle and skin stretched before the final fixed-volume implant placement. An expander is inserted under the muscle and then gradually filled through a valve with a saline (salt water) solution every few weeks for 3 – 6 months. The surgeon injects about 50-cc of saline at each filling, causing slight discomfort for about 24 hours until the body adjusts to the new size. This gradual filling stretches the muscle and skin before the final implant placement. Additional surgery is required to remove the expander and position the fixed-volume implant.

A new combination expander and implant model allows the gradual expansion of the muscle and skin and does not have to be removed when the desired size is reached. The expander also serves as the permanent implant. Ask your physician about this type of implant.

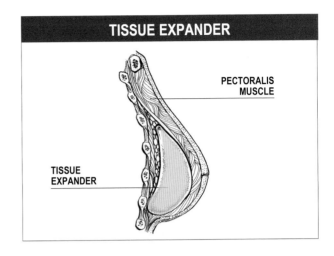

TISSUE EXPANDER

PECTORALIS MUSCLE

TISSUE EXPANDER

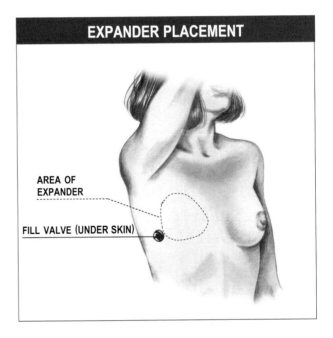

EXPANDER PLACEMENT

AREA OF EXPANDER

FILL VALVE (UNDER SKIN)

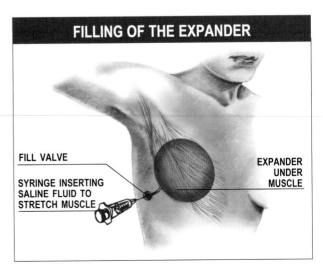

FILLING OF THE EXPANDER

FILL VALVE

SYRINGE INSERTING SALINE FLUID TO STRETCH MUSCLE

EXPANDER UNDER MUSCLE

2. Implant (fixed volume implant)

A soft shell filled with silicone gel or saline fluid or a combination of both is implanted under the skin and chest muscle. Surgery is either outpatient or inpatient and lasts approximately an hour. Local or general anesthesia may be used.

Ask your reconstructive surgeon which implant procedure is recommended for you.

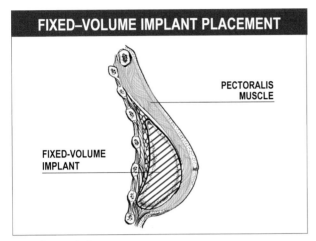

FIXED–VOLUME IMPLANT PLACEMENT

PECTORALIS MUSCLE

FIXED-VOLUME IMPLANT

Implant Advantages:

- Decreased surgical time for implant procedure
- Less pain after surgery than autologous body tissue reconstruction
- Decreased recovery time after surgery
- Decreased potential for surgical complications during and after surgery
- Less expensive surgery initially

Implant Disadvantages:

- An expander is usually needed to stretch out the muscles and skin before final implant placement. This requires several visits to the surgeon for injections of saline into the expander before final implant placement. During this time the surgical breast gradually matches the size of the other breast, unlike autologous (using your own body tissues) reconstruction where the breast matches the other breast in size immediately after surgery.

- Final implant may leak or rupture, requiring replacement
- Difficult to match a large remaining breast with implants
- Radiation therapy after implant placement increases risk of complications
- Capsular contracture risk (tissues around implant harden and distort its shape)
- Contracture may cause pain, as well as visual change in shape
- Severe contracture may require removal of implant and placement of new implant
- Difficult to get reconstructed breast with implant to hang symmetrically on chest wall with opposite breast (implant cannot match natural droop of other breast)
- Implants will stay same size with weight gain or weight loss, unlike natural breasts
- Implants have a limited lifespan of between 10 to 15 years; they deteriorate and need replacement (potentially requiring future surgical procedures)

Saline Versus Silicone Implants

For your final implant you will have to decide between a saline-filled or silicone-filled model. To help with the decision we will discuss the differences.

Saline Implants:

- Saline implants are filled with sterile saline (saltwater) water that has the same concentration of salt as most body fluids, causing it to have no adverse impact on the body if it leaks or ruptures. The problem is that if it ruptures, it deflates within hours, causing your chest to appear flat.
- Ruptured implants have to be replaced in an additional surgical procedure.
- Saline implants are firmer when touched than silicone implants.

Silicone Implants

Silicone implants have been in use for over forty years. In the early 1990s, reports that ruptured implants might be causing autoimmune disorders caused the Food and Drug Administration (FDA) to investigate them, and for a period of time they were available only to breast cancer patients for reconstruction and not to women who simply wanted to increase the size of their breasts. The final conclusion by the FDA in 2006, after the Institute of Medicine researched the charge, was that there was no evidence of a link between currently available silicone implants and health disorders. Two brands of silicone implants were made available to anyone. Unlike the early implants where the filling was the consistency of oil, the present implants' filling is very thick, like uncooked egg whites.

- Silicone implants are filled with a thick silicone filling that causes them to feel most like the human breast—softer to touch.
- Ruptured silicone implants can go undetected for years because the thick filling causes any leaks to be very slow—unlike saline leaks which are immediate. Surgical removal and replacement is recommended for leaking implants.
- The FDA recommends that women undergo magnetic resonance imaging (MRI) every few years to evaluate their silicone implants to detect any ruptures.

Comparison of Silicone and Saline Implants

	SALINE IMPLANTS	SILICONE IMPLANTS
Feels Natural	- Less able to mimic the feel of a natural breast	- Feels more like the normal breast
Size Variations	- Implant size can be increased or decreased after surgery during filling stage.	- Implant size cannot be changed after final implant placement. Implant is a fixed volume and is not filled by the surgeon.
Implant Rupture Potential	- Equal chance of rupture	- Equal chance of rupture
Ruptured Implant Symptoms	- Reconstructed breast deflates quickly as saline leaks into surrounding tissues and is absorbed. Patient is aware immediately that the implant has ruptured. - Replacement is required.	- Silicone gel leaks into the surrounding tissues but is not absorbed. Breast volume remains the same. Silicone implant ruptures may take longer to detect. - Replacement is required.
Replacement of Ruptured Implant	- Replacement is usually required at time of rupture, requiring an additional surgical procedure.	- Replacement is usually required at some point, requiring an additional surgical procedure.
Implant-Related Conditions	- Fibrosis or hardening of the tissues around the implant—called capsular contraction—may require surgery. - Infection - Pain - Nerve damage	- Fibrosis or hardening of the tissues around the implant—called capsular contraction—may require surgery. - Infection - Pain - Nerve damage

Autologous Reconstruction

Breast reconstruction using a woman's own body tissues (autologous) has many advantages, even with increased surgical complexity.

Advantages of Autologous Reconstruction:
- Avoids many complications relating to future surgical procedures for revision or replacement of implant
- Autologous tissues feel more like normal breast tissue, unless a woman is extremely thin
- Normal ptosis (drooping of breast) and inframammary crease (where the wire in an under-wire bra would be positioned) can be better matched by surgeon
- Surgeon can add additional skin flaps to avoid having to stretch skin if mastectomy scar is tight
- Post-surgical deformities or irregularities can be corrected with additional autologous tissues
- Donor sites (abdomen or hips) can have improvement in contour with reduction of body fat
- Lower cost over time because of fewer future complications and surgical revisions
- Volume and shape of autologous tissues follow body weight changes
- Return of breast sensation is possible with certain types of reconstruction
- Breast feels warm when touched
- Provides solution for partial mastectomies or wide lumpectomies because of flexibility of tissues
- Preferred reconstruction if radiation therapy is to be part of cancer treatment

Disadvantages of Autologous Reconstruction:
- Requires sacrificing another body part to reconstruct your breast
- Additional time required for surgery
- Increased recovery time
- Increased pain after surgery
- Potential for tissue necrosis (cell death) of reconstructed breast from lack of blood supply to newly transplanted tissues requiring removal and total loss of transplanted body part (Note: After surgery, you will be closely monitored for adequate blood supply to the newly transplanted tissues to detect any problems early and prevent loss of tissues.)
- Increased weakness in abdomen may limit physical activities and increase risk of hernia/bulge if abdominal muscles are used

Autologous Tissue Retrieval Sites And Reconstruction Types
- **Abdomen:**
  1. TRAM (Transverse Rectus Abdominis Myocutaneous muscle)
  2. DIEP (Deep Inferior Epigastric Perforator)

- **Back:**
  1. LD (Latissimus Dorsi)
  2. TAP (Thoracodorsal Artery Perforator)

- **Buttock:**
  1. Free superior or inferior gluteus
  2. S-GAP (Free-Superior Gluteal Artery Perforator)

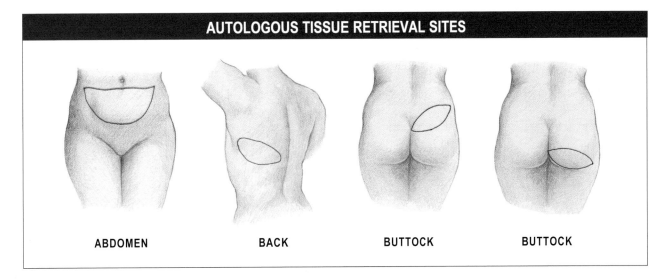

AUTOLOGOUS TISSUE RETRIEVAL SITES

ABDOMEN   BACK   BUTTOCK   BUTTOCK

CHAPTER 7

Types of Reconstruction Flaps

If you are using your body tissue for reconstruction, your donor tissues will be moved to the breast area with the blood supply left intact (pedicle flap) or the blood supply may be cut and reattached to the breast area (free flap).

- **Pedicle flap** is a procedure that moves the tissues, along with their own blood supply, to the breast area.

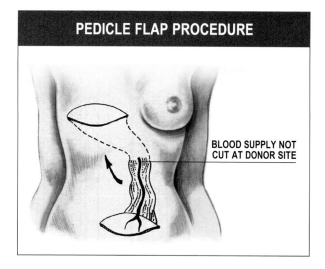

PEDICLE FLAP PROCEDURE

BLOOD SUPPLY NOT CUT AT DONOR SITE

- **Free flap** procedure cuts the tissues of the selected area from their blood supply and reattaches them through microsurgery to blood vessels in the breast area. Free flaps are the most complex of all reconstructive procedures, requiring a surgeon with expertise in microsurgery.

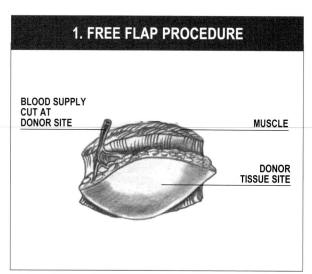

1. FREE FLAP PROCEDURE

BLOOD SUPPLY CUT AT DONOR SITE

MUSCLE

DONOR TISSUE SITE

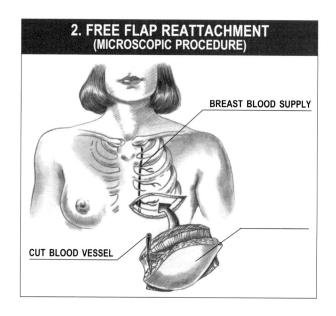

2. FREE FLAP REATTACHMENT (MICROSCOPIC PROCEDURE)

BREAST BLOOD SUPPLY

CUT BLOOD VESSEL

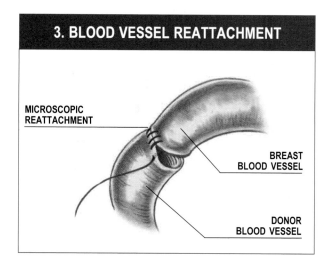

3. BLOOD VESSEL REATTACHMENT

MICROSCOPIC REATTACHMENT

BREAST BLOOD VESSEL

DONOR BLOOD VESSEL

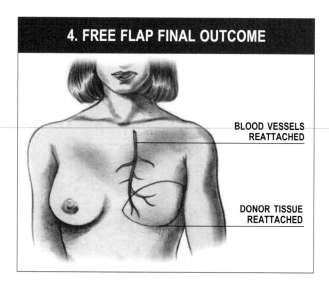

4. FREE FLAP FINAL OUTCOME

BLOOD VESSELS REATTACHED

DONOR TISSUE REATTACHED

Muscle-Sparing Reconstruction Flaps

Perforator flaps are recent refinements of conventional flaps where **none** of the underlying muscle is used. Perforator flaps can be taken from the abdomen (DIEP), back (TAP) or the buttocks (S-Gap). These procedures are relatively new. Ask your healthcare team if your reconstructive surgeons are skilled in these newer techniques.

Advantages of Perforator Flaps:
- Preserves muscle, which decreases the potential for future problems in donor site (weakness or restriction on activities)
- Preserving underlying muscle allows usual activities of daily living (sports, activities) as before surgery

Disadvantages of Perforator Flaps:
- Reconstructive surgeon experienced in new procedure is needed
- Prolonged operating time because of complexity of procedure

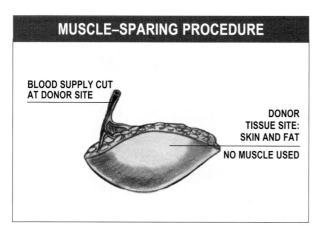

MUSCLE–SPARING PROCEDURE

BLOOD SUPPLY CUT AT DONOR SITE

DONOR TISSUE SITE: SKIN AND FAT

NO MUSCLE USED

Three Major Types of Autologous Reconstruction

There are three major areas of tissue used for autologous reconstruction: abdomen, back or buttocks. Each of these sites may be left attached to the original blood supply (pedicle flap) or cut from blood supply (free flap). In addition, the muscle may or may not be used from each of the three sites.

Abdominal Tissue Procedures
1. TRAM Flap (Transverse Rectus Abdominis Myocutaneous muscle)

The transverse rectus abdominis myocutaneous muscle (major stomach muscle) is moved to the breast area with fat and skin and is attached to form a breast. This procedure is most commonly called a tummy tuck. This is the most common type of autologous flap used at present and is excellent for women with additional abdominal fat.

Tram Flap Procedures:
- The transplanted tissue usually remains connected to its blood supply (called a pedicle flap), but occasionally tissues and muscle will be cut loose (free flap) and reconnected by microsurgery.
- Inpatient surgery with general anesthesia is required, lasting three to five hours and requiring several days of hospitalization.
- The procedure is moderately painful, causing difficulty in standing up straight for several days or weeks because of the cut muscle.

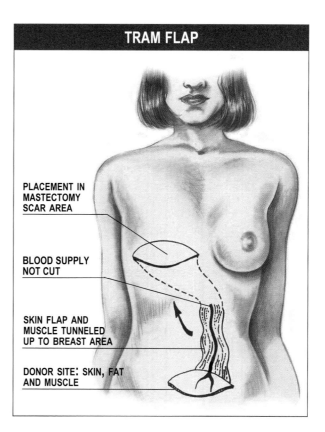

TRAM FLAP

PLACEMENT IN MASTECTOMY SCAR AREA

BLOOD SUPPLY NOT CUT

SKIN FLAP AND MUSCLE TUNNELED UP TO BREAST AREA

DONOR SITE: SKIN, FAT AND MUSCLE

- Drains are usually removed after one week, but may be left in place for several weeks.

- A scar is left on the abdomen where the flap is removed.

- Disadvantages are an increased weakness of the abdominal muscle and wall, limiting strength and making some activities difficult, along with an increased potential for hernias.

2. DIEP (Deep Inferior Epigastric Perforator)

This procedure uses abdominal tissues without the abdominal muscle (rectus abdominis). The fat is harvested with local blood vessels (free flap, cut loose from local blood supply). Nerves can also be harvested along with the flap and used to restore sensation to the tissues when reattached in the breast area. Recovery time is reduced in this procedure compared to the TRAM flap because the muscle is not being moved, allowing earlier mobilization and return to normal activities.

Back Tissue Procedures

1. Latissimus Dorsi (back flap)

The back muscle (latissimus dorsi) and an eye-shaped wedge of skin are moved from the back and sewn in place on the breast area. The transplanted tissues are left attached to their original blood supply (pedicle flap). This is an inpatient procedure with general anesthesia lasting two to four hours and requires several days of hospitalization. The procedure is moderately painful, and a scar is left on the back. Drains may be left in place for several weeks. An implant, in addition to your own tissue, may be required to match the opposite breast because of the size of the latissimus muscle moved. Some procedures can be performed endoscopically (using special instruments under the skin) without leaving a scar on the back. This procedure is excellent for small, non-drooping breasts or for partial, outer-quadrant reconstruction.

2. TAP (Thoracodorsal Artery Perforator)

This procedure is an alternative to the latissimus dorsi flap; it does not move the muscle, but uses the fat of the upper and lower areas around the muscle. Because some women do not have a lot of additional fat in this area, it may not be the preferred procedure.

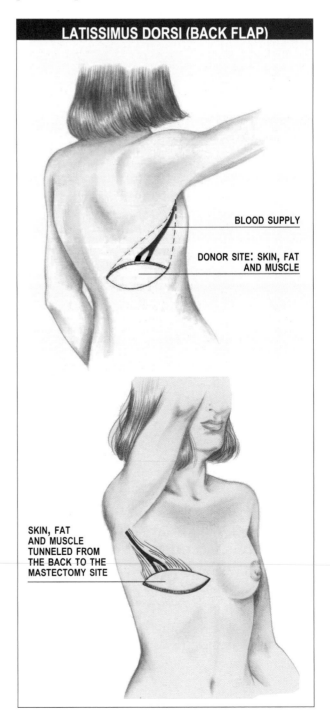

LATISSIMUS DORSI (BACK FLAP)

BLOOD SUPPLY

DONOR SITE: SKIN, FAT AND MUSCLE

SKIN, FAT AND MUSCLE TUNNELED FROM THE BACK TO THE MASTECTOMY SITE

Buttock Tissue Procedures
1. Inferior (lower) Gluteus (buttock) Flap

This procedure uses a patient's own tissue from fat and muscle in the buttocks. The tissue is detached (cut free) from its blood supply and reattached to the breast area blood supply using microsurgery. This is an inpatient procedure that includes general anesthesia. Surgery can range from three to eight hours, according to the degree of microscopic reattachment necessary. The scars on the buttocks are easily covered with underwear. Most women, except extremely thin ones, have tissue to spare.

INFERIOR GLUTEUS FLAP (BUTTOCK FLAP)

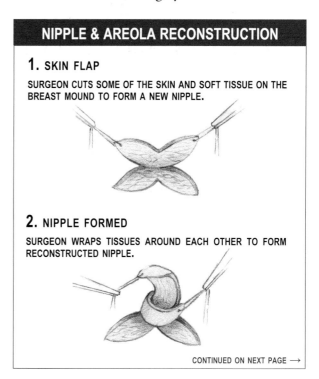

BLOOD
SUPPLY CUT

DONOR SITE:
SKIN, FAT
AND MUSCLE

AREA PREPARED FOR
DONOR TISSUE

DONOR SITE
SCAR

2. S-GAP
(Free-Superior Gluteal Artery Perforator)

This is an upgrade of the gluteus flap; it requires no muscle to be harvested and only the fatty tissue and an artery for blood supply are moved to the breast and reattached using microsurgery. The tissue is removed from the upper portion of the buttocks (superior). This area has the potential to remove and transfer nerves to restore sensation to the new breast.

Nipple and Areola Reconstruction

The nipple and areola are usually reconstructed from existing skin and fat on the breast itself, or occasionally from tissues removed from other areas of the body such as the groin. The skin is molded to form the shape of the nipple and attached to the breast mound. Areola reconstruction may be done by tattooing a dark pigmented color to match the other areola. Surgery is outpatient and pain is minimal. The procedure is usually performed about six months after reconstruction when breast symmetry is satisfactory. Some women choose not to have their nipple and areola reconstructed after breast reconstructive surgery.

NIPPLE & AREOLA RECONSTRUCTION

1. SKIN FLAP
SURGEON CUTS SOME OF THE SKIN AND SOFT TISSUE ON THE
BREAST MOUND TO FORM A NEW NIPPLE.

2. NIPPLE FORMED
SURGEON WRAPS TISSUES AROUND EACH OTHER TO FORM
RECONSTRUCTED NIPPLE.

CONTINUED ON NEXT PAGE →

← CONTINUED FROM PREVIOUS PAGE

NIPPLE & AREOLA RECONSTRUCTION

3. SUTURES
SURGEON SUTURES NEW NIPPLE IN PLACE.

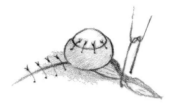

4. TATTOOING
AFTER THE NIPPLE HEALS, THE AREOLA IS ADDED BY TATTOOING TO MATCH THE OPPOSITE BREAST.

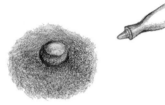

VARIOUS OTHER TECHNIQUES, INCLUDING SKIN GRAFTS FROM OTHER PARTS OF THE BODY, MAY BE USED. MOST OFTEN, THOUGH, SURGEONS USE A LOCAL SKIN FLAP. ASK YOUR SURGEON WHICH TECHNIQUE WILL BE USED.

What to Expect After Autologous Reconstruction

Recovery Timeline:
- Someone will need to stay with you for several days when you return home after your surgery.
- Most patients can plan to return to work in 4 – 5 weeks unless their job requires physical exertion.
- Swelling in the reconstructed breast and donor site where tissues were removed will persist for 1 – 2 months.
- Numbness in the reconstructed breast, donor site and sometimes the inner arm may occur for 6 – 12 months.
- Emotional letdown is normal for most women after breast reconstruction recovery and subsides when mobility returns.

Report to Physician:
- Temperature elevation above 100.5°
- Swelling that occurs quickly in breast or donor site
- Infection (redness, pus) in the area of incision or drain insertion site
- Change in color or temperature of reconstructed breast
- Pain that suddenly increases in the breast or donor site

Self-Care After Reconstruction:
- Sponge baths only until drains are removed. After drains are removed, you may shower. Water and mild soap are safe for your incision; however, do not scrub with a washcloth. No tub baths for two weeks.
- After a shower or bath, pat skin around surgical incisions to dry before applying clothes or bandage. A blowdryer set on "cool" can speed the drying process.
- Change bandage as ordered by physician to keep area clean and dry.
- Take prescribed antibiotics until all tablets are taken.
- Take prescribed pain medication as needed, switching to extra strength Tylenol® or ibuprofen as soon as you are comfortable. Do not drive while on prescribed pain medications.
- Do not drink alcohol while on prescription medication.
- No smoking.
- No lifting of objects over 5 pounds for three weeks.
- Do not sleep on the reconstructed breast or donor tissue site for three weeks; get out of bed on the side opposite your reconstruction.
- Daily walks are recommended.

Comparison of Breast Reconstruction Procedures

TYPE	ADVANTAGES	DISADVANTAGES	RECOMMENDED FOR	NOT RECOMMENDED FOR
Tissue Expander and Implant	▪ Short surgical time ▪ Low initial cost	▪ Multiple fillings of expander with saline ▪ 2nd surgery for implant ▪ Capsular contracture ▪ Leakage or rupture	▪ Medium size breast (400 – 800 cc) ▪ Lumpectomy defect ▪ Tight skin from radiation therapy	▪ Previous radiation therapy may limit size
Fixed-Volume Implant Only (Saline or Silicone)	▪ Short surgical time ▪ One-step procedure ▪ Lower initial cost	▪ Capsular contracture ▪ Leakage or rupture	▪ Small breast (200 – 400 cc)	▪ Thin skin flaps ▪ Radiation therapy
Latissimus Dorsi Flap (Pedicle Flap) Muscle and Tissue	▪ Autologous tissues: skin, fat and muscle transfer ▪ Small donor scar on back	▪ Muscle weakness ▪ Potential seroma ▪ Flap necrosis risk (1%)	▪ Small to medium size breast (200 – 600 cc) ▪ Lumpectomy defect ▪ Tight skin from radiation therapy	
TAP Thoracodorsal Artery Perforator (Free Flap) Tissues Only	▪ Autologous tissues: skin and fat only ▪ No muscle removed ▪ Small donor scar	▪ Potential seroma ▪ Flap necrosis risk	▪ Small to medium sized breast (200 – 600 cc) ▪ Lumpectomy defect ▪ Tight skin from radiation therapy	▪ Extremely thin women
TRAM Flap Transverse Rectus Abdominis Myocutaneous (Pedicle Flap)	▪ Autologous tissues: skin, fat and muscle ▪ Pedicle flap ▪ Tummy tuck	▪ Scar on abdomen ▪ Muscle weakness ▪ Extended operative time ▪ 6 – 12 wks. recovery ▪ Abdominal wall hernia ▪ Flap necrosis risk	▪ Mastectomy	▪ Previous abdominal surgery or liposuction ▪ Certain physical conditions ▪ Cigarette smokers (some physicians)
DIEP Deep Interior Epigastric Perforator (Free Flap)	▪ Abdominal tissues: skin and fat only ▪ Potential return of nerve sensations in area ▪ No muscle removed	▪ Additional scar on abdomen ▪ Extended operative time from microscopic reattachment ▪ Flap necrosis risk	▪ Mastectomy	▪ Previous abdominal surgery or liposuction ▪ Certain physical conditions ▪ Cigarette smokers (some physicians) ▪ Extremely thin women
Inferior Gluteus Flap (Free Flap)	▪ Autologous tissues: muscle, fat and blood vessels removed from lower buttocks	▪ Scar at donor site ▪ 6 – 12 weeks recovery ▪ Extended surgical reattachment time ▪ Flap necrosis risk	▪ Mastectomy	▪ Cigarette smokers (some physicians) ▪ Extremely thin women
S-GAP Superior Gluteal Artery Perforator (Free Flap)	▪ Autologous tissues: skin and fat only ▪ No muscle removed ▪ Potential return of nerve sensations in area	▪ Scar at donor site ▪ Shorter recovery ▪ Extended surgical reattachment time ▪ Flap necrosis risk	▪ Mastectomy	▪ Cigarette smokers (some physicians) ▪ Extremely thin women ▪ Excessively heavy women

Complications and Risks of Reconstruction Procedures

COMPLICATION RISKS	MUSCLE–SPARING (FREE-TRAM OR DIEP)	NON MUSCLE–SPARING	IMPLANTS
Abdominal bulge or hernia	2 – 4%	5 – 10%	
Abdominal weakness	Virtually eliminated	30 – 60%	
Delayed Healing	Less than 5%	Less than 5%	Less than 5%
Second surgical procedure necessary to remove or replace due to contracture, spontaneous rupture, damage to implant or patient dissatisfaction.			Up to 40% within first 5 years
Free flap failure	2%	2%	

*most common with previous radiation or smokers

Remember

Reconstruction is an option that all breast surgery patients need to know about, but not a procedure that all patients necessarily need to have.

Costs of reconstruction for women having a mastectomy are now covered by law. Cost should not be of concern when making your decision.

If all of this information overwhelms you, you do not have to make a decision now. Reconstruction can be performed at a later date, even years later. Make decisions based on what you feel best meets your needs.

To read explanations of DIEP and SGAP procedures, check timelines and see before and after photos, visit:
www.mauricenahabedian.com
www.diepflap.com

Tear-out Worksheets
Questions for Reconstructive Surgeon - Page W • 11
Reconstructive Surgery Options - Page W • 12

CHAPTER 8

The Surgical Experience

"I had the normal fear of adjusting to the loss of my breast, but by now I was more angry than afraid. My worst nightmare had become a reality."

—Harriett Barrineau

Prior to your surgery, you will need to have a pre-admission physical assessment that is usually performed in the facility where your surgery will take place. Lab work includes a profile of your blood components and body chemistry, urinalysis, possibly a chest X-ray or electrocardiogram and any other tests your physician may think are necessary. Remember to take your insurance card when going for this assessment, which usually takes one to two hours.

If you have a living will, healthcare directives or any special instructions, take them with you to be attached to your chart the day of surgery. It is now customary for everyone entering a hospital to be asked if they have a living will before any admission. This is asked of all patients and has nothing to do with your type of treatment or diagnosis. Also, take a list of any prescription or non-prescription medications that you regularly take. This also includes all herbal products.

A registered nurse will conduct an interview asking questions about your physical and medical history. You will be asked dates of previous surgeries or major illnesses and to list any allergies that you have experienced. Don't dismiss any detail as too insignificant or embarrassing to mention. It is better that the medical team be aware than be surprised by some complication.

Prior to your surgery, tell the nurse or physician if you are under the care of another specialist, such as a cardiologist or pulmonologist. Be sure that your surgeon is aware of their names and telephone numbers. Also inform your healthcare team if you have a physical limitation that would prevent you from being able to care for yourself at home. A home health service or aide may be ordered to assist you for a short period of time after your return home.

"Probably the most alone I have ever felt was the five minutes after my husband left my side before I went into surgery. Alone, scared of the unknown, so afraid. I felt like my heart was going to beat out of my chest. But then the anesthesia took effect and I went to sleep, and what seemed like minutes later, my surgeon was waking me up. In reality it was 8 hours later! Brian also says this was the hardest time for him."

—Anna Cluxton

You will be given instructions about any special preparations before surgery. For example, you will be told not to eat or drink after midnight before your surgery and to stop smoking as early before surgery as possible. Ask the nurse if you should take any of your regular medications the morning of surgery. The time you should arrive before your surgery and the scheduled time of your surgery will be provided during your pre-admission visit. Ask if there are any restrictions on the number of people allowed to wait in the surgical waiting room. Ask if cell phones are allowed in the waiting room.

Blood transfusions are rarely needed with lumpectomy and mastectomy surgeries. Occasionally, some types of reconstruction may require that blood be available if needed. Your reconstructive surgeon will inform you if you may possibly need to have blood available for your type of surgery. Information on how to arrange to have your blood collected and stored can be provided by your doctor.

Overnight Stay Packing Reminders:

- Personal hygiene items such as your comb, brush, toothbrush, toothpaste, deodorant, makeup and shampoo

- Robe and gown or pajamas (two to three changes—better if they are front-opening)

- Undergarments

- Bedroom shoes

- Reading material

- Telephone numbers of family and friends

- Pencil and note paper

- A small travel pillow to elevate your arm while in the hospital and to use with your seat belt on your ride home.

- Clothes to wear home. Some women find that large, soft sweatshirts or loose-fitting, front-opening tops are comfortable. Flat, comfortable shoes are recommended.

- Some surgeons and reconstructive surgeons place a special post-operative surgical bra on a patient immediately after surgery. Ask if they use surgical bras. If not, you may wish to be prepared by talking to your surgeon about recommendations.

- Lumpectomy patients need to ask their surgeon about recommendations for a well-fitting, soft, front-closing bra to wear after surgery. It is recommended that you purchase two or more before surgery to have another available if one gets soiled or wet.

- Mastectomy patients need to ask the surgeon about recommendations for a bra and how to restore their body image if they have a mastectomy without reconstruction. Local prosthetic stores have soft fiber puffs that will fill the surgical side of the bra cup until you are healed and can purchase a prosthesis. You don't have to wear a bra; this is a decision for women who want their body image restored as soon as possible. Many women choose to obtain this fiber puff before surgery so that it can be matched to the size of their breast.

- Reconstructive patients need to ask the surgeon for recommendations on purchasing a special type of bra to wear after surgery.

Outpatient Surgery Preparation:

- Wear loose-fitting, front-opening, comfortable clothing along with comfortable shoes that are suitable for your return home.

- Pack a bag with a comb or brush, mirror, toothbrush and toothpaste.

- Take a bra to wear after surgery as discussed above.

It will be psychologically and physically helpful to have someone plan to be with you on the day of surgery. A trained nurse is not necessary because mastectomy and lumpectomy surgeries are usually relatively simple and do not involve extensive assistance after surgery. A family member or friend will be able to assist you and make this time more comfortable (for example, by helping you to the bathroom or getting you something to drink).

Informed Consent

Sometime before your surgery, you will be asked to sign an informed consent form. Consent forms will also be presented for your signature before chemotherapy, radiation therapy or reconstructive surgery. Your physician or an assistant will explain the procedures that will be performed and the possible risks involved. This explanation will occur before you are given sedation. Read the consent form carefully.

Information Includes:

- Type of surgery and treatment you will receive
- Name of the doctor who will perform the surgery or treatment
- Risks of the surgery or treatment
- Benefits of the surgery or treatment
- Identification of any experimental treatments
- When the treatment will begin and end

By signing this form, you acknowledge that you understand and have no other questions. Discuss with the surgeon what type of post-operative pain management will be used and if the medication will be given on request. If you do not understand and would like more information, this is the time to request it.

Day of Your Surgery

On the day of surgery you will need to report to the surgery area at the assigned time. Do not wear jewelry (watches, rings, earrings) or contact lenses. Eyeglasses may be needed to read and sign admission forms. Dental bridges or false teeth can be worn and removed just prior to your surgery. The nurse will place them in a special storage container during surgery and they will be made available to you as soon as you are alert. Do not bring money, credit cards or a checkbook. Leave these with family members or at home.

You will be interviewed by your anesthesiologist (the physician who administers the anesthesia)

before going to surgery. Some anesthesiologists may prefer an interview prior to the day of surgery. Your medical history will be reviewed before surgery. Inform your nurse if any changes in your health have occurred since the initial assessment (cold, fever, diarrhea, etc.).

You will be taken to a room where you will undress and begin preparation for surgery. Your underarm area will be shaved. An intravenous needle to be used for medications and fluids will be inserted into the arm opposite the surgical site. A medication will be administered to keep you calm.

After entering the surgical suite, you will be positioned upon a surgical table. A blood pressure cuff will be placed on your arm to monitor your pressure, a device will be placed on your finger to measure the oxygen in your blood and an electrocardiogram machine will be hooked up to monitor your heart. The surgeon will cleanse a large area surrounding the site of the surgical incision. You will be given your anesthesia sometime during this process. After you are asleep, you will have a tube placed in your throat to facilitate your breathing. Your surgery will then be performed.

When the surgical procedure is completed, you will be transferred to a post-anesthesia (recovery) room. Your blood pressure, oxygen level and heart rate will be monitored while in this room. Usually, you are in recovery for two or more hours according to the type of anesthesia you received. When you are awake and your vital signs are in normal range, you will be transferred to your room or allowed to return home if you are having outpatient surgery. Your family members will be able to join you at this time. If you are to leave the same day, you may be transferred to an outpatient recovery room and monitored for several more hours before being dismissed. If staying in the hospital, your blood pressure, pulse and breathing rate will be monitored at regular intervals.

After you wake up, you may also have a slight headache or nausea from the residual anesthesia. This is not unusual and often may be caused by the long period of time you have been without food or caffeine. Resume eating by taking fluids first, then adding light foods and finally progressing to your normal diet as you desire. Nausea can be increased by eating heavy foods.

Your throat may feel sore from the tube inserted during surgery. Soreness in the back or shoulder area is very common because of the position you were required to be in during surgery. This soreness will last for several days.

Dressing and Drain Bulbs

You will have a dressing on your chest and may have one or more bulb drains to avoid fluid collection in the surgical site. Some surgeries may not require a drain. At first the drainage will be bright red from blood, but it will gradually change color over the next few days. If at any time you notice that your bandage feels wet or you see bright red blood coming through your bandage, notify your healthcare team. The drain(s) may remain in place after you return home.

Discomfort After Surgery

Most women are surprised at the small amount of pain they experience after their surgery. Pain medication has been ordered by the physician to control any pain you experience. If you are an inpatient, you must request it from the nurse. If you have pain, use your nurse call button to let your nurse know so the medication can be administered. If you return home, take the prescribed pain medication as ordered. Always take pain medication when you begin to feel uncomfortable. Pain can increase other postoperative symptoms. Medication is most effective when taken early, so do not deny yourself medication if you experience pain. Your goal is to take what you need to be as comfortable as possible. Remember, there are no rewards for suffering unnecessarily.

The pain experienced after breast surgery has been described by women as a discomfort in the breast area, accompanied by numbness or tingling in the arm. Others say that they felt pain in the removed breast that felt like a heaviness or sensations from the nipple. Doctors call this phantom pain because even though the breast is gone, the brain perceives the sensation of pain from the remaining nerves. Some of the nerves on the chest wall may be irritated or cut during the surgical procedure, and this causes a feeling of numbness across the chest. Most women state that most discomfort is under the arm where the lymph nodes were removed. This pain often radiates down the arm, and you may feel as if needles or pins are pricking you. The arm may also feel numb. The numbness is not unusual, and the pricking sensations may or may not improve in the coming months. Incisional pain is usually over in about a week to ten days, and the arm sensations will improve as arm mobility is restored. The surgical staff's goal is for you to experience the minimum amount of pain, and they will provide you with the amount of medication required to keep you comfortable.

Personal Hygiene After Surgery

For the next few days, you may need to take sponge baths in order to keep your dressing dry. Ask your doctor when you have permission to take a shower or a tub bath. The dressing should always be kept dry. If at any time the dressing becomes wet, you need to have it changed. Dressings that are damp and remain over the incision can cause a local infection.

Your physician will tell you when you can use your surgical arm to shampoo your hair. Do not use deodorant under the surgical arm for the first six weeks. However, you may wipe the area with an alcohol pad if you feel a need to cleanse the area. Avoid allowing the alcohol to run into the surgical area and cause stinging.

Post-Surgical Arm Care:

- Continue to use your hand on the side of your surgery to feed yourself, comb your hair and wash your face. These activities will help reduce the soreness.

- When lying down, keep your surgical arm propped up on a pillow above the level of your heart to prevent fluid accumulation and swelling in the arm and to reduce pain.

- Place a small pillow between your surgical arm and body to keep the arm from pressing tightly against the body. This position also promotes drainage and reduces swelling.

- Do not lift anything heavy (over 1 – 2 pounds) or begin any exercises until your physician gives you permission.

- Get in and out of your bed on the side opposite your surgery.

- Elevate your arm above the level of your heart for 45 minutes twice daily for the first six weeks after surgery.

Rest After Surgery

The time spent in the hospital will be only a day or a few days. During this time you may feel sleepy and tired from the anesthesia and all the stress that accumulated prior to the surgery. If you don't feel up to having many visitors, ask your nurse to place a "No Visitors" sign on your door. If you return home the same day of surgery, you may also want to have your family members monitor visitors so that you can get the amount of rest you need.

You may also take the telephone off the hook or turn the ringer off when you are trying to rest. Ask family members or friends to speak to visitors or answer the telephone if you feel you need rest. Remember to ask for or take medications to keep you comfortable. During a hospital stay, pain and nausea medications are not given automatically. They must be requested by the patient.

The Surgical Incision

Your first dressing change will occur before you leave the hospital unless you have outpatient surgery—in which case, you will return to the physician's office. Some women report it was difficult to view the incision for the first time, but afterward they were glad they did. Viewing the incision may also be difficult for your partner. Many women feel that viewing the incision together the first time was helpful in their future adjustment. Postponing the viewing does not make it easier or help either of you.

It is important that you observe the incision area carefully at this time to learn what is normal for the scar area. This will help as you monitor the incision for changes after you return home. A mastectomy scar is one long scar. You may have sutures or staples to close the incision. A lumpectomy will have an incision on the breast and another under the arm if lymph nodes were removed. Your doctor or nurse will provide instructions at this time on how and when to change the dressing and on changes to report to the medical staff. It will be helpful if a family member is present during these instructions to help you understand and be able to assist you with dressing changes and managing drains.

Care of Your Surgical Dressing

The goal while caring for your incision is to keep a clean, dry dressing in place and monitor the area for changes that might indicate an infection. Types of dressings vary with physicians, but all dressings need to remain dry. A wet dressing will set up an environment for bacteria to breed and may cause an infection. If your dressing becomes damp, follow your physician's instructions for changing it. Sutures or staples are removed five to ten days later in the doctor's office.

Your surgeon or nurse will discuss care of your dressing prior to discharge. It may help to have a family member assist with dressing changes because of the soreness you will experience and the difficulty of working on your own chest. Ask your nurse for dressing supplies to take home. Follow special orders from your physician for dressing changes. If you do not receive orders, the steps for changing a dressing are listed below.

Dressing Change Instructions

1. Gather all dressing supplies: disposable bag, dressing (gauze), tape, scissors, alcohol wipes or gauze pads.

2. Wash your hands.

3. Pre-cut tape into strips to apply to new dressing.

4. Remove the old dressing and note the color, odor and amount of drainage on dressing.

5. Dispose of the old dressing by placing it in the bag.

6. Wash your hands thoroughly with soap.

7. Observe incision carefully as you wipe off any old blood or tape residue with an alcohol wipe. Always start wiping near the incision and wipe away from the incision, not back over it.

8. Place clean dressing on the area and tape it into place.

9. Dispose of the bag containing old dressing and alcohol wipes.

10. Wash your hands.

Monitoring Your Incision

When changing your dressing, observe the old bandage for signs of drainage. Normal drainage is a blood-tinged, watery discharge. Discharge that is thick and yellowish to greenish in color may indicate infection. Often this type of discharge will have a foul odor. If you notice this occurring, notify your healthcare provider.

Carefully observe the incision site. An increase in tenderness, warmth, redness, swelling and signs of discharge anywhere along the incision line may indicate a potential infection. Call your physician's office and ask for instructions. Often, early intervention may require a local antibiotic to the area.

Ask your physician when you may take a shower or tub bath and use soap and water on the area. Some physicians allow showers first because of the constant flow of clean water over the incision. After your bath/shower, pat the area dry or use a hairdryer on low heat to thoroughly dry the area. Apply a soft dressing or covering to prevent irritation and rubbing by your clothing. Some find that a soft tee shirt or a long-line cotton sports bra, sold in department stores, serves this purpose. Special camisoles sold in prostheses shops, boutiques and online are designed for the post-surgical patient. These garments are soft and have pockets to accommodate the soft fiber puff on either side if you have had a mastectomy without reconstruction. The camisole can be worn without a bra after a dressing is no longer required and during radiation therapy treatments when the skin becomes sensitive. Post-reconstruction camisoles are also available. These camisoles are often reimbursed by your insurance provider if you get your surgeon to write an order. You can view these products on-line.

It is important not to allow any powder, deodorant, lotions or perfumes to come in contact with the surgical incision site. These products should be avoided for six weeks past surgery or until the site has healed completely. You may wipe the area with an alcohol wipe to further cleanse after your bath.

Care of Your Drain Bulbs

Instructions will also be given on how to care for your drain(s) if you have one. Drains are inserted to collect fluid accumulating at the surgery site and to reduce swelling and pain. The tubing is anchored to your tissue during surgery. At the end of the tubing is a soft plastic bulb with a plug that allows the fluid to be emptied.

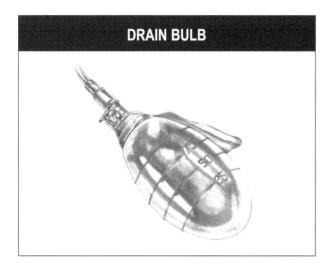

DRAIN BULB

The fluid that accumulates in the drain bulb is a mixture of blood cells and lymphatic fluid. During surgery, the lymphatic system vessels are cut, causing the microscopic vessels to empty their fluid into the area. The drainage will be dark red at first because of the large amount of blood cells in the area. It will gradually change to pink-tinged and finally to a yellow straw color. The amount of drainage varies, and there is no way to predict how much drainage any woman will accumulate. Some women have large amounts and others have a minimal amount. Gradually, these small vessels seal themselves off, and the fluid stops accumulating. The time this takes varies among women. Neither body size nor age seems to determine the amount; however, the amount of drainage during the first 24 hours often predicts the accumulation volume later.

Physicians remove the drains when the amount of drainage is reduced to between 20 to 50 ccs (½ to 1½ ounces or 4 to 10 teaspoons) per drain, per 24 hours. Some women have very little drainage and have their drain(s) removed within the first week. Others may need their drain(s) for several weeks and, occasionally, longer. If the drain(s) are removed too soon, the fluid can accumulate under the skin, forming a seroma (collection of fluid), and become painful by putting pressure on the surgical site. Neither the amount of fluid produced nor the length of time you are required to have drains has anything to do with your cancer. Fluid and drains are only related to the amount of fluid your lymph system produces.

Your nurse will discuss care of your drains. It is important not to allow the drains to hang loosely. Always secure them to your clothing and empty them when they become heavy. (Some post-surgical camisoles have drain holders.) The first day your drains may require emptying every several hours. Later, twice a day will be sufficient. Pressure from a heavy drain that is not pinned to your clothing and pulls on your incision site can cause pain and scar formation at the drain insertion site. The scar will heal but will be thick and have an uneven appearance. Be careful not to allow drains to drop away from your body.

Emptying and Recording Drainage

Empty drains when they become heavy or over half-filled with fluid. When your drainage has decreased to a small amount, empty twice a day.

1. If you have more than one drain, place a piece of tape on each, and mark them with numbers (drain 1 or drain 2). Refer to the amounts emptied, and record by number designation.

2. Gather your supplies: a drain record (found on page W • 15), pencil or pen and a measuring cup.

3. Open one drain by removing the plug in the drain bulb and empty drainage into a measuring cup.

4. Squeeze the air out of the empty bulb and keep the bulb squeezed as flat as possible as you replug the drain. This compression of the bulb encourages the flow of fluid from the surgical site into the bulb.

5. If any of the drainage spilled onto the outside of the bulb, wipe it off with a damp cloth using soap and water or an alcohol wipe.

6. Secure the bulb by pinning it to your clothing or placing it into a surgical drainage bulb bag or holder. Do not allow the bulb to hang freely.

7. Measure the drainage in the cup.

8. Observe the color of the drainage. If you notice that the fluid has changed color, becoming a darker red, or if fresh blood reappears after the color had changed to a light pink, contact your physician's office and inform them of the change.

9. Empty the drainage into the toilet and flush. Do not save the drainage.

10. Wash your hands with soap and water.

11. Record drainage under the appropriate column, documenting the time and amount emptied.

12. If you have a second drain, repeat the process.

13. Take the written drainage record to the surgeon on your return visit. An accurate record will assist the physician in determining when to remove your drain(s).

Potential Post-Surgical Problems

Fluid Leakage at Drain Site
Occasionally, a small amount of fluid will leak from the insertion site of the tubing. This is not dangerous. However, you should change the dressing when it becomes damp and apply a sterile dressing. Do not allow a wet dressing to remain in place. The dressing should be changed as often as needed to prevent irritation and breakdown of the skin. A wet dressing will allow bacteria to grow. If large amounts of fluid begin leaking from the site, call your surgeon or nurse and ask for instructions.

Clogged Drains
Bulb drains may clog because of the formation of small clots in the tubing. This is not an unusual occurrence. If you notice that there is no fluid in the bulb, check the tubing for a possible blockage caused by a clot.

Instructions for Opening a Clogged Drain:
1. Wash your hands with soap and water.

2. Gently squeeze the area in which the clot is located to dislodge it.

3. After squeezing the clot, begin near the insertion site on your chest and squeeze downward the entire length of the tubing toward the drainage bulb. Do not pull on the tubing. Repeat the process several times, squeezing the entire length of the drainage tubing.

4. Secure drains to prevent hanging loosely.

5. Monitor the drain bulb for fluid accumulation. If no drainage has accumulated after several hours, notify your physician for further instructions.

Monitoring Drains for Infection
It is very rare for infections to occur with bulb drains. However, if you notice the insertion site begins to have an increased redness, discharge of pus (thick yellowish or greenish fluid) or foul odor, notify your physician of these changes. The main prevention for infection is to keep the area clean and dry.

Drain Removal
Drains are removed by the surgeon or an assistant during an office visit. Women report a pulling feeling with a moderate amount of pain lasting for a few seconds when the drain is removed. A small bandage is placed over the drain removal site. This site will also need to be monitored for infection for the next several days. Any increase in redness, swelling, discharge or pain should be reported to your surgeon's office.

Seromas
Before or after your drains are removed, if you have a painful accumulation of fluid at the incision site, below the incision site or in the underarm area, notify your physician. This fluid accumulation is called a seroma. The accumulation of fluid forms a soft lump and feels like a water balloon under the skin. If a seroma continues to increase in size and puts pressure on your incision, it can become painful.

Seromas are the most common complication after surgery. Painful seromas may require the withdrawal (called aspiration) of the fluid from the area using a small needle and an empty syringe by the physician. This procedure is performed in the physician's office. Withdrawal of the fluid is relatively painless, and removal of the fluid relieves the pain. However, as with any invasive procedure, the potential for infection increases. You will need to monitor the area and report any redness, swelling or pain to your physician. Occasionally, the fluid will continue to accumulate, requiring several aspirations by the surgeon. This fluid accumulation has nothing to do with your cancer. It is related only to lymphatic fluid accumulation in the area.

Hospital Discharge Instructions

Prior to leaving the hospital or surgical center, your nurse will provide you with verbal and written instructions concerning your care and a list of symptoms that might occur and need to be reported to the doctor. Write down any questions as they occur.

Ask Your Physician:

- To clarify anything you do not understand about your diagnosis or surgery.

- What activities can I do with my surgical arm until my next appointment?

- Are there any special exercises or recommendations regarding use of my arm?

- Are the numbness or tingling sensations I am experiencing temporary or permanent?

- What kind of pain is normal after my type of surgery?

- What medications will I take for pain?

- Will I be given any prescriptions for medication to take at home?

- Do I resume previous medications (especially estrogen-type medications)?

- When can I shampoo my hair?

- When can I shower or take a tub bath?

- When can I remove my dressing?

- When can I drive?

- When and how do I make my next appointment?

- Will I be referred to any other doctors or have any other treatments? If so, when will I see these doctors?

- When will my final pathology report be available?

- Is there anything special that I can do to ensure a speedy recovery?

Ask Your Nurse:

- To write down any appointment dates or names of doctors to whom you will be referred for further evaluation.

- For a telephone number that you can call after you return home if you have any questions regarding your discharge instructions.

- If surgical dressing supplies are provided to take home with you in case you need them.

Seat Belt Use After Surgery

On your ride home after surgery have a small travel pillow to place over your chest and the area of your incision so that you will be able to wear your seat belt in the car. The pressure of a seat belt during sudden stops can cause pain and potential injury to new mastectomy or lumpectomy surgical sites. The protection provided by the pillow can prevent this type of injury or discomfort and make wearing your seat belt more comfortable. Using the pillow for protection when wearing a seat belt is helpful for the first several weeks after your surgery if the seat belt crosses your incision.

Recovering at Home

Your discharge instructions from the hospital give you information about when you need to call the physician, how to manage your drains and how to change your bandage. Recovery from surgery for breast cancer usually requires two to three weeks. Discomfort in the incisional area(s) will improve daily, usually resolving within ten days. In five to six weeks, most women report that they have resumed their normal activities. Remember, we are all different. Listen to the cues from your body, rest when needed and resume your normal activities when you feel up to them.

Your incision will change color as it heals; this is normal. The scar will be red and raised initially and for several months past surgery. The redness is caused by the additional blood flow to promote healing in the area. The redness and thickness of the scar will subside over the next one to two years, and the area will become less obvious and very faint in color.

Plan to begin your exercise program to restore your normal range of motion in the surgical arm as soon as the physician gives you permission. Report any problems you have when performing the exercises to your physician.

It is important that you keep your follow-up appointments with the surgeon and any other physicians. You will be monitored for proper healing and the return of proper range of motion in your surgical arm. Your remaining breast will also be closely checked on following visits.

Uncommon Post-Surgical Problems

Most women have very few problems after breast surgery. However, there are some uncommon problems that may arise from the surgical procedure that you may need to be aware of. These problems have nothing to do with the cancer and are only due to the surgery.

Phlebitis

Occasionally some women will have very little pain after their surgery only to experience a pain that begins days after surgery. The pain may radiate down the arm, usually to the elbow, but sometimes to the wrist. This occurs when the basilic vein in the arm has become inflamed after the surgery. This inflammation, called phlebitis, is not serious; it causes pain that can be helped with an analgesic such as aspirin or ibuprofen. Phlebitis is not a common occurrence and will resolve in several days to a week. This pain may limit your ability to perform your exercises. Inform your physician if this should occur.

Breast Sensations

In some women, various breast sensations may occur in the surgical site after mastectomy with or without reconstruction. Some physicians refer to these sensations as "phantom breast sensations." These are the same types of feelings experienced after limb amputation in other areas of the body and are caused by nerves that were cut during surgery. During the surgical healing process, the brain interprets the signals from the remaining nerves on the chest wall and may cause some women to experience a variety of sensations.

Phantom Sensations May Include Feelings Of:
- Pins and needles
- Itching
- Pressure
- Extreme sensitivity of skin to clothing touching the area

If you experience these sensations after mastectomy and they become bothersome, inform your physician. Sometimes ice packs are helpful. Check with your physician about their use. Physical therapists are trained to treat these symptoms with a procedure called "desensitization," which decreases the sensations from the nerve endings left in the area causing the problem. The therapist can instruct you on how to perform the procedure at home if needed, and this then becomes part of your daily exercise routine. Massage of the area may also be recommended. If the sensation does not decrease, medications may be prescribed by your physician. This is a time-limited problem that usually resolves as healing progresses.

Frozen Shoulder

Failure to use your arm after the physician has given you permission to begin exercises to restore normal range of motion can result in a condition called a "frozen shoulder." This condition causes pain and inability to move the shoulder freely; however, it is a rare occurrence. Any complication that can keep you from proceeding with your exercise program should be brought to the surgeon's attention. Restoring full range of motion is accomplished by gradually increasing the movements of the arm and using exercises such as the ones in Chapter 18.

Post-Surgical Products

www.softeeusa.com

1-866-605-8585

Site offering a wide selection of after-breast surgery products for recovery including reconstruction camisoles and fiber-filled breast forms.

Refer to Tear-out Worksheets

Drain Bulb Record - Page W • 15

Surgical Discharge Questions - Page W • 13

Remember

Surgery for breast cancer is usually not very physically painful, but it may be very emotionally painful.

Ask your healthcare team for what you need to make this time as easy as possible for you—additional information or instructions, pain medication, privacy, access to a chaplain, etc. You are employing them to meet your needs.

Tell your support partner, family or friends what you need from them during this time. Be honest.

Do not hesitate to call your physician if any problems arise when you return home.

Use the time of your surgery to rekindle your emotions and energy. Rest when needed. Be good to yourself. Think about any changes you would like to make in your life. At no other time in life will people give you as much permission to make changes.

What is it you have always wanted to do—begin a new hobby, go on a trip, take a class, get a pet or start an exercise program? You decide what will give you the most happiness, and GO FOR IT.

Breast cancer is not a valid excuse to forego planning for events and activities that will bring you happiness. Plan your exciting new future. Use breast cancer as the reason and not the excuse!

Survivorship

Life has hurts, pains and disappointments for everyone. It's a part of the human experience. Expecting losses and disappointments as a normal part of life keeps us from being overwhelmed when they occur. The secret is to take your hurts, pains and disappointments and use them to learn how to build a better life. Since you can't avoid them, learn to use them as tools for refining and redesigning your life.

—Judy Kneece

Going through loss and grief is like going through a tunnel. The bad news is the tunnel is dark. The good news is once you have entered into that tunnel, you're already on your way out.

—Dr. Robert Jeffress

Understanding Your Pathology Report

"I asked for and kept copies of my pathology reports. Over the years, I have found this to be helpful."

—Anna Cluxton

The preliminary pathology report you received after your biopsy contained a lot of information about your cancer. A final pathology report will be prepared after any additional surgery that will give additional information about your cancer and the status of cancer in your lymph nodes. Your treatment plan is based on both the preliminary and the final pathology reports. From this series of reports, your physicians will determine which course of treatment is best suited for your individual case. The most common treatments are surgery, chemotherapy, radiation therapy and hormonal therapy. Your treatment may consist of one or more types of treatment. For some women, no further treatment may be needed beyond close observation by the physician. A brief explanation of each type of treatment will be discussed. Because of the wide variety of treatment plans, your physician will provide you with specific information regarding your planned treatment.

Your Pathology Report

Because treatment decisions will be based on the pathology reports on your tumor, it may be helpful to understand how the reports are used in determining your treatment options. However, it is not essential that you understand all of the following information. Some people feel that this is more information than they want to know. Feel free to skip this section. It is included in case you need to have some questions about your pathology report clarified.

After your tumor was removed from your breast, it was sent to a pathology laboratory where it was carefully processed. There, a pathologist (a physician who specializes in diagnosing diseases from tissue samples) analyzed your

"I was serious about wanting to know about breast cancer. I wanted to be a part of my treatments. I wanted to know what was being done and why. The secrets to my individual tumor lay in my final pathology report."

—Harriett Barrineau

"My doctors explained and then gave me my report. I looked over it, but I wasn't really interested in what was on that piece of paper. There was nothing there that was going to change my circumstances in life one bit. I was more interested in what we were going to do to take care of it."

—Earnestine Brown

tissues by careful, naked-eye dissection as well as under a microscope and issued a pathology report to your physician. This report contains the unique characteristics of your individual tumor. This report will help your physicians determine if you need additional treatment. If additional treatment is needed, the pathology report will be used as a guide for all of your physicians to develop a treatment plan for your cancer.

The slides and tissue blocks prepared by the pathologist to study your tumor and interpreted in your pathology report may remain available for additional consults and future studies if future research unfolds with new tissue diagnostic tests.

Characteristics of Cancer Cells

- **Normal Cells**—Normal ducts and lobules are lined with one or more layers of cells in an orderly pattern.

- **In Situ Cancer**—It is called "in situ cancer" when these normal cells become abnormal and cancer develops and grows. In situ cancer does not break through the wall but remains in the duct or lobule where it began. This type has a good prognosis.

- **Invasive (Infiltrating) Cancer**—Cancers that have broken through the wall of the duct or lobule and have begun to grow into surrounding tissues in the breast are considered invasive or infiltrating cancers. "Microinvasive" means that just a small amount of cells have grown through the duct or lobular walls.

Types of Breast Cancer

The most common types of breast cancer are listed below. There are also various other rare types of breast cancer and combinations of the following types.

- Infiltrating (invasive) ductal (approximately 52% of patients)

- In situ ductal (intraductal) (approximately 21%)

- Invasive lobular (approximately 5%)

- In situ lobular (intralobular) (approximately 2%)

- Medullary (approximately 6%)

- Mucinous or Colloid (approximately 3%)

- Paget's disease with intraductal (approximately 1%)

- Paget's disease with invasive ductal (approximately 1%)

Remaining Cancers Occurring in 1% or Less:

- Tubular
- Cribiform
- Papillary
- Micropapillary
- Apocrine

- Adenocystic
- Inflammatory
- Carcinosarcoma
- Squamous
- Sarcoma

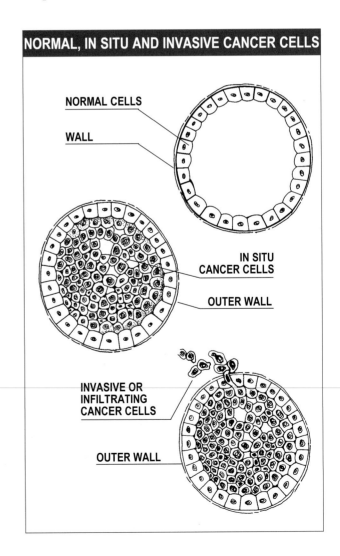

NORMAL, IN SITU AND INVASIVE CANCER CELLS

NORMAL CELLS

WALL

IN SITU CANCER CELLS

OUTER WALL

INVASIVE OR INFILTRATING CANCER CELLS

OUTER WALL

Tumor Size

Tumor size is the measured size of the tumor. Results are reported in millimeters (mm) or centimeters (cm).

- 10 mm equals 1 cm
- 1 cm equals ⅜ inch
- 1 inch equals 2.5 cm

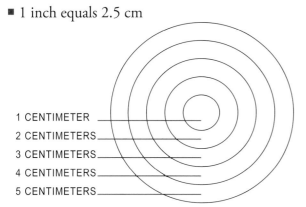

1 CENTIMETER
2 CENTIMETERS
3 CENTIMETERS
4 CENTIMETERS
5 CENTIMETERS

Tumor Shape

The report may also state the shape of a solid tumor as being round, spherical or having irregular contours such as stellate or spiculated.

Margins

Margins are the area cut by the surgeon's knife surrounding your tumor.

Terms to Describe Pathology Margins:

- **Negative, clear, clean or uninvolved:** means there was no evidence of cancer cells in the margins
- **Positive, involved or residual cancer:** means that cancer was found in the margins.
- **Indeterminate:** means the pathologist could not determine and make a definite statement about the margins.

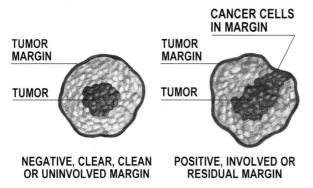

CANCER CELLS IN MARGIN

TUMOR MARGIN

TUMOR

NEGATIVE, CLEAR, CLEAN OR UNINVOLVED MARGIN

TUMOR MARGIN

TUMOR

POSITIVE, INVOLVED OR RESIDUAL MARGIN

Node Status

If surgery included lymph node removal using sentinel node or axillary dissection, the report will state how many nodes were removed, a description of the area from which the nodes came and how many nodes tested positive for cancer cells.

- **Lymph node negative** means no cancer was found in the lymph nodes.
- **Lymph node positive** means that cancer was present in the lymph nodes.

Nuclear Grade

Nuclear grade evaluates the size and shape of the nucleus in tumor cells and the percentage of tumor cells that are in the process of dividing or growing. Cancers with a low nuclear grade (Grade 1) grow and spread less quickly than cancers with a high nuclear grade (Grade 3).

Grading of Tumor

The general grading of cells is a microscopic examination of the cells that shows the degree of change from normal. The pathologist observes how much the cells resemble the original cells.

Tumor Cells Are Graded or Classified As:

- **Undifferentiated cells**—These cells have an abnormal appearance and have changed greatly from the cell from which they originally developed. Usually most aggressive. High grade (Grade 4).
- **Poorly differentiated cells**—These cells have lost most of the characteristics of the cell from which they came. Usually aggressive. High grade (Grade 3).
- **Moderately differentiated cells**—These cells have changed but still resemble the parent cell. This term is used to describe cells between the well differentiated and poorly differentiated stages. Moderately aggressive. Intermediate grade (Grade 2).
- **Well differentiated cells**—These cells are very similar in appearance to the cell from which they evolved. Usually least aggressive. Low grade (Grade 1).

USC/Van Nuys Prognostic Pathologic Classification — Ductal Carcinoma in Situ

Treatment for ductal in situ carcinoma (DCIS) is undergoing change. Some physicians use the USC/ Van Nuys Prognostic Pathologic Classification to determine if a patient could be a candidate for breast conservation rather than mastectomy according to various pathological studies performed on the tumor. In this pathologic evaluation, four categories are observed and a score is given to each category. The total score is used to determine who may qualify for various treatments. Ask if your physicians use this method of evaluation for DCIS. Many experts use other means of evaluation.

1. Nuclear Grade **Grade Value** Non-high grade without necrosis 1 point Non-high grade with necrosis 2 points High grade with necrosis 3 points		Evaluates size and shape of nucleus of cells
2. Tumor Size **Grade Value** 1.5 cm and under (<14 mm) 1 point 1.6 cm to 4.0 cm (15 – 40 mm) 2 points 4.1 cm or greater (>40 mm) 3 points		Evaluates size of the area where DCIS is found
3. Tumor Margins **Grade Value** 1.0 cm or greater (>10 mm) 1 point 0.1 – 0.9 cm (1 – 9 mm) 2 points 0.1 cm or under (<1 mm) 3 points		Evaluates distance from DCIS to margins of surgical specimen
4. Age at Diagnosis **Age Value** Over 60 1 point 40 – 60 2 points Under 40 3 points		Factors in age at diagnosis
Final Cumulative Total 4 – 6 points = no difference in survival-free local recurrence lumpectomy with/without radiation therapy 7 – 9 points = significant decrease in local recurrence with radiation therapy 10 – 12 points = high rate of local recurrence; mastectomy recommended		**Total of the scores in the above four areas determines final grade**

The Scarff/Bloom/Richardson/Elston Grading Scales

Some pathologists use the Scarff/Bloom/Richardson scale or a slight modification called the "Elston Grade" for grading invasive tumors. These grading systems give a number from 1 to 3 according to aggressiveness of three different characteristics of the tumor: (1) tubular formation, (2) nuclear size/shape and (3) cell division (or proliferation) rate.

The numbers from each characteristic are then totaled to determine the aggressiveness of a tumor. The higher the number, the more aggressive the characteristics of the tumor.

1. Tubular Formation Majority (>75%) Moderate degree (10 – 74%) Little or none (0 – 9%)	**Grade Value** 1 point 2 points 3 points	Evaluates cell arrangement for characteristics of looking like a small tube
2. Nuclear Shape/Size Uniform, small nuclear shapes Moderate increase in size and varying shapes Marked abnormalities (often large nucleus)	**Grade Value** 1 point 2 points 3 points	Evaluates size and shape variation of cells and nucleus of cells
3. Cell Division Rate Low (0 – 5) Moderate degree (6 – 10) High (>11) ***Cell Division Rate** (Elston Grading Scale Modification) Low (0 – 9) Moderate degree (10 – 19) High (>20)	**Grade Value** 1 point 2 points 3 points **Grade Value** 1 point 2 points 3 points	Determines how many cells are visible in the dividing stage in an area of the tumor *These numbers vary according to the Elston Grading Scale.
Final Cumulative Total Grade 1 – well differentiated Grade 2 – moderately differentiated Grade 3 – poorly differentiated	**Points** 3 – 5 points 6 – 7 points 8 – 9 points	**Total of the scores in the above three areas of evaluation determines final grade**

Prognostic Tests

Various tests may be performed on your tumor by your pathologist to look at specific characteristics of the tumor cells.

- **Flow Cytometry**—A test that looks at the genetic material found in the DNA of a cell. Normal DNA of a cell has two sets of chromosomes. **Diploid** means having two sets of chromosomes, which is normal. **Aneuploid** refers to the characteristic of having either fewer or more than two sets of chromosomes.

- **Cell Proliferation Rate**—Flow cytometry can also identify the number of cells dividing, called the S-phase fraction. This information allows a physician to know approximately how rapidly the cancer was growing (mitotic rate) at the time of surgery. A high S-phase fraction means the tumor is more aggressive. Other tests that may be ordered to measure the rate of growth are **thymidine labeling index (TLI), mitotic activity index (MAI)** and **Ki67.** These tests measure cell proliferation and may also be referred to as **cell kinetics.**

- **Hormone Receptor Assay**—Hormone receptor assay is a test that measures the presence of estrogen (ER) and progesterone (PR) receptors in the tumor cell nuclei. It tells the physician whether the tumor was stimulated to grow by female hormones and is very important in determining what type of treatment will be used after surgery. If a tumor is positive, that means it was stimulated by estrogen or progesterone and usually carries a more positive prognosis.

Tumors May Be:
- ER positive (+) PR positive (+)
- ER positive (+) PR negative (-)
- ER negative (-) PR positive (+)
- ER negative (-) PR negative (-)

- **Blood Vessel or Lymphatic Invasion**—A microscopic examination of the tumor will show if the surrounding blood vessels (vascular) or lymphatic vessels have been invaded by the tumor. No invasion offers a better prognosis.

- **HER2/neu**—A prognostic indicator that is over-expressed or amplified in about 25 to 30 percent of breast cancers. Elevation of HER2 indicates a more aggressive cancer. However, identification of elevation indicates that a drug called Herceptin® which targets the HER2/neu receptor is an appropriate treatment choice.

- **p53**—Determines elevation of oncogenes (substances within cells that promote tumor development) to predict potential recurrence.

- **Tumor necrosis**—Observes the death of cancer cells inside the tumor.

Triple Negative Breast Cancer

Recently, the term "triple negative" breast cancer has been used to describe a woman's cancer when tests for three different breast cancer receptors are all negative. A triple negative breast cancer is one that is negative for estrogen receptors (ER), progesterone receptors (PR) and HER2 receptors (human epidermal growth factor receptor 2). Many drugs used in cancer treatment are designed to target one of these positive receptor sites, thus a triple negative breast cancer diagnosis limits the use of some medications. Triple negative women, however, are typically responsive to chemotherapy drugs that are not targeted at ER/PR or HER2 receptor sites.

Final Pathology Report

There are many other diagnostic tests being used to evaluate tumors. Your physician will discuss with you the tests selected to evaluate your tumor. Each of these tests helps to collect pieces of the puzzle needed for the oncologist to determine your best treatment.

The pathologist prepares a written report that is sent to your physician. Time varies as to when the final report will be available. The pathologist's findings help the physician determine which surgery and treatment will be needed. Further diagnostic tests, such as additional blood work, a bone scan, liver scan, chest X-ray, CT scan or an MRI (magnetic resonance imaging), may be ordered.

Breast Cancer Stages 0 – 4

When the results are received from the tests, your cancer will be **staged** on a scale from zero (in-situ cancer) to four (a cancer with distant metastasis). A stage zero cancer is the earliest form of breast cancer and has the best prognosis. Staging is an estimate of how much the cancer has spread and is important in the selection of appropriate treatment (refer to pages 72 – 73).

Three Basic Factors Considered in Staging Are (TNM):

- **T**umor size (T)
- Lymph **N**ode involvement (N)
- **M**etastasis to other areas (M)

When you return to the physician for your pathology results, you may want to ask the following questions and write down the answers. (Some doctors will provide a copy of your pathology report for your records, and some pathologists will be happy to talk with you.) Early in your diagnostic work-up, all the answers to the following questions may not yet be available.

Pathology Report Questions:

- What is the name of the type of cancer I have?

- Was my tumor in situ (inside ducts or lobules) or infiltrating (invasive—grown through the duct or lobule walls into surrounding tissues)?

- What size was my tumor? (The size is in millimeters (mm) or centimeters (cm). 10 mm equal 1 cm. 1 cm equals ⅜ inch. 1 inch equals approximately 2.5 cm.)

- Was the cancer found anywhere else in my breast tissue? The term multifocal means additional cancer was found in the same quadrant of the

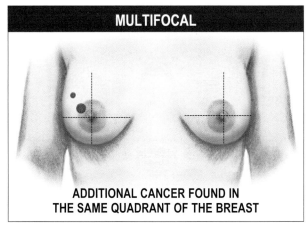

MULTIFOCAL

ADDITIONAL CANCER FOUND IN THE SAME QUADRANT OF THE BREAST

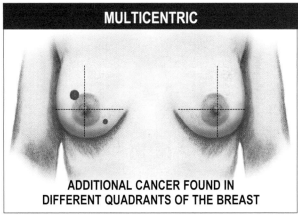

MULTICENTRIC

ADDITIONAL CANCER FOUND IN DIFFERENT QUADRANTS OF THE BREAST

breast; multicentric means that it was found in another quadrant of the breast distant from the tumor.

- How many lymph nodes were removed? Sentinel node biopsy alone usually removes from one to three nodes. (Approximately 75 percent of tumors have two sentinel nodes). How many levels of lymph nodes did you sample or remove? (You have three levels of nodes. Most axillary dissection removes levels one and two.)

- Were any nodes positive for cancer cells?

- Were my tumor receptors for estrogen or progesterone positive or negative?

- What was my cell proliferation status? (Indicator of how fast cancer is/was growing at the time of surgery.)

- Was my tumor positive for HER2?

- Is there anything else that I need to know about my cancer?

Breast Cancer Stages

STAGE 0

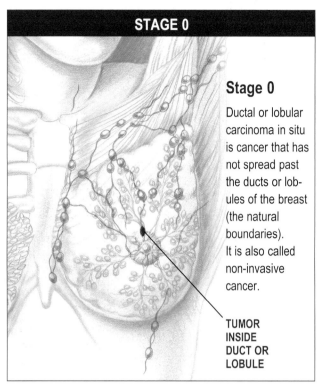

Stage 0

Ductal or lobular carcinoma in situ is cancer that has not spread past the ducts or lobules of the breast (the natural boundaries). It is also called non-invasive cancer.

TUMOR
INSIDE
DUCT OR
LOBULE

STAGE 1

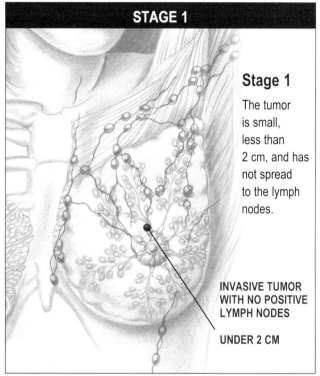

Stage 1

The tumor is small, less than 2 cm, and has not spread to the lymph nodes.

INVASIVE TUMOR
WITH NO POSITIVE
LYMPH NODES

UNDER 2 CM

STAGE 2

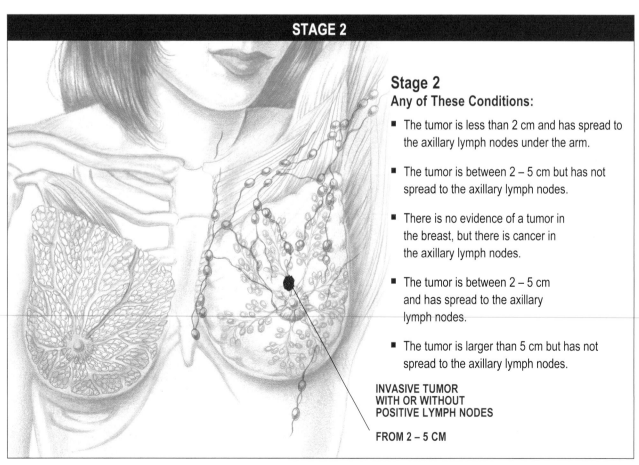

Stage 2
Any of These Conditions:

- The tumor is less than 2 cm and has spread to the axillary lymph nodes under the arm.

- The tumor is between 2 – 5 cm but has not spread to the axillary lymph nodes.

- There is no evidence of a tumor in the breast, but there is cancer in the axillary lymph nodes.

- The tumor is between 2 – 5 cm and has spread to the axillary lymph nodes.

- The tumor is larger than 5 cm but has not spread to the axillary lymph nodes.

INVASIVE TUMOR
WITH OR WITHOUT
POSITIVE LYMPH NODES

FROM 2 – 5 CM

Breast Cancer Stages

STAGE 3

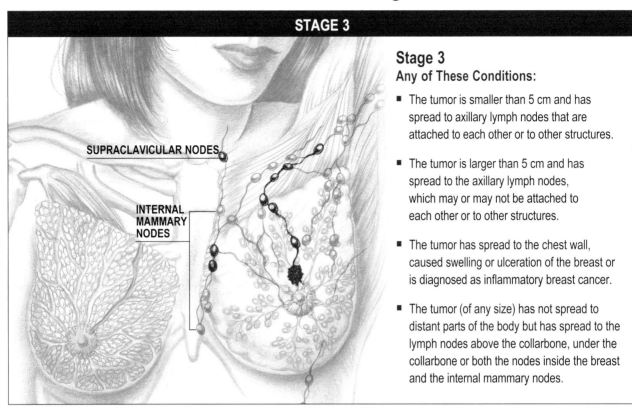

SUPRACLAVICULAR NODES

INTERNAL MAMMARY NODES

Stage 3
Any of These Conditions:

- The tumor is smaller than 5 cm and has spread to axillary lymph nodes that are attached to each other or to other structures.

- The tumor is larger than 5 cm and has spread to the axillary lymph nodes, which may or may not be attached to each other or to other structures.

- The tumor has spread to the chest wall, caused swelling or ulceration of the breast or is diagnosed as inflammatory breast cancer.

- The tumor (of any size) has not spread to distant parts of the body but has spread to the lymph nodes above the collarbone, under the collarbone or both the nodes inside the breast and the internal mammary nodes.

STAGE 4

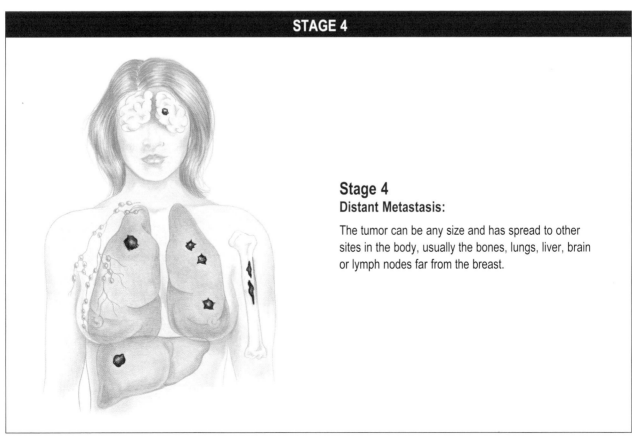

Stage 4
Distant Metastasis:

The tumor can be any size and has spread to other sites in the body, usually the bones, lungs, liver, brain or lymph nodes far from the breast.

73

Major Pathology Factors

Reading a complete pathology report can be overwhelming because of all of the medical language. As a patient, there are just a few major facts that you need to understand. The main components of the report that determine your final treatment plan are the stage of the cancer, hormone receptor status, HER2 status, lymph nodes status and whether the cancer has metastasized to other parts of your body. If you have a copy of your pathology report, you can find these characteristics by looking for the answers to the following questions. If you are unable to identity these major facts, mark the characteristic and ask your physician to clarify the results. (Check the boxes that apply.)

Pathology Report Information:

1. Hormone receptor status
☐ ER positive (+)   PR positive (+)

☐ ER positive (+)   PR negative (-)

☐ ER negative (-)   PR positive (+)

☐ ER negative (-)   PR negative (-)

☐ Could not determine; ask doctor for test results

2. HER2 receptor status
☐ HER2 positive (HER2+)

☐ HER2 negative (HER2-)

☐ Could not determine; ask doctor for test results

3. Lymph node status
☐ Lymph node positive

☐ Lymph node negative

☐ Could not determine; ask doctor for test results

Surgical Information:

4. Stage of your cancer
☐ Stage 0

☐ Stage 1

☐ Stage 2

☐ Stage 3

☐ Stage 4

☐ Ask doctor for information

5. Has your cancer metastasized?
☐ Yes

☐ No

☐ Ask doctor for information

6. If yes, where has your breast cancer metastasized?
☐ Bones

☐ Lungs

☐ Liver

☐ Brain

☐ Other

☐ Ask doctor for information

Tear-out Worksheet
Tumor Location & Size - Page W • 7

Remember

Breast cancer is a treatable disease. It certainly is not an illness you would choose, but it is an illness with many proven treatments.

Acquire an understanding of the treatment options. This will allow you to communicate with your healthcare team and become an active participant in decisions. Understanding will serve to alleviate many irrational fears and restore a sense of control to your life.

Employ the best of all medicines—your attitude. The most productive approach that you can bring, and one that the physician cannot provide, is a positive, cooperative attitude. Determination, combined with optimism, creates a healing environment that only you can provide.

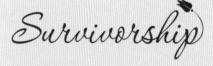

Survivorship

Loss in our lives causes us to stop and review what we have and where we are. At this point, we can learn how we can grow and how we can make our lives more rewarding as a result of the experience.

—*Judy Kneece*

Survivorship

As survivors, we fight adversity with a desire to grow and learn.

We find resources to give us the skills to handle what life has brought our way.

We put priority on learning about the challenges rather than fleeing in panic.

We read, listen and reach out to those who can give us understanding.

—*Judy Kneece*

Appreciating all of life, we can see painful events as opportunities, for those are the moments that truly stretch us and expand us to grow and deepen beyond who we think ourselves to be.

In what may seem the worst of times, when we face loss, or tragedy, we discover our heroism, our courage, our love, our creativity, and our power.

These seemingly catastrophic experiences are occasions to stretch ourselves beyond whoever we have been up to now and to play life full-out. These are profound challenges.

—*Judy Tatelbaum*

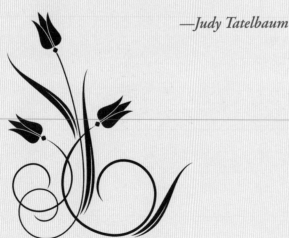

Understanding Chemotherapy Treatments

You have had your surgery and received your final pathology report, and your cancer has been staged. The next step will be determining the need for additional treatment of your breast cancer. For a few, it will be observation only. However, the majority of women receive some type of additional treatment—radiation therapy, chemotherapy or hormonal therapy. These treatments are often called **adjuvant** (additional) **therapy**. Adjuvant therapy is given to prevent a recurrence of cancer by killing any undetected cancer cells that may remain in your body. Adjuvant therapy may be local (radiation therapy, which targets only the radiated area to kill microscopic cancer cells) or systemic (chemotherapy or hormonal therapy, which travel throughout your body to control or destroy microscopic cancer cells). Your physicians will study your pathology report and tell you which treatments are indicated to be most advisable for your type and stage of cancer. They will determine which one or combination of adjuvant therapies will work best for you.

Your First Oncologist Visit

It is very important when planning your first visit to the oncologist to carry a list of any medications that you take. Include all nonprescription medicines, such as cold or sinus pills, aspirin, antacids, laxatives, vitamins and herbs. Many drugs can alter the response of the treatment, and your oncologist will need to evaluate if you can continue the medication. Check with your oncologist before starting any new medication.

Your oncologist will carefully review your pathology report and any other tests, perform a thorough physical exam and then prescribe a treatment plan.

Your Treatment Plan Will Be Designed According To:
- Cancer cell type
- Size of tumor
- In situ or invasive cancer

"I kept a binder notebook with all my reports and labs, along with a calendar of my appointments. I asked ahead what kind of treatments they predicted would be prescribed so I could look them up. I read everything I could about the type of treatment that was being recommended. I wanted to be prepared to ask the appropriate questions before they were given. This gave me a sense of being involved in my treatment decisions."

—**Anna Cluxton**

"My doctor told me, 'If you can't remember everything you want to ask me about, write it down.' That's what I did. I had so many questions, and he would sit down there and answer every last one of them."

—**Earnestine Brown**

- Growth rate of tumor
- Evidence of cancer in other parts of the body
- Lymph node involvement
- How much the cells have changed from original cells
- Estrogen and progesterone hormone receptor status
- HER2 status
- Your menopausal state
- Your medical history and general health

Remember, there is more than one kind of breast cancer, and different types of cancers may require different treatments. Do not compare your treatment with another patient's treatment because you will probably be comparing two completely different cases. Also, the information you can get from newspapers, magazines, radio and television may not be applicable to your cancer. Many are reports of experimental treatments that have not been tested extensively. Rely on your physician and staff to make sure you are receiving accurate information that is relevant to your treatment.

Oncotype DX®

In the past several years, a new test, Oncotype DX, has become available for women with early stage breast cancer to predict the potential for recurrence and whether chemotherapy is likely to benefit the patient. The test analyzes 21 different genes in the tumor sample that are known to predict a higher rate of recurrence. This information helps physicians and patients make more informed treatment decisions about chemotherapy based on a woman's individual cancer.

Who Qualifies for the Test:
- Stage I and II cancer (refer to page 72)
- ER (estrogen receptor) positive
- Negative (cancer-free) lymph nodes or have nodes showing micrometastases. Certain patients with cancer in only one to three lymph nodes may benefit. Ask your physician.
- HER2 negative or equivocal status

Oncotype DX is not appropriate for use in women with ductal or lobular in situ cancer or for women with later stage disease.

How Is the Test Performed?
You do not have to undergo any additional testing or procedures. A pathology slide of the tumor that was removed during surgery (biopsy, lumpectomy or mastectomy) is shipped for testing. Your physician (surgeon or oncologist) may order the test if you qualify.

Oncotype DX Recurrence Score® Report
Results of the test are returned to the physician with a Recurrence Score from 0 to 100. The Recurrence Score corresponds to the potential for breast cancer recurrence within a period of 10 years from the time of diagnosis and correlates with the likelihood of benefiting from chemotherapy.

Women with lower Recurrence Scores have a lower risk that their cancer will return. These women are also less likely to benefit from chemotherapy. It is important to note that a lower Recurrence Score does not mean that there is no chance that a woman's cancer will return. Women with higher Recurrence Scores have a greater chance that their breast cancer will return. These women may also gain a larger benefit from chemotherapy. A higher Recurrence Score also does not mean that a woman's breast cancer will definitely return. The test analyzes the genes and serves as a prediction, not an absolute fact. It is based on the latest scientific methods known in determining cancer treatment appropriateness.

Knowing the genomic profile of a cancer allows your physician to plan and tailor a treatment plan for you and your cancer. Ask your physician if you are a potential candidate for the test if you have early stage breast cancer.

Chemotherapy

Chemotherapy is a compound of two words that mean "chemical" and "treatment". We have all experienced treatment with chemicals, such as antibiotics and cold medicines, for other illnesses. The word chemotherapy usually refers to treatment of cancer through the use of drugs. This is systemic treatment that travels to all parts of the body through the bloodstream. A combination of several drugs may be used to fight your cancer. The drugs selected will have different side effects and work in different ways to kill or control growth of any cancer cells that may be left in the body. Most often people think of the drugs that cause hair loss and nausea when they think of chemotherapy; however, anti-hormonal drugs that alter the hormonal environment of the body and cause few side effects are also included in this category.

The Goals of Chemotherapy Drugs:

- Destroy cancer cells in other parts of the body
- Stop cancer from spreading to other parts of the body
- Slow cancer growth
- Relieve symptoms of cancer

Hormonal Therapy

Hormonal therapy may be recommended by your oncologist. This type of additional anti-cancer therapy is prescribed after surgery for some women if their cancer pathology reports revealed that tumor growth was dependent on the female hormones estrogen and progesterone. Tumors that have a significant number of estrogen receptors (ER) are considered "ER positive," and tumors that have a high number of progesterone receptors (PR) are considered "PR positive." The receptor status of the tumor determines what treatments will best affect your cancer. The use of hormonal drugs often depends upon whether you are pre-menopausal (having your monthly menstrual periods) or post-menopausal (not having your monthly menstrual periods). Patients who have estrogen receptor positive (ER+) and/or progesterone receptor positive (PR+) cancers are often given hormonal therapies as part of treatment.

Tamoxifen Citrate (Nolvadex®)

Hormonal therapy may be recommended if the studies performed on the tumor prove that it is stimulated by estrogen or progesterone. The most commonly used drug is tamoxifen citrate (Nolvadex®). While doctors don't know exactly how tamoxifen works, they acknowledge that it blocks the effects of estrogen on breast cancer cells. It does not kill, but it may control, any remaining cancer cells that have been left in the body after surgery. It does not cause the side effects of chemotherapy. There is no hair loss or fatigue.

Tamoxifen is given by pill once or twice a day. The most frequently reported side effects are hot flashes (80 percent on tamoxifen and 68 percent on placebo) and vaginal discharge (55 percent on tamoxifen and 35 percent on placebo).

In studies of tamoxifen, the risks for cancer of the lining of the uterus and for blood clots in the lungs and legs increased two to three times compared to numbers recorded for the placebo group, although they occurred in only one percent of women. Women who have a history of blood clots or who require anti-coagulant medication should not take tamoxifen for reducing the risk of breast cancer. Strokes and cataracts also occur more frequently with tamoxifen therapy. In addition, if you are pre-menopausal and sexually active, it will be necessary to ask the physician about appropriate non-hormonal birth control. Women who are pregnant or expect to become pregnant should not take tamoxifen. New drugs (SERMs) similar to tamoxifen, Evista® (raloxifene) and Fareston® (toremifene), may be prescribed by your physician if an anti-hormonal therapy is needed.

Aromatase Inhibitors

A newer class of drugs called aromatase inhibitors, Aromasin® (exemestane), Femara® (letrozole), and

Hormonal and Biological Response Modifier Drugs

BREAST CANCER CLASS OF DRUGS	DRUG ACTION	DRUG NAMES
SERMs (Selective Estrogen-Receptor Modulators)	Drug binds to estrogen receptors in breast, controlling cancer growth	**Nolvadex**® (tamoxifen) **Evista**® (ralosifene) **Fareston**® (toremifene)
Aromatase Inhibitors	Reduces or prevents estrogen production in adrenal glands	**Aromasin**® (exemestane) **Femara**® (letrozole) **Arimidex**® (anastrazole)
Biological Response	Drug binds with certain estrogen proteins on breast cancer cells preventing growth in HER2 positive women	**Herceptin**® (trastuzumab)
Miscellaneous Hormonal	Used for breast cancers that are estrogen dependent	**Zoladex**® (goserelin acetate) **Faslodex**® (fulvestrant) **Lupron**® (leuprolide)

Chemotherapy Drugs

CHEMOTHERAPY CLASS OF DRUGS	DRUG ACTION	DRUG NAMES
Anthracyclines (antibiotic-based)	Alters the structure of cellular DNA	**Adriamycin**® (doxorubicin) **Ellence**® (epirubicin) **Doxil**® (doxorubicin HCl liposome)
Taxanes	Prevents cancer cells from dividing	**Abraxane**® (plasma bound paclitaxel) **Taxol**® (paclitaxel) **Taxotere**® (docetaxel)
Alkylating Agent	Interferes with cellular metabolism and growth	**Cytoxan**® (cyclophosphamide)
Antimetabolites	Interferes with cancer cell division	**Gemzar**® (gemcitabine) **Methotrexate**® **5-FU**® (5 fluorouracil) **Xeloda**® (capecitabine)
Miscellaneous Anti-Neoplastic	Interferes with microtubule assembly	**Navelbine**® (vinorelbine tartrate)
Platinum Analog	Binds with DNA	**Paraplatin**® (carboplatin)

Arimidex® (anastrazole), show promise in the treatment of many breast cancers in women who are naturally or are chemically made post-menopausal. The data shows that they may be slightly more effective than tamoxifen, which has been the standard hormonal treatment for breast cancer for thirty years. Aromatase inhibitors work by depriving hormone dependent cancers (ER or PR positive) by blocking or preventing estrogen production in the adrenal glands. Your physician will tell you if your cancer treatment will include an aromatase inhibitor.

Biological Response Modifier

A biological response modifier is a drug that binds with certain proteins on a tumor to prevent their growth. For women whose tumors test positive for over-expression of HER2 receptors, the drug Herceptin® (trastuzumab) may be used. Herceptin® attaches to the HER2 protein found on the cancer cell to prevent the cell from growing or dividing. Your pathology report will show if your tumor is HER2 positive. This drug is only indicated in treatment when a tumor tests positive for over-expression of HER2.

How Chemotherapy Drugs Work

Chemotherapy works by killing cells that are dividing in your body, unlike the hormonal and biological response modifier drugs that prevent or slow growth. The cancer cells are constantly dividing until something disrupts this cycle, which is the role of chemotherapy. Even when the surgeon thinks all of your tumor has been removed, you may receive adjuvant chemotherapy because there is a possibility that some cells may have broken away from the original site and moved through the lymphatic or blood vessels to other parts of your body (metastasis) where they cannot be detected; this is called micrometastasis (the cells are too small to be detected). Adjuvant chemotherapy helps destroy these cells. Chemotherapy and hormonal therapy are effective in all parts of the body.

Because chemotherapy works by killing only dividing cells, most of the side effects will be on the cells in your body that are constantly dividing to produce new cells. These cells are found in your bone marrow, where your blood components are made, resulting in lowered blood cell counts; in the gastrointestinal tract, resulting in a possible sore throat, sore mouth or diarrhea; and in hair follicles, which could result in hair loss. Most of these cells are able to recover quickly when treatment is over. Therefore, these side effects are temporary. Some people experience very few side effects and are able to continue to work throughout treatment.

Don't listen to anyone else and their stories about the side effects of chemotherapy. Instead, ask your nurse for the names of the drugs prescribed for you and the side effects of those particular drugs. There are many drugs being used to treat cancer, and there are about 100 types of cancer, including approximately 15 different types of breast cancer. Therefore, it would be difficult to get accurate information from anyone but medical professionals involved with cancer treatment.

How Chemotherapy Is Given

Chemotherapy drugs may be given by mouth, as an injection into the muscle or fatty tissues, or into a vein by an I.V. (intravenous) needle. Most chemotherapy for breast cancer is given intravenously. If your veins are hard to locate or you are to receive certain types of chemotherapy drugs, some doctors may request the insertion of a permanent I.V. device (referred to as a vascular access device or a port—"life port" or "port-a-cath"). This is a device inserted by a surgeon under the skin, usually on the chest opposite your surgery site or, occasionally, on the arm. This device may be used to draw your blood for blood studies as well as to administer chemotherapy and other medications. It prevents repeated needle sticks to your arm. You are able to bathe and swim as usual with a port.

Chemotherapy may be administered in the doctor's office, a hospital or in a clinic. Most breast cancer patients take treatments in a physician's office or clinic.

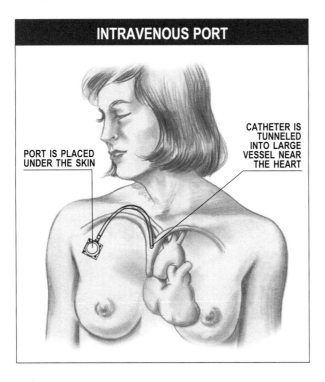

INTRAVENOUS PORT

PORT IS PLACED UNDER THE SKIN

CATHETER IS TUNNELED INTO LARGE VESSEL NEAR THE HEART

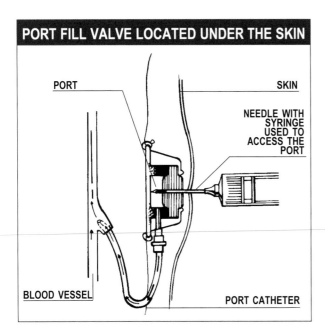

PORT FILL VALVE LOCATED UNDER THE SKIN

PORT

SKIN

NEEDLE WITH SYRINGE USED TO ACCESS THE PORT

BLOOD VESSEL

PORT CATHETER

Chemotherapy Scheduling

The frequency of treatments may vary, just as doses will vary from patient to patient. It will depend on the kind of cancer, the drugs being used and how your body responds to them. Some drugs are given by mouth daily. Others may be scheduled biweekly, weekly, every three weeks or by other schedules. Traditionally, most breast cancer chemotherapy administered through a vein or port is given every three weeks. Recently, the schedule for some women has been shortened to a two-week interval and is called "dose-dense chemotherapy." The same dose (amount) of chemotherapy may be given every two weeks when drugs are given to support the blood cells' repopulation after chemotherapy administration.

In a dose-dense schedule, Neupogen® (filgrastim) or Neulasta® (pegfilgrastim) is administered to support the white blood cells' return to normal range more rapidly. Red blood cells are supported with Procrit® (epoetin) or Aranesp® (darbepoetin alfa) to bring hemoglobin back up. Other drugs, Emend® (aprepitant) or Aloxi® (palonosetron), may also be given. Chemotherapy treatments can be given every two weeks if the newer drugs are used in combination with the chemotherapy drugs when needed.

Your oncologist will be able to advise you on a treatment plan and schedule after your case has been evaluated. This schedule may be readjusted to meet your individual responses and treatment needs. Treatments usually begin after surgery; however, some types of cancer require chemotherapy administration before surgery.

Neoadjuvant Chemotherapy

Sometimes several doses of chemotherapy may be given before surgery to shrink a tumor; this is called neoadjuvant chemotherapy. Giving chemotherapy before surgery may shrink a large tumor to a size that allows for breast conservation in a woman with a smaller breast. Chemotherapy may also be given before surgery for inflammatory breast cancer or advanced stage tumors.

What Is Chemotherapy Nadir?

Nadir is the time in your treatment when chemotherapy drugs that impact your blood counts cause blood values to fall to their lowest level. Different drugs impact different blood components. Your physician will tell you the expected side effects of the drugs in your treatment protocol and when the nadir is expected. During this time you will feel most fatigued if red blood cells are impacted, be most susceptible to acquiring an infection or virus if white blood cells are lowered and have the highest potential for spontaneous bleeding if platelets are decreased. Usually this is midway between scheduled treatments. Blood values are allowed to come back to near normal before your next treatment is given.

Chemotherapy Side Effects

You have probably heard horrible stories about cancer treatments. Times have changed. There are new drugs that have changed many treatment side effects. Newer drugs for nausea have greatly reduced vomiting as a side effect. Drugs can now be given to elevate your immune response during treatment, preventing many of the infections traditionally experienced from extremely low white blood counts. Ask your nurse or doctor to tell you about the side effects of your treatment plan. Do not rely on well-meaning friends or family. Chemotherapy has been repeatedly successful in increasing breast cancer survival.

Additional Information

Chemotherapy Drugs - Pages 193 – 202

Nausea and Vomiting - Pages 159 – 160

Hot Flashes

Hot flashes are sensations of increased body temperature. A hot flash usually begins in one region of the body and spreads quickly. A sudden wave of warmth in the face, neck and chest occurs and usually lasts between a minute and several minutes. Researchers attribute hot flashes to irregular expansion and contraction of the small blood vessels of the skin, which produce perspiration and blushing. Hot flashes are usually caused by a lack of estrogen. The sensation from a hot flash is unexpected and can be very bothersome. Most women, however, notice that their hot flashes tend to occur during certain times of the day. Most chemotherapy drugs, including anti-hormonal drugs such as tamoxifen, cause hot flashes.

The best management technique is to control body temperature and the immediate environment. Hot flashes can also be associated with nausea, dizziness, headache, irregular heartbeat pattern and sweating. Hot flashes are not a disease, even though they may feel that way.

Suggestions for Coping With Hot Flashes:

- Notice a time or pattern for your hot flashes. Expecting them can give you a sense of control.

- Dress in light, layered clothing so that outer garments can be removed during a hot flash. Avoid turtleneck sweaters. Wear slip-on shoes that can be quickly removed so you can place your feet on the cold floor.

- Avoid hot environments, if possible.

- Drink cold liquids; avoid hot drinks. When a hot flash starts, try drinking cold water to reduce the sensation and keep yourself hydrated.

- Sleep in a cool room. Use cotton sheets and bed coverings that can be quickly removed. Select cotton pajamas or nightgowns.

- Turn on an electric fan.

- Avoid highly seasoned foods, alcohol and drinks with large amounts of caffeine (coffee, tea, soft drinks).

- Avoid stressful situations that can stimulate you emotionally.

- Avoid activities that can increase body temperature, such as hot baths, saunas and sunbathing.

- Learn mental visualization techniques that can reduce the intensity of the sensation.

Medications for Hot Flashes

If your hot flashes are interfering with your quality of life and are not managed with the above suggestions, talk to your doctor. Several of the selective serotonin reuptake inhibitor medications (SSRIs) have proven effective in reducing hot flashes. If you are taking tamoxifen, recent clinical studies show that these medications do not interfere with its effectiveness: citalopram (Celexa®), escitalopram (Lexapro®), venlavaxine (Effexor®) and fluvoxamine (Luvox®).

Hair Loss

Chemotherapy for breast cancer produces temporary alopecia (hair loss) that varies from thinning to complete baldness. Some medications damage the hair cells, causing the hair follicle to produce weak, brittle hair that either breaks off at the surface of the scalp or falls out. Only the growing hair is lost. Dormant hair (about 10 percent of all scalp hair) does not fall out. Hair loss is usually preceded by scalp tingling. The kind of drug and the length of time the drug is administered will determine how long alopecia will last. Most hair loss occurs 7 – 21 days after the administration of drugs. The amount of hair loss varies according to the drug and the dosage of the drug. However, the amount of hair loss may also vary among patients even when they are given the same dosage and number of chemotherapy treatments. It is an individual response. Ask your healthcare provider when you should expect to lose your hair. Hair loss may also occur in other body sites such as the eyebrows, eyelashes and pubic and facial hair. These hair follicles have a slower growth rate, though, and seem to suffer less damage.

Hair re-growth starts during or shortly after treatments are completed. When the hair grows back, it may have a different texture and slightly different color. Very often the hair has a wavy pattern or is curly and darker. Most women like the texture and manageability of their new hair.

Drugs Causing a High Degree of Hair Loss:

- Doxorubicin (Adriamycin®)—hair loss usually in 7 – 21 days; 90% average loss

- Methotrexate—3 to 4 weeks; 33% average loss

- 5-Fluorouracil (5-FU®)—minimal hair loss

- Epirubicin (Ellence®)—total hair loss; 7 – 21 days

- Cyclophosphamide (Cytoxan®)—partial to total hair loss with thinning (with oral version)

- Taxol® and Taxotere®—total hair loss; 7 – 21 days

Hair loss is sometimes more difficult to face than the loss of all or part of a breast. Hair loss is obvious, visible evidence of the cancer process and the first public indication of the battle with cancer. Hair loss further compounds the change in body image and sense of diminished femininity. When hair loss occurs, acknowledge the loss and grieve, but don't feel guilty. In focus groups held by EduCare in 2002, women who took chemotherapy and lost their hair were asked which was more emotionally painful—their surgical experience or loss of their hair. The answer was overwhelmingly hair loss—74 percent said hair loss was more difficult; only 26 percent said that their surgery was more difficult emotionally.

Some people may try to offer consolation and support by pointing out how insignificant hair loss is compared to battling a life-threatening disease, but most can say this because they have never lost their hair. After grieving, talk about your feelings with people whom you trust and feel comfortable. Remind yourself that hair loss is visible proof that chemotherapy is killing cells—good and bad. Talk with and visit other women who have suffered alopecia and now have their own hair back. Support such as this may be found in breast cancer support groups in which women are in all stages of breast cancer treatment. Some women have had great fun buying different colors and styles of wigs, scarves and turbans. Sporty hats and caps worn with scarves are another way many women look and feel fashionable during treatment. The American Cancer Society offers a catalog called *tlc* which combines helpful articles with products for women coping with any cancer treatment that causes hair loss. To request a copy of *tlc*, call 1-800-850-9445 or visit *tlc* online (www.tlcdirect.org). Plan to buy or order your turbans or scarves as soon as you find out that you will have hair loss from treatment.

Before hair loss begins, you can do several things to minimize the trauma. A short, easily managed haircut minimizes the appearance of thinning hair and makes complete hair loss somewhat less alarming. Some women prefer to let someone shave their head if they know that their chemotherapy will cause complete hair loss.

Select a wig prior to losing your hair when your natural hair color and style can be closely matched. Wear the new wig occasionally before you have significant hair loss to help in the adjustment. In addition, the change will not be as noticeable to other people. If you have long hair, you can have it made into a set of bangs or a ponytail to wear under turbans or hats. Ask a cosmetologist if she can refer you to companies that provide this service. Some insurance companies may cover the cost of a wig if your physician writes a prescription. Wigs are tax deductible as a medical expense.

Turbans or hair nets worn at home will help control the loose hairs as they fall out. Turbans are excellent to sleep in at night. Hats, turbans and scarves are good when wigs become too hot.

Hair Care to Minimize Loss and Thinning:

- Shampoo hair with protein-based shampoo and follow with a conditioning rinse.

- Shampoo less often, every three to five days.

- Gently dry hair with towel; pat hair dry.

- Dry hair on low temperature setting or allow it to dry naturally.

- Minimize use of electric curlers and curling irons; a curly perm prior to treatment may be helpful.

- Avoid use of hair clips, barrettes and ponytails with elastic bands.

- Use hair spray sparingly.

- Avoid hair dyes that further weaken hair.

- Avoid excessive brushing and combing of hair.

- Purchase a satin pillowcase to reduce hair tangling while sleeping.

- Once treatment begins, wear a hair net or turban at night to prevent falling hair from getting on bed linens.

Skin Care

During chemotherapy your skin may become dry and sensitive to chemicals or products you have used for years. You will also be more sensitive to sun exposure.

Special Steps to Protect Your Skin:

- Eat more protein to promote faster skin healing.

- Drink at least eight 8-ounce glasses of water daily.

- Bathe or shower with warm rather than hot water.

- Bathe with soaps that have no perfumes like Dove®, Cetaphil® or Ivory®.

- Don't scrub the skin when bathing. Pat dry gently with a towel.

- Moisturize your skin with gentle moisturizers such as Cetaphil®, Aveeno® or Nexcare Advanced Healing®.

- Apply a sun block of at least SPF 30 thirty minutes before going outside. Be sure to apply under your makeup as well. Zinc or titanium oxide sunscreens scatter ultraviolet light and are less likely to be irritating to sensitive skin. Check the label or ask your dermatologist. Research has shown that the best protection from the sun is tightly woven garments. Polyester is better than cotton, linen or acetate at blocking harmful rays. UV protective clothing specifically designed to block the sun is available if you spend extended periods of time outside.

Cosmetics

During treatment you may find that you require a change in makeup because of sensitivity of the skin and changes in skin color. Patients recommend trying a bronzing powder or lotion to help maintain a healthy glow instead of using a make-up base. Bare Minerals® and similar products are natural and are usually well tolerated when your skin becomes sensitive.

The American Cancer Society offers a program called "Look Good, Feel Better" at most large cancer centers. These sessions, led by licensed professionals, provide makeup techniques specifically for cancer patients and information on ways to wear hats, scarves and head coverings to make you look and feel better. Call your cancer center and avail yourself of this wonderful, free opportunity to deal with the changes chemotherapy brings to your grooming.

Stomach and Mouth Irritation

Chemotherapy irritates cells in the gastrointestinal system of your body because it damages healthy cells that are in the dividing stage as well as cancer cells. The main complaints are gastritis (stomach irritation) and stomatitis (sore mouth). These conditions are temporary and are relieved when treatment is over. Other factors that increase the potential for irritation are excessive stomach acid caused by stress, alcohol, excessive caffeine, smoking, eating fatty, acidic or spicy foods that are not easily digestible and medications such as aspirin, non-steroidal anti-inflammatory medications (Motrin®, Advil®, etc.), cortisone and some antibiotics.

Gastritis Signs and Symptoms:

- Burning, gnawing sensation in the stomach
- Dull, annoying pain in the chest
- Abdominal pain and cramps; swollen abdomen
- Acid taste in the mouth; belching or gas
- Appetite loss
- Vomiting (occasionally)

- Bleeding—often identified as dark, tarry stools or vomit that resembles coffee grounds. (Notify your physician immediately if any blood is seen in stool or vomit.)

Gastritis Treatments:

- Take non-prescription antacids on a regular basis, according to directions on the bottle, until symptoms improve.
- Do not take aspirin or ibuprofen for pain; instead take acetaminophen (Tylenol®).
- Eat a bland diet until symptoms improve—no spicy, hot, acidic or fatty foods.
- The first day of the attack, take antacids and try a liquid diet to allow the stomach to rest. Resume normal, healthy diet slowly with bland foods.
- Keep a small amount of bland food in your stomach and avoid large meals.
- Stop smoking. Do not drink alcohol during stomach irritation.
- Medications that irritate your stomach should be taken with food.
- If symptoms do not improve, inform your healthcare provider. Medications may be ordered to reduce or block the secretion of stomach acid.

    Acid Reducers: famotidine (Prevacid®), nizatidine (Axid®) or ranitidine (Zantac®). Recent studies show cimetidine (Tagamet®) may interact with some chemotherapy drugs.

    Acid Blockers: omeprazole (Prilosec®), lansopraxole (Prevacid®), esomeprazole (Nexium®), pantoprozole (Protonix®) or rabeprazole (Aciphex®).

Notify Healthcare Provider If:

- Pain persists after several days of antacids and diet modification.
- Vomit looks like coffee grounds or bowel movements appear dark and tarry because of bleeding.
- Pain becomes severe.
- You cannot eat or drink anything for 24 hours.
- You cannot take prescribed medication because of pain or vomiting.

- Prescribed medications for stomach irritation do not bring pain relief within a week.

Stomatitis

Stomatitis is a condition that refers to an inflammation of the lining of the mouth and throat, causing discomfort or pain. Your mouth and throat hurt when you eat or drink. Mouth sores or ulcers may occur. Cells in the mouth completely replace themselves every seven days. Usually, a sore mouth from chemotherapy administration will improve and cells repair themselves in a week, if additional chemotherapy is not given during that time.

Early Stomatitis Signs and Symptoms:
- Redness and swelling of the mouth or lips

- Sensations of dryness

- Sensations of mild burning or discomfort when eating or drinking

Early Interventions:
- Cleanse mouth thoroughly after every meal; brush with a very soft toothbrush, being careful not to injure gums; soak your toothbrush in hot water to soften bristles to prevent irritation to gums; use a non-irritating toothpaste or baking soda.

- Rinse your mouth with water to remove food particles if you cannot brush after a meal.

- Prepare a mouthwash solution of 1 tablespoon baking soda in 2 cups water, or ½ teaspoon salt and 1 teaspoon baking soda in 4 cups water. Avoid commercial mouthwashes containing alcohol; alcohol-free mouthwashes (such as Biotene®) can promote healing and prevent infection by stimulating the body's own immune system in the mouth and saliva.

- Keep your lips moist with lip balm or K-Y Jelly®.

- Avoid tobacco and alcohol.

- Avoid foods that are too hot or too cold; avoid foods that are spicy, acidic or have a coarse, irritating texture.

- Floss between teeth, but avoid any contact with gums. Stop flossing if it causes pain.

- Swish an over-the-counter medication, such as Kaopectate®, between meals to relieve some of the discomfort and promote healing.

- If sores develop, pour an antacid into a dish and allow the liquid to come to the top; discard this liquid and swab the concentrated part of the solution, which will be pasty, onto inflamed areas using a cotton-tipped applicator.

- Apply Orabase®, an over-the-counter oral protective paste, to irritated areas to relieve discomfort.

- Apply vitamin E oil to the irritated area by puncturing a capsule and applying with a cotton swab.

- If your pain prevents you from eating or drinking, ask your physician for a prescription for a topical analgesic to deaden the area before eating or drinking. Swish these products around in the mouth and swallow or spit out to relieve pain temporarily.

Severe Stomatitis Interventions:
- Call your healthcare provider—medication may be required. Ask your physician about Carafate®, a prescription drug which protects not only your mouth and throat, but also the entire upper gastrointestinal tract.

- Report signs of infection, such as temperature greater than 100.5° F.

- Cleanse your mouth thoroughly. Mix one part hydrogen peroxide to four parts water and use immediately; swish around in your mouth and hold for several minutes; spit the mixture out and follow with a rinse of water or salt water mixed (½ teaspoon salt to 4 cups water).

- Do not wear dentures.

- Avoid brushing teeth if it irritates gums; wrap clean gauze around your fingers and rub your teeth clean; avoid dental floss.

- Increase your fluid intake.

- Use Tylenol® or whatever medication your physician recommended to control pain.

- If white or yellowish patches develop on your tongue, inside cheeks or throat and they do not come off after rinsing your mouth with salt water, notify your healthcare provider. This may be thrush, a fungal infection that requires a prescription medication.

Chemo Brain

Some chemotherapy patients complain that their treatments cause changes in their ability to concentrate. They struggle to find the right words, and their short-term memory seems unreliable. Some people refer to this as "chemo brain," and, recently, the phenomenon patients have been reporting for years has been validated by research.

Many factors can contribute to the "fuzzy thinking" women experience during chemotherapy treatment. One of the major causes is the decrease of female hormones caused by chemotherapy. Other conditions that can contribute to "fuzzy thinking" are stress, anemia, fatigue, anxiety, depression, side effects of anesthesia and medications. For most, these symptoms resolve after treatment is over, and pre-treatment thinking ability returns. Some doctors recommend taking B-Complex vitamins to combat chemo brain, but be sure to consult your healthcare team to get their best advice for you.

If you find that your thinking still feels fuzzier than usual, purchase a calendar or PDA to keep track of dates and appointments. Write lists and leave yourself notes. Keep a family calendar with everyone's schedule—several online sites offer free programs. Most of all, remember that your clear thinking should improve when your treatments are complete.

Report to Your Doctor

During cancer treatment with chemotherapy, your blood cell counts will be lowered, putting you at higher risk for infection if your white blood cells are affected. If your platelet count is lowered, you will be at higher risk for bleeding. If your red blood cells are lowered, you will have increased fatigue. Be sure to track your symptoms and side effects so that you know what to report to your doctor during your next visit. A tear-out sheet is located in the back section (page W • 29) to help you keep track.

There are some symptoms that you should report immediately to your healthcare provider so an appropriate evaluation can be made for treatment.

Symptoms to Report:
- Fever greater than 100.5°F
- Shaking chills with or without fever
- Sore throat; mouth sores; swallowing problems because of pain
- Cough with sputum (saliva mixed with mucus) production
- Pain or burning when urinating; sudden increase in frequency; inability to control urine
- Redness or discharge from any wound, incision or sore
- Clear blisters on the skin
- Bleeding from any site not controlled after 20 minutes of pressure to the area
- Vomit that has a coffee ground appearance; urine that has a dark tea color; spitting up blood or sputum that is blood tinged
- Racing or irregular heart beat
- Fainting or sudden onset of dizziness
- Severe headache
- Shortness of breath; difficulty catching your breath; chest pain
- Sudden vision changes
- Sudden onset of severe pain in any area of the body
- Nausea not controlled in 24 hours with medication
- Diarrhea not controlled in 24 hours with medication

Ask your physician if there are any symptoms specific to your care that you should report.

Treatment Response Terminology

Remission or Cancer Free or Disease Free

No signs of cancer can be found based on your symptoms, physical exam, radiology scans, X-rays or lab tests. This does not mean you will never have recurrence. It means that with the current studies we have today there is no evidence of cancer seen and that treatment was successful.

Incomplete Remission or Residual Disease

Your cancer has been reduced after treatment, but there are still some signs of cancer based either on physical exam, radiology scans, X-rays or lab tests. Your healthcare team may recommend additional treatment or observation to see if the disease remains stable and does not progress.

Disease Progression

Scans, X-rays or lab tests show that your disease did not respond to treatment but continued to increase, indicating the need for a different drug or treatment.

Clinical Trials

Occasionally, as part of treatment decisions, some women may have the opportunity to participate in new treatments called clinical trials. These are new investigational studies that research effective treatment and prevention strategies. Thousands of research studies are currently underway in the United States. Most trials are conducted by the National Cancer Institute, major medical centers or pharmaceutical companies. If a new treatment is determined safe and effective at the completion of the trial, the U.S. Food and Drug Administration (FDA) grants approval for its widespread commercial use by patients.

Four Phases of Clinical Trials

1. **Phase I** trials test new treatments to determine the acceptable dose and administration method.

2. **Phase II** trials study the safety and effectiveness of the drug and how it affects the human body.

3. **Phase III** trials require that a large number of patients receive either the newer therapy or the standard therapy in order to compare beneficial survival results and quality of life during treatment. If the newer drug is found to be more effective than the standard one, the trial is stopped and all participants are eligible for the more successful treatment. If there is any evidence that the newer drug is inferior or has unusual toxic side effects, the experimental medication is discontinued.

4. **Phase IV** trials are conducted to further evaluate long-term safety and effectiveness of the trial drug after approval for standard use.

Clinical Trial Informed Consent

Your doctor or nurse will explain in detail the type and purpose of the trial. You will be given an informed consent form to read and sign. This form must include the expected benefits, the negative aspects, other treatment options, assurance that your personal records will be kept confidential and a statement indicating that your participation is voluntary and that you may withdraw at any time.

Participating in the trial does not prevent you from getting any additional medical care you may need. If you decide to participate in the trial, you will need to contact your insurance provider to ask if it covers any charges. Be sure the researchers are aware if your plan does not cover the costs of clinical trials. Some trials are simply a comparison of two drugs or timing of administration to determine which is more effective. Your physician will explain the details of the trial.

Clinical Trial Questions:

- What phase is the clinical trial now in?

- Who is sponsoring the study? (Needs to be approved by a reputable national group like the National Cancer Institute, a major teaching institution or the FDA.)

- What is the purpose of this study?

- What advantage does this trial have compared to standard recommended treatment?

- How long will the clinical trial last?

- Where will treatments be given and evaluated while on the trial?

- Is the drug or combination of drugs available outside the clinical trial?

- How will the success of the treatment be evaluated (blood tests, scans, etc.)?

- How much additional time will participating in the trial require over standard treatment?

- Will there be any extra expenses or will all costs of the trial be covered?

- Will my insurance cover the cost of the trial?

- What type of follow-up will continue after the trial is completed?

Understanding Clinical Trials

If you want to know more about clinical trials, the most obvious place to start is with your oncologist. The Cancer Information Service (CIS), a program supported by the National Cancer Institute, can compile information about the latest nationwide cancer treatments for a specific type and stage of cancer. For more information on clinical trials, you can access www.cancer.gov and search "PDQ" for access to the Physician's Data Query.

Patient advocacy groups such as the American Cancer Society (ACS), at 1-800-ACS-2345 or online (www.cancer.org), also have patient information about participating in clinical trials and other relevant information on new trials.

To Participate or Not to Participate

The decision is often not an easy one to make. This decision is very personal and one that can only be made after you discuss the advantages and disadvantages with your physician and clinical trial nurse. When the final decision is made, you need to feel that you have chosen what is best for you. Some women prefer the "tried and true," while others feel that they are getting an even

better chance by taking a newer drug or drug combination. Some feel that by their participation in clinical trials they will be helping other women in the future. Remember, no one has the right answer to the question of whether or not you should participate; there is not an absolute answer. That is why it is called a "trial."

Questions to Ask Your Oncologist:

- What kind of treatment will I receive (chemotherapy, hormonal, immunotherapy)?

- On what schedule will I receive these treatments?

- How long will I receive treatments?

- How long will each treatment take?

- Where will I receive my treatments (office, clinic, hospital)?

- Will any other tests be given before or while I receive my chemotherapy?

- Can someone come with me when I receive my treatments?

- Will I feel like driving myself home after my treatment or do I need a driver?

- Will I need radiation therapy?

- Do you have written information on my cancer or treatment plans?

- Should I eat before I come for my treatments?

- Can I take vitamins or herbs if I choose?

- What kind of precautions about skin protection should I take during chemotherapy (exposure to sunlight)?

- What side effects will I experience from the treatments (nausea, hair loss, changes in blood cell counts, etc.)?

- Will I be given medications to treat the side effects?

- After I complete my treatments, how often will I return for checkups?

- How will you evaluate the effectiveness of the treatments?

- What are the names of the drugs?

- Are the drugs given by mouth or into a vein?

- Will I need a port (device implanted under the skin) to receive any I.V. medications or will you use a vein in my arm?

- Will I continue to have menstrual periods? If not, when will they return?

- Should I use birth control? What type do you recommend?

- Will I be able to conceive and bear a child after treatment?

- Can I meet with a fertility specialist before we start treatment?

- What physical changes should I report to you or your nurse during treatment?

- Can I continue my usual work or exercise schedules, or will I need to modify them during treatments?

- Are there any precautions my family should take to limit exposure to the chemotherapy during my treatments (shared eating utensils, bathroom facilities)?

Remember

Chemotherapy has significantly contributed to the increase in survival from breast cancer this past decade.

Surgery removes cancerous cells, and radiation therapy destroys cancer cells that might be left in the breast. Chemotherapy is systemic treatment (throughout the body) designed to kill or control any microscopic cancer cells that may have escaped from the breast via the blood or lymph systems.

Chemotherapy decisions are not cookie-cutter. Your treatment plan is designed by an oncologist according to all of the unique factors of your cancer pathology. It is unwise to compare your treatments with other patients because of the wide variations among patients. Only your healthcare team knows all the variables of your cancer.

Be proactive; ask your healthcare team how to manage side effects of treatment.

Communicate openly with your healthcare team about the side effects you are experiencing.

Survivorship

"Instead of thinking about how bad treatment was, I would sit with the needle in my arm, look out the window, and think about how chemo was going to save my life. I had no complaints."

—*Earnestine Brown*

Tear-out Worksheets

Personal Treatment Record - Page W • 23
Questions for Medical Oncologist - Page W • 17
Healthcare Check-Up Worksheet - Page W • 29

Survivorship

As survivors, we learn that survivorship is an attitude we adopt.

It is the one component of recovery that no one else can do for us. We have to decide for ourselves how we intend to respond to our illness and how we will approach our recovery. We, alone, decide to become survivors.

—Judy Kneece

Each individual decides whether and how he or she will grow from an experience of suffering. Perhaps your decision already has been clearly made. Perhaps you've said to yourself, "I am determined that I'm going to learn from my loss."

If you have made such a decision, your healing is not just underway—it's a foregone conclusion!

—Anne Kaiser Stearns

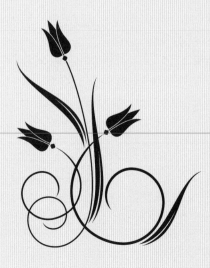

CHAPTER 11

Radiation Therapy

adiation therapy involves delivering X-rays to the breast area to destroy any remaining microscopic cancer cells. Radiation treatment is designed and administered under the care of a radiation oncologist—a physician who specializes in using radiation to treat diseases. During surgery, cells so small they can't be seen with the human eye may remain in the body. The goal of radiation therapy is to destroy those remaining cells to prevent future recurrence. Radiation destroys cancer cells by making them unable to divide and multiply. When these cells die, the body naturally eliminates them. Healthy tissue is able to repair itself in a way that cancer cells cannot.

Lumpectomy patients usually have radiation therapy to the breast for six to seven weeks. Mastectomy patients may also receive radiation therapy if their pathology report shows certain characteristics such a large tumor, positive lymph nodes or a tumor close to the chest wall. Your radiation oncologist will review your pathology report and, working with a physicist, will write a prescription for the dose of radiation and the exact area to be treated. Radiation therapy is usually given after chemotherapy is completed. If you do not require chemotherapy, radiation starts about three to six weeks after surgery or when the breast has healed. If you require chemotherapy, radiation usually starts about four weeks after your last chemo treatment is given.

When Is Radiation Therapy Not a Treatment Option?

You may not be a candidate for radiation therapy if:

- You had previous radiation to the chest area on the same side

- You are pregnant and cannot safely deliver within six weeks

- You have connective tissue disease such as scleroderma

- You cannot commit to the daily schedule for receiving radiation therapy

- You cannot lie on your back with your arm positioned above your shoulder for about 15 minutes if receiving external beam radiation

> *"I actually looked forward to my treatments every day, because I knew I was taking care of what I needed to do. Each day was a day that was behind me until I got through my thirty-three treatments."*
>
> —*Earnestine Brown*

> *"For seven weeks I made daily trips to the hospital for radiation therapy. There were four breast cancer patients scheduled within the same hour. We became good friends and still meet for lunch periodically. We bonded with the healthcare personnel as well and almost hated to see 'graduation' come!"*
>
> —*Marilyn Rej*

Radiation Therapy Treatments

There are two methods to deliver radiation therapy for breast cancer—external and internal. External beam radiation is the most common type. Internal breast radiation, also called brachytherapy or partial breast radiation, is a newer method being used after lumpectomy. It is still being compared to whole breast radiation in clinical trials. There are several types of internal breast radiation under study.

External Beam Radiation

External beam radiation therapy is delivered by a machine called a linear accelerator that produces high-energy X-rays with the use of microwaves. The treatments are painless and are delivered in a series of daily sessions, Monday through Friday, for six to seven weeks.

Before treatment begins, you will be scheduled for an appointment to map out the area being treated. This visit will involve having X-rays and/or a CT scan to precisely identify the area for the therapy. When the area is identified, your therapist will make tiny marks, similar to a tattoo, to mark the area so that the radiation therapist can precisely position you for the treatments. These marks may or may not fade.

During external radiation therapy, you will lie on your back on a table with your arm above your head. The radiation device that delivers your treatment will be overhead, and the therapist will use the marks on your chest to properly align the machine with the planned area of treatment. You will be alone in the room during the treatment, but a two-way communication system allows you and your technologist to talk. The therapist views your procedure on a screen from outside the room. Each treatment usually takes only 10 – 15 minutes in the treatment room but requires that you allow approximately 30 minutes for each visit. During the course of treatment, you will see your radiation oncologist weekly.

Internal Breast Radiation

Internal breast radiation may be given using a procedure called MammoSite® partial breast irradiation. During lumpectomy surgery, a small, soft balloon is placed in the site of the removed tumor. The balloon has a thin catheter (tube) that is later used to insert a tiny radioactive source (seed) that delivers radiation therapy to the internal site. The radiation source is removed after each treatment. Between treatments you are not radioactive. Treatments are usually given on an outpatient basis, twice a day for five days. The balloon is removed when treatments are completed. Side effects to the skin are minimal. This type of radiation is for patients who meet strict criteria for the treatment including tumor size, size of the breast and location of the tumor in the breast. MammoSite® is now available in some centers. Your physician will inform you if you meet the criteria and if this treatment is available in your facility.

Another method of internal breast radiation uses a series of catheters placed into the breast surrounding the area where the tumor was removed. Treatments are also given twice a day over five days. Other modalities, such as electrons, are also being studied.

Side Effects of Treatment

Radiation therapy does not make you radioactive, nor does it make you a danger to your family. Throughout radiation therapy your therapist and radiation oncologist will monitor side effects from treatment. The side effects from radiation are usually mild and well tolerated.

Radiation Side Effects:

- Skin redness similar to sunburn causing sensitivity and itching during treatment
- Potential for blisters and breaks in the skin, called wet desquamation, which may require that you stop radiation for a short period of time (more common after mastectomy)
- Tanning of radiated area after redness subsides

- Mild to moderate breast swelling with potential for arm swelling

- Mild fatigue that begins during the third or fourth week and generally gets better a month or two after treatment ends

- Potential sore throat

- Potential cough occurring six weeks to several months after treatment (uncommon)

- Increased risk for future lymphedema of arm if underarm lymph node area is radiated

- Increased risk for future breast lymphedema

Skin Care During Radiation Therapy:

- When bathing, avoid extremely hot water and use only mild soaps (Tone®, Dove®, Basis® or baby soap) in the area being treated.

- Avoid scrubbing or vigorous wiping with a washcloth or towel.

- Avoid washing the marks off; if the marks should come off, inform your technologist.

- Avoid extremes of hot or cold to the skin: no heating pads, ice packs, hot-water bottles, sun lamps, tanning beds or sunbathing.

- Wear loose-fitting, soft cotton clothing over the treated area. A 100 percent cotton bra, tee shirt or camisole is recommended.

- Do not wear a tight-fitting bra or a prosthesis that rubs the area. (Some women sew a light-weight prosthesis into a tee shirt or a loose cotton camisole to wear during radiation treatments if radiation therapy is required after mastectomy. Cancer boutiques have cotton camisoles with temporary prostheses for sale.)

- Wait until two weeks after treatment to wear your regular bras or prosthesis. However, if you have a breakdown of the skin, you will need to wait until you are completely healed.

- Do not shave under your arm with a razor blade; use an electric razor.

- Do not use deodorant products on the side being treated during therapy.

- Do not use any powder, perfumes, lotions or other scented or alcohol-containing skin preparation on the treated area.

- If dryness and peeling occur, ask your nurse if you may apply pure aloe vera gel or Lubriderm® lotion to the area. Avoid petroleum jelly since it is insoluble and hard to remove.

- If the area becomes painful and blisters occur, report this to your nurse or physician. If the blisters burst and the skin is irritated and painful, ask if you can apply cool compresses moistened with water or normal saline (salt) water. If the area is being rubbed by clothing, ask about applying a sterile dressing such as Op-Site® or Tegaderm® (available in a pharmacy) while it heals. Expose covered area to air for 10 – 15 minutes 2 or 3 times per day. Moist desquamation usually heals in 1 – 2 weeks after treatment ends.

- Avoid sun exposure to the treated area. Outside activity in the sun is possible with protective clothing and high grade sunscreens.

Ask Your Radiation Oncologist:

- How many radiation treatments will I receive?

- On my first visit, how long will it take to mark the area that will be radiated during treatment?

- How do you mark the area that will be radiated?

- Can I wear a bra or my prosthesis?

- What kind of soap and bathing do you recommend during the treatments?

- Is there anything that I cannot use during my treatment (deodorant, perfume, lotions to the chest or back, etc.)?

- Do you have written information on radiation therapy for the breast area?

- What side effects are considered normal during therapy?

- What side effects, if they occur, should I report immediately?

Success Evaluation for Any Treatment

Absolute Risk Reduction or Relative Risk Reduction

One of the challenges in making treatment decisions is understanding how a treatment will increase longterm outcomes in survivorship. Often there is a great source of confusion. When percentages are used to describe a benefit of a treatment or drug, it can cause confusion because there are two ways that percentages can describe the outcome. Both ways are truthful, but the percentage is derived in two very different ways. Therefore, it is essential to understand these two terms, **absolute risk reduction** and **relative risk reduction,** and their implications on your decisions.

Study Example: New drug to prevent breast cancer, two groups of 10 women each. One group is given a new drug and the other is given a placebo (dummy pill). At the end of five years the findings are: 1 woman has breast cancer in the new drug group and 2 women in the placebo group have breast cancer.

The same data from the study could be reported as either:

1. "New drug reduces breast cancer by 50 percent."
2. "New drug results in a 10 percent drop in breast cancer."

Both are accurate. How can this be? The first is reported using **relative risk reduction** percentages and the second is reported using **absolute risk reduction** percentages. This distinction is very important to understand if you are a patient making a decision about your healthcare. Let's look at how these figures are derived.

Study with two groups of ten women. Women in the first group get a new treatment. Women in second group get a placebo (dummy pill).

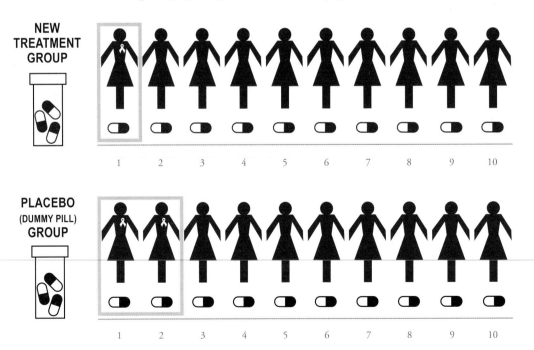

At the end of the study, two women (20 percent) in the placebo group have been diagnosed. The group that got the new treatment only has one diagnosis (10 percent).

Two Ways to Report the Outcome of the Study:

Absolute Risk Reduction

20% – 10% = 10%

"The new treatment reduces breast cancer diagnoses by 10%." OR "After treatment, 1 woman in 10 was diagnosed instead of 2 in 10."

Relative Risk Reduction

One diagnosis in the New Treatment Group is half as many as the two diagnoses in the Placebo Group, and that equals 50%.

"After treatment, only half as many women got breast cancer." OR "New treatment reduces breast cancer diagnoses by 50%." The media often reports **Relative Risk Reduction.**

Both statements are true, but **Absolute Risk Reduction** allows you to make better choices. Be sure to always ask your doctor for your **Absolute Risk Reduction.**

Not knowing if your healthcare provider is quoting you absolute risk reduction figures or relative risk figures can be very misleading and confusing. If percentages are used, ask if these are absolute risk reduction figures or relative risk reduction figures. It is best to always know the absolute benefit from a drug or treatment in order to make an informed decision. Simply ask, "What is the actual number of women out of 100 that benefited from taking the drug/treatment?"

Tear-out Worksheet
Questions For Radiation Oncologist - Page W • 19

Remember

Radiation therapy is used to destroy any cancer cells in the area that is radiated.

Radiation treatments are painless during delivery of the treatment.

Radiation therapy does not make you radioactive. You are not a danger to those with whom you come in contact.

Ask your healthcare provider about how to care for the radiated area.

Survivorship

If you insist on seeing with perfect clarity before you make a decision, you'll never decide. The future always looks like fog; only when you are on the other side can you see what was previously hidden from view.

—Judy Kneece

CHAPTER 12

Complementary Therapies

> *"I did a lot of meditating. I did a lot of praying."*
>
> —*Earnestine Brown*

In the treatment of cancer, there are proven and unproven treatments. The doctors, nurses and other healthcare providers involved in your cancer care are referred to as practicing conventional, Western, mainstream or biomedicine. You will also hear about other types of treatment called CAM (complementary, alternative medicine). CAM therapy is a group of diverse medical and healthcare systems, practices and products, some of which are used by conventional medicine.

After a diagnosis of cancer, you will hear about treatments for cancer from many sources—friends, family and the media. Some of the information will sound very appealing, especially when you are faced with choosing between treatments that have unpleasant side effects and those that do not. It is true that chemotherapy and radiation therapy have some unpleasant side effects; however, these treatments have proven results. They have been found effective in fighting your type of cancer. The treatments recommended by your physicians have many years of scientific study and clinical trials supporting their effectiveness. Many of the alternative therapies have never been the subjects of scientific studies, and their effectiveness has

not been proven. Some healthcare organizations, including hospitals, cancer clinics and physicians, however, are engaged in clinical trials to test the effectiveness of some alternative therapies. Choosing to forego conventional therapy and replace it with an alternative treatment calls for a critical, thorough and wise investigation.

Alternative Therapy Questions:

- What and how much scientific evidence from clinical studies on humans has been published that explains the effectiveness of this treatment on my type of cancer?

- Are the testimonials from reputable, trained healthcare professionals or are they only anecdotal reports?

- Are the claims validated with clinical data such as X-rays or laboratory tests?

- Is the person promoting the therapy benefiting personally?

- Do the promoters claim that if the products fail, it is because of "lack of faith"?

- What will the treatment cost? Will insurance cover it?

- Can you continue your regular treatments and try the alternative therapy at the same time?

Internet as a Source of Information

The Internet is an easily accessible source of helpful information. Be careful, though, because the Internet can also be a source of misinformation.

Internet Guidelines:

- Select Web sites created by major medical centers, universities, government agencies and well-known advocacy groups like Susan G. Komen for the Cure and Young Survival Coalition. You will find that they offer advice that has been clinically proven effective for the treatment of cancer.

- Look for a board of qualified professionals who review information before it's published. What expertise do they have?

- Avoid commercial sites or personal testimonials that push a single point of view or sell miracle cures.

- Avoid sites that don't clearly distinguish between scientific evidence and advertisements.

- Always ask your healthcare team if you find medical advice that conflicts with their recommendations.

- Beware of scams and healthcare frauds. Many make their alternative treatments sound very persuasive. Remember, if it sounds too good to be true, it probably is.

Cancer Treatment Terminology

Various terms associated with healthcare therapies, including medical or clinical, investigational, complementary, integrative, unproven, alternative and quackery are often used to describe methods of diagnosing, preventing or treating conditions and diseases. As a patient, it is important to understand what the terms mean, which approaches are considered safe and where you can find accurate information about various types of treatments.

Medical Treatments

Medical or clinical treatments are those that have been clinically tested for years following a strict set of guidelines and are found to be safe and effective. The results of such studies have been published in medical journals and peer reviewed by other doctors and/or scientists in the field. The Food and Drug Administration (FDA) grants approval for the treatments or procedures to be used in mainstream medicine.

Investigational Treatments

Investigational treatments or research treatments or therapies are studied in a clinical trial. Clinical trials are research-based projects that determine if a new treatment is effective and safe and, if applicable, the optimal dose for treatment. Before a drug, device or other treatment can be widely and responsibly used to treat patients, it is studied and tested, first in a laboratory setting, usually with test tubes, and then in animals. If these studies prove successful and safe, it is then tested on patients in a clinical trial. Patients are recruited to participate in a clinical trial and are monitored as to their response to the investigated therapy. A significant number of patients must participate in order to validate the results. If clinical trials prove the effectiveness of the treatment or drug, the FDA may approve it for regular use by healthcare providers. Only then does the treatment become part of the standard, recommended collection of proven methods used to treat or diagnose disease in human beings.

Integrative Therapy

Integrative therapy is a term that refers to the combination of both evidence-based or mainstream medicine and complementary therapies.

Complementary Therapies

Some complementary therapies are encouraged by physicians. Complementary therapies and activities may enhance your recovery. These may include meditation, relaxation, stress management, acupuncture, yoga and some diets and vitamin supplements which do not compromise your nutrition. Discuss with your physician which complementary therapies will not interfere with your treatment and may be beneficial to you.

Many healthcare organizations, including hospitals and cancer centers, have included these types of therapies in their treatment protocols in an attempt to provide a more holistic and balanced approach to treatment.

Unproven or Untested Methods

Unproven or untested therapies refer to treatments with little basis in scientific fact, or they may also be treatments or tests that are currently under investigation. Adequate scientific study and evidence is not yet available to support their use.

Alternative Therapies

Alternative is a term that refers to treatments that are used in place of conventional medical therapies and may often be promoted as cures. Most often alternative treatments have never been scientifically tested according to US standards. They may also have been tested and found to be ineffective. Choosing alternative therapies instead of traditional medical treatments may cause a patient to put her health at risk.

Quackery

Quackery refers to the treatments, drugs or devices that claim to prevent, diagnose or cure diseases or health conditions, including cancer, that are known to be false or have no proven scientific evidence on which to base their claims. These methods are most often based on a few patient testimonials or so-called "doctor" recommendations as evidence for their effectiveness and safety. Often the treatment is claimed to be effective for multiple diseases as well as cancer. The elderly or chronically ill are often targets of quackery therapies.

FDA Clues to Identify Fraudulent Web Sites:

- Red-flag words: "satisfaction guaranteed," "miracle cure" or "new discovery."

- Pseudomedical jargon terms such as "purify," "detoxify" and "energize."

- Cure-all claims suggesting the product treats a wide range of symptoms and cures or prevents a number of diseases. No single product can do all of this.

- Anecdotal evidence. Testimonials are no substitute for solid scientific documentation. If the product is scientifically sound, it's actually to the manufacturer's advantage—and ultimately yours—to promote the scientific evidence.

- False accusations. The manufacturer of the product accuses the government or medical profession of suppressing important information about their product's benefits. Neither the government nor any medical profession has any reason to withhold information that could help people.

Selecting CAM Providers

When selecting a complementary or alternative treatment provider, your best sources of information about the provider's qualifications are:

- **Medical centers.** CAM practitioners often work in medical centers or by referral from conventional physicians. Ask your physician, nurse navigator or social worker.

- **National associations.** The local affiliates of national associations can usually provide you with the names of certified practitioners in your area.

- **Friends and family.** Ask for advice from someone who has received the treatment you're considering.

Making the Right Choices

After a cancer diagnosis, you deserve every opportunity to restore your health to optimal levels. Choosing appropriate treatments is the foundation for your recovery. Many people find that it is helpful to combine complementary therapies with treatment recommended by their healthcare providers, but they feel reluctant to share this decision with their physician. However, it is important to tell your healthcare providers about any treatments, therapies, drugs, vitamins or herbal products you are considering. There are many therapies that you can safely use along with standard medical treatment to relieve symptoms, reduce side effects, ease pain and enjoy your life more. However, there are also some therapies that could interfere with traditional treatment and even cause harmful side effects. Recovery is a partnership between you and your physician. You must communicate to receive the best care possible.

Types of Complementary Therapies:

- nutrition
- aromatherapy
- herbal therapy
- art and music therapy
- journaling
- counseling
- psychotherapy
- spiritual practices
- prayer
- meditation

- biofeedback
- hypnotherapy
- healing energy
- massage therapy
- chiropractic therapy
- t'ai chi
- exercise
- reflexology
- yoga

Journaling

Writing in a journal is an effective way to handle the emotions that living with cancer has triggered. Journal writing empowers you to express your difficult feelings in a safe and private way. It allows you to come to terms with cancer at your own pace and in your own way. Your journal is always there to receive your thoughts and feelings. It helps you make sense of life events, find meaning in them and learn the lessons they have to teach. Because journal writing forces you to look inward, it helps clarify your fears and thoughts. By writing, you will realize that your illness is only a part of you, not the whole person. It helps you put your illness in perspective.

Prepare by getting a notebook or using your computer and select a time for daily journaling.

Ideas for Journaling

1. Record your feelings, fears and what blessings you enjoyed or discovered each day.

2. Start a list of 50 ways cancer has changed your life; 50 things that can help you cope; 50 things you have always wanted to do; 50 ways to nurture yourself. Add to the list gradually.

3. Write down your prayers if you are spiritual.

4. Collect inspirational sayings and poems. Read these when you are feeling depressed or overwhelmed.

Reputable Internet Sources

The following is a list of reputable sites providing information you may find helpful.

Alternative and Complementary Medicine:

- American Cancer Society: www.cancer.org
- CancerGuide by Steve Dunn: www.cancerguide.org
- National Cancer Institute: www.nci.nih.gov
- National Center for Complementary and Alternative Medicine (NCCAM): www.nccam.nih.gov

Herbal and Food Supplements:

- American Botanical Council: www.herbalgram.org
- Medical Herbalism: A Journal for the Clinical Practitioner: www.medherb.com
- US Pharmacopeia Consumer Information (Botanicals): www.usp.org
- Office of Dietary Supplements (ODS), NIH: www.ods.od.nih.gov
- U.S. Food and Drug Administration (FDA): www.cfsan.fda.gov

Research on Alternative/Unproven Methods:

- National Council Against Health Fraud: www.ncahf.org

Complementary and Alternative Therapies:

- American Cancer Society's Guide to Complementary and Alternative Cancer Methods, Foreword by David S. Rosenthal, M.D., book available: www.cancer.org

Remember

There are proven and unproven breast cancer treatment therapies.

Ask for data on alternative treatments to see if they have proven human results available on effectiveness of the therapy.

Keep your healthcare team informed of any additional treatments you receive.

Ask your healthcare team about therapies that will complement your treatment and add to the quality of your life.

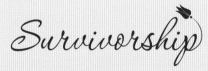

Survivorship

The storms of life cause the oak trees to develop deeper roots. Life's problems cause us to become stronger and more sensitive human beings, if we take the opportunity to grow and learn from our experiences.

—Judy Kneece

Survivorship

Worry is taking our past negative experiences and projecting them into the future. This becomes self-torture and does not prevent anything we worry about from happening. We have to say "no" to our negative, defeating thoughts or we will spend our time in a mental prison built from our own thoughts.

As survivors, we refuse to carry along old resentments, grievances, axes to grind or injustices to remember. We know that harbored memories grow increasingly heavy and slow our journey to recovery. Instead, we decide not to waste our lives by permanently losing ourselves in sorrow, defeat, anger, fear or guilt. We lighten our recovery load by unloading these energy drainers.

—*Judy Kneece*

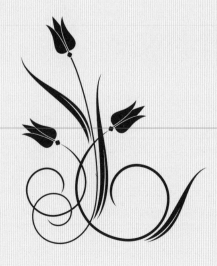

CHAPTER 13

Prosthesis Selection

"The day I was fitted with my prosthesis was a major step in my road to recovery. For the first time in weeks, I began to feel that life just might return to normal again."

—Harriett Barrineau

Restoring your body image after breast surgery is an important part of recovery. A prosthesis is a form molded as a breast and worn inside your bra. Prostheses vary from a soft fiber filling placed in your bra to a custom-made form of your breast. Some women prefer to leave the hospital with a balanced body image. To make this possible, a temporary soft prosthesis, a fabric form that can be filled with fiber filling to match the size of the remaining breast, can be placed into a bra. When the incision is healed, a permanent prosthesis can be selected.

Temporary Prosthesis

Ask your nurse where to find a temporary soft prosthesis. Some hospitals or the American Cancer Society's *Reach to Recovery* program provide patients with a temporary soft prosthesis.

If you desire to purchase your own temporary prosthesis, check with your local prosthesis fitter. You can find the names located in your phone book under Prosthetic Devices, or you can ask your surgeon's staff for recommendations. Prosthetic shops specialize in custom forms, and you can purchase soft, front-opening bras and a form

you fill with a soft fiber puff to match the size of your remaining breast. Some women have found it helpful to purchase these items before their surgery. This allows them to restore their body image soon after a mastectomy and before they can be fitted with a prosthesis.

Wearing a Bra

Women who have breast-conserving surgeries (lumpectomies) usually are more comfortable wearing a bra immediately after surgery to prevent movement of the remaining breast tissue. A well-fitted bra can prevent discomfort caused by excessive movement of the breast tissues. Sleeping in the bra can also be helpful.

Mastectomy patients often find that wearing a bra right after surgery is uncomfortable and tends to rub the incision area. They feel more comfortable braless while wearing a large, soft cotton sweatshirt until their incision heals. Some find a man's cotton tee shirt is a good choice and can be worn under their clothing. A cotton exercise bra, found in any department store, is comfortable for some. Others are comfortable wearing a lightweight bra with a temporary prosthesis of fiber filling.

Some choose to go braless at home and wear their lightweight bra and prosthesis when going out. You be the judge of what best suits your needs, either a soft bra or going braless. However, **do not** wear any bra that rubs or causes irritation to your incision while it is healing. Reconstructive surgery patients need to ask their reconstructive surgeon for recommendations on wearing a bra during the weeks following surgery.

The lightweight temporary prosthesis presents a problem—the bra rides up and causes the prosthesis to be higher on the chest wall. You can hold the bra down in position by anchoring the bra to other undergarments (panties) with a piece of elastic which is pinned or sewn on and attached by snaps or Velcro. Weights, such as those used in curtains and found in fabric shops, may also be sewn into the bra cup on the prosthesis side to add weight and prevent the bra from riding up.

Post-Mastectomy Bras

Special post-mastectomy bras are available, but many women prefer to purchase a prosthesis that fits into their favorite bra. This bra should not have underwires and must fit well. The fitter can help you decide if it is possible to use your existing bras. She can show you how to create a pocket in which to place the prosthesis in order to prevent it from falling out.

Permanent Prosthesis Selection

When your incision has healed, usually four to six weeks following surgery, your physician will give you a prescription for a prosthesis, which allows you to file for insurance coverage. Do not be fitted until your surgical site has healed. For some patients this may take longer.

When ready to shop for a prosthesis, it is best to make an appointment for a fitting with a trained prosthetic specialist. The specialist will help you decide on a prosthesis according to your breast size, the weight you need in a prosthesis and your lifestyle. Plan to go when you have time to look

carefully at all she has to offer so you can find the prosthesis that best suits your needs. A fitting usually takes between one and two hours. When you go for your fitting, take or wear a close-fitting garment so that you can see what your body looks like with the prosthesis. Some women have found a man's cotton tee shirt is easily accessible. If possible, take a friend or your partner with you—someone who can see how the prosthesis looks and who will give you an honest opinion.

Types of Permanent Prostheses

Breast forms, like our breasts, come in many shapes and sizes. They may feel rubbery and very much like your own skin. They may be covered with a soft fabric, polyurethane or a silicone envelope. Some are filled with foam rubber, chemical gels, polyethylene material, polyurethane foam or silicone gel.

Like natural breasts, prostheses vary in weight, and their consistency varies from soft and pliable to relatively firm. They are also designed for the right and left side. Some have nipples that will appear much like your remaining breast. Prostheses are designed to fit into special pockets inside mastectomy bras to prevent them from falling out.

There is also a model that attaches to your skin with a sticky adhesive or a tape that is applied to the skin so that when you move, it moves. This model also prevents the riding up of the prosthesis and bra, which is a problem for many women. If you feel this would be appropriate for your lifestyle, you should ask to try the adhesive and tape. Wear it for several days to be sure that you do not have an allergic reaction. This prosthesis can be worn with your regular bras, and you can also go braless.

If you have reconstruction and do not have the nipple reconstructed, there are nipple prostheses. The nipple prostheses from ReForma are reusable, hypoallergenic and self-adhering. They cost about $60 and are covered by most major insurance providers.

Women who have a wide-excision lumpectomy may need a prosthesis called an equalizer, which is designed to fill in the section of tissue removed from the breast.

Altering Clothing for Prostheses

You can also learn from the fitter how to alter your swimsuits for use with your prosthesis. Extremely lightweight forms are available for use with your nightgown or leisure clothes. Many clothing items such as sportswear, lingerie and swimsuits that accommodate prostheses are also sold in prosthetic shops. Some women buy silky, lacy camisoles and sew lightweight prostheses inside to wear under their nightclothes and when they do not want to put on their regular prosthesis.

Ask Your Prosthesis Fitter:

- How do I clean my prosthesis?

- Can I get it wet?

- How long will it take to dry?

- Does perspiration damage the prosthesis?

- Will pool chemicals cause any damage?

- Is there an exchange policy if I decide it does not meet my needs?

- How long should the prosthesis last?

- How much will my insurance provider pay toward the cost?

- Does my insurance provider pay for mastectomy bras?

- If yes, how many bras will my insurance pay for at my initial purchase?

- How often will my insurance provider pay replacement costs of my prosthesis?

- How often will they pay for replacement bras?

- If I alter them, can I wear my regular bras with my selected prosthesis?

- Do you bill the provider for the cost, or do I pay and bill my provider?

What Prostheses Cost

Prices range from a few dollars for fiber filling up to around $350 for a permanent prosthesis. Most women spend around $250 for a prosthesis. Custom-made prostheses and prostheses that adhere to your body are more expensive. Bra costs start at $20 and go up.

Most professional shops will assist you in finding out how much your insurance company or Medicare will pay on your prosthesis and bras. Some insurance policies state that they will only pay for **either** a prosthesis or reconstruction. If you plan to have reconstruction later, your provider may not cover the cost of your surgery if you have already filed for the cost of a prosthesis. Check your policy or call your provider if you plan for later reconstructive surgery.

When You Cannot Afford a Prosthesis

If you cannot afford a prosthesis, some local American Cancer Society units have loan closets. Women who have had reconstruction may donate their prostheses to be given to other women who cannot afford one. Call your local cancer treatment center to ask if anyone provides this service.

The Breast Cancer Network of Strength organization (1-800-221-2141) has a Prosthesis and Wig Bank to provide women who have financial needs with a free breast prosthesis or a wig, if they have the appropriate size of prosthesis or color of wig available. A small handling charge is requested, and the product is mailed anywhere in the United States.

Ask your healthcare team if they know of any sources that assist women in the purchase of a prosthesis after surgery. Some local organizations may offer this type of support for patients who cannot afford to purchase needed prosthetic devices.

Remember

Plan to shop for a prosthesis when you have time to carefully evaluate which breast form best suits your need. Make an appointment with a specialized fitter.

Take someone with you who will be supportive and honest in helping you evaluate how it looks. Take a tee shirt or tight sweater to try on over the new form to see how it looks under clothing.

Do not try to save a few dollars on a prosthesis you do not like or feel comfortable wearing. Restoring your body image is a very important part of recovery.

CHAPTER 14

Monitoring Your Emotional Recovery

"My physical recovery went well. At first, it seemed, so was my mental and emotional state. After three or four months, things began to change. I knew people still cared, but the initial interest and concern began to wane. I was still surrounded by so much love, yet I was feeling totally alone."

—Harriett Barrineau

"My one-year diagnosis anniversary date blindsided me a little bit. My mother sent a huge bouquet of pink roses to work and I broke down crying. But I still reflect back upon the entire thing as a gift of change. Going to a support group, even if there are no other young women in the group, is incredibly helpful. I found an online "virtual" support group with discussion boards. Later I joined the organization as a volunteer. Getting involved in breast cancer advocacy work has helped me with the need to give back and continue the fight."

—Anna Cluxton

The unexpected diagnosis of breast cancer can serve as a threat to your self-esteem, body image, sexuality, social life and career. That's a lot of unexpected threats and changes to deal with after diagnosis. During this time, you may experience many confusing emotions—things you may have never felt—as these threats are individually worked into your life. The biggest surprise for many women was the struggle they had emotionally—they thought dealing with treatment would be their biggest challenge, but they found that the hardest part was dealing with their emotions.

The problem they had dealing with their anxiety and depression threw them a curve ball. One patient shared about her emotional struggles:

I had always been so strong and able to handle anything that came my way ... until now, and now I feel as if I am falling apart many days. My doctor assures me I am doing great and have a good prognosis. I know that this should make me happy, and I should be grateful, but somehow I can't feel that way. I feel so alone in my struggle to make sense of this. What is happening to me?

"I actually started taking care of ME after my diagnosis—the way you're supposed to. I had to realize that there are only 24 hours in a day and not 99 like I thought there were before."

—Earnestine Brown

If you have had difficulty with your emotional recovery, you are not alone. Somehow the emotional struggle is seldom talked about. It may not be discussed by your healthcare team because they are trained to treat your cancer and that is their main focus. You may have to approach the topic with them to find the same good treatment for your emotional struggles as you do for your cancer.

This is the reason for this chapter—to share insights to help you understand the normal emotional challenges you may or may not face, what you can do about them and when you should seek help from a professional to deal with your emotions.

Major Emotional Challenges

Anxiety and depression are the major challenges patients deal with. Anxiety is a signal that you are under too much stress and is defined as the time spent fighting the problem. Depression, on the other hand, signals that you have stopped struggling with a problem, have given in to it and have given up the fight.

During the diagnostic period, you may experience a high level of anxiety. This is normal. Cancer is a new experience for most and brings many unknowns for the future. When you're faced with a new challenge, anxiety is expected. For many, anxiety gives way to depressed feelings, which are also normal for short periods of time. For some, though, anxiety and/or depression continues to linger too long and can impact recovery. This is when trained professionals can help if you reach out to them.

Anxiety

Anxiety occurs throughout life when someone is faced with a new challenge and feels frightened or threatened by it. A breast cancer diagnosis is certainly one of these times. High anxiety is expected during the diagnostic period, immediately after a diagnosis and anytime a new "stressor" (an event that is frightening and perceived to be a threat) happens.

Signs and Symptoms of Anxiety:

- Nervousness and shaking inside; lips quiver; hands shake and speech is rapid
- Racing heart; tightness in chest; choking sensation; palpitations (heart skips a beat)
- Rapid breathing; lightheadedness; tingling or numbness in arms, hands, legs and feet
- Pacing, can't sit still; lack of concentration and memory about event; confusion
- Difficulty falling asleep and staying asleep; restless, unsatisfying sleep

Anxiety symptoms are real and show that you are dealing with something that is frightening to you. Anxiety can rob you of your ability to make decisions, cause you to be fatigued and irritable and, if experienced for a long period of time without relief, can impede your recovery. Anxiety may be a short-term problem that resolves itself and only reappears when a new challenge arises. When anxiety is a daily experience that doesn't let up, it's called chronic anxiety.

Depression

Depression results when you give in to a situation—life is just too hard, so you withdraw. It often follows an extended period of anxiety. Depression symptoms manifest themselves differently than anxiety. Depression varies in degree of severity from a short period of feeling down and "blue" to a debilitating depression that continues day after day. It is essential to understand the difference between a normal reaction of feeling depressed for a short period of time and prolonged clinical depression, which needs intervention by health professionals.

Reactive Depression

After breast cancer, most women suffer from an expected short-term depression called a reactive depression. Your diagnosis was a real loss that has to be incorporated into your life. Scattered throughout the months after your surgery and during treatment, sometimes for unknown reasons, you may find yourself feeling "blue," down or depressed. If the feeling lasts for several days and then you begin to feel better, this is a normal reaction (reactive depression) after a loss in your life.

Common Times for Reactive Depression:

- **Treatment conclusion:** Many women feel depressed at the conclusion of all their chemotherapy or radiation treatments. This depression is referred to as post-treatment depression and is very common.

- **Check-ups:** This same depression may occur around the time for a return visit to your physician for a check-up after breast cancer. We refer to this normal reactive depression as check-up anxiety. Most women are anxious the week or days surrounding their check-up, wondering if anything new will be found. If the exam is negative, the "blue" mood lifts.

- **Anniversary dates:** Dates of diagnosis, surgery or treatments can cause an anniversary reaction. These dates may bring back vivid memories and the feelings you experienced during the original event. It is normal for these dates to create a sad reminder of the experience, but anticipating and planning can significantly reduce the emotional strain.

It can be helpful if you anticipate these times and plan your activities to accommodate for your "blue" feelings. Plan a time away from your routine duties to do something special, spend time with friends or arrange a light schedule of work. At the conclusion of treatment, set new goals to do things that you have always wanted to do.

Depression That Needs Intervention

For some women, incorporating the changes a cancer diagnosis brings into their lives becomes a problem. Their depression and tears do not cease; they continue for extended periods of time during or long after surgery and treatments are completed. These periods may occur often or remain as a constant companion. This is a sign of clinical depression that needs intervention by a professional. Clinical depression is a serious condition with real symptoms that affect the mind, body and relationships. Symptoms are prolonged, severe and increasingly incapacitate your ability to return to normal functioning.

The first step in distinguishing the difference between feeling "blue" and clinical depression is to know the warning signs and not feel uncomfortable about seeking appropriate help. Women can be helped to overcome depression and live normal, healthy lives. Feeling "blue" or periodic depression means that one may feel sad but can still enjoy and look forward to parts of life, such as a family gathering, a movie or seeing a friend.

Clinical Depression Is Often Manifested By:

- Continuous (week after week) feelings of sadness during or after surgery and treatment
- Social withdrawal from friends or family
- Feelings of worthlessness
- Excessive feelings of guilt
- Excessive fear of the future
- Slowness in physical movement or speech
- Constant jitters or nervousness with no apparent reason
- Low energy level; feeling tired all the time
- Inability to make decisions
- Negative thinking; constant anger or mistrust
- Imaginary health problems
- Obsessions about health and cancer
- General disinterest in food or eating excessively
- Disinterest in work or day-to-day activities (things which used to interest you)
- Disinterest in intimacy or sex
- Insomnia (inability to sleep, waking early or being unable to go to sleep)
- Hypersomnia (sleeping too much, wanting to sleep all the time)

■ Suicidal thoughts (If you have suicidal thoughts and feel that death would be an easy choice, please call your physician or nurse immediately.)

If you find that you are experiencing several of these symptoms (some experts say five) for a period of two weeks or longer during or after treatment completion, your physician should be notified. Breast cancer patients who take chemotherapy also have to deal with hormonal fluctuations caused by treatment, greatly increasing the potential for mood changes and other side effects that increase stress and contribute to the potential for depression. It is essential to understand that seeking help for your depression is not a sign of weakness; it is a sign of strength.

Is It Anxiety or Depression or Both?

Sometimes it is difficult to determine if you are suffering from anxiety, depression or a combination of both. A quick assessment may help you determine. Answer the questions below by marking a yes or no for each question to help determine whether your struggle is with anxiety, depression or both.

Assessment Score

Total up the yes and no answers to each set of questions. Generally, if you answered yes to more of the questions in Set I, you are experiencing anxiety. If you answered yes to more of the questions in Set II, you are experiencing depression. If you answered yes to more than three in each set, you are suffering from both depression and anxiety. Discuss this questionnaire with your physician or someone on your healthcare team. This guide can help you ask for the correct interventions.

Treatments for Depression and Anxiety

The good news is that there is good treatment for acute or chronic anxiety and clinical depression. Both are easily treated through learning personal coping skills, seeking professional counseling and drug therapy.

Counseling

In some cases, counseling—talking to a professional—may be all that is needed. Counseling identifies weaknesses in coping skills and works to strengthen them. Often talking to an understanding person accomplishes a lot for a depressed or anxious person. Counseling therapy, often called

---

IS IT ANXIETY, DEPRESSION OR BOTH?

Set I

1. Do you feel nervous or edgy most of the day for no reason?	Yes	No
2. Do you sometimes panic when something happens?	Yes	No
3. Do you often feel scared, as if something bad is going to happen?	Yes	No
4. Are you sometimes too nervous to do anything?	Yes	No
5. Do you constantly feel stressed out?	Yes	No
Totals	___	___

Set II

1. Do you no longer feel confident in yourself to handle problems?	Yes	No
2. Do you feel hopeless about what is happening in your life?	Yes	No
3. Do you feel helpless about what is happening in your life?	Yes	No
4. Do you feel worthless as a person?	Yes	No
5. Do you sometimes think life is not worth living?	Yes	No
Totals	___	___

"talk therapy" or psychotherapy, allows a person to talk about her past and present experiences, relationships, feelings, thoughts and behaviors that may be contributing to the problem. The counselor's aim is to identify major causes of stress and then help you determine the best approach to solve your problems. Ask your nurse or physician for local counseling resources. Most often, counseling after breast cancer is short-term.

Drug Therapy for Depression and Anxiety

Medication may be needed to assist the therapeutic process and requires a prescription from a medical physician or an advanced care practitioner. Some people feel there is a societal stigma to taking anti-anxiety or antidepressant medications. However, taking medications for depression or anxiety is no different from taking medication for diabetes. Both conditions are uninvited and attack the body, and both can be successfully managed with medication. Denying yourself medication to help with your acute anxiety or depressed mood is like denying yourself insulin to treat diabetes.

Anxiety Medication

Anti-anxiety drugs are used to calm your nervousness or agitation; they begin to work immediately. They are called benzodiazepines. Many women diagnosed with acute anxiety find that taking an anti-anxiety drug allows them to regain their composure, concentrate to make needed treatment decisions and sleep much better. When taken correctly, symptoms of anxiety are reduced within 30 to 90 minutes. If you are experiencing a lot of anxiety after your diagnosis, do not hesitate to ask your physician for help. This will allow you to get the rest you need and make decisions in a more timely, informed manner.

Your doctor will usually prescribe these medications only for a short time to help you get through a particularly rough period of anxiety. Long-term anxiety is better controlled with other medications. Anti-anxiety drugs for acute anxiety may be

prescribed on a regular schedule or to be taken as needed (prn) during periods of high anxiety. Don't drive while taking these drugs; they cause drowsiness. Remember, your healthcare team does not know what you are experiencing or need unless you tell them.

NAMES OF ANXIETY MEDICATIONS

The most commonly prescribed anti-anxiety medications:

- Alprazolam (Xanax®)
- Lorazepam (Ativan®)
- Chlordiazepoxide (Librium®)
- Clonazepam (Klonopin®)
- Diazepam (Valium®)

Depression Medications

Antidepressants are often prescribed to stabilize your mood and will take approximately two to three weeks to become effective. There are numerous categories of antidepressants to treat depression. Both the drugs and the dosages must be carefully matched with a patient's symptoms and overall health. This is not a "one-size-fits-all" approach. Physicians consider numerous factors. For example, if you are experiencing depression accompanied by fatigue, the selective serotonin reuptake inhibitors (SSRIs) will help with the fatigue and some will reduce hot flashes. The SSRIs are the most commonly prescribed group of antidepressants. Remind your physician if you are taking tamoxifen. Some SSRIs have shown in recent studies to reduce tamoxifen's effectiveness.

If you are experiencing anxiety with your depression and are not able to fall asleep or stay asleep, another type of antidepressant may be a better choice because of its sedating effect. Wellbutrin® is another antidepressant for patients who do not have anxiety with their depression. Wellbutrin® has no sexual dysfunction associated with use.

It is important to understand that not all drugs are effective in all people. It may take several attempts before your physician finds the most effective medication for your needs. Remember, it takes time for antidepressant medication to build up in your body before you feel the full effects. For this reason, it is important to contact your physician when you first recognize symptoms of depression.

Antidepressants are usually prescribed for an extended period of time and are withdrawn gradually when you and your physician feel you are ready. They need to be taken as prescribed, without skipping doses or stopping when symptoms are controlled. Anti-anxiety medication and an antidepressant may initially be prescribed at the same time. When the antidepressant begins to take effect, the anti-anxiety drug is reduced, discontinued or used only when needed. Talk to your healthcare team about the help you need to regain control of your emotions and improve the quality of your life.

MEDICATIONS FOR DEPRESSION
■ Bupropion (Wellbutrin®)
■ Citalopram (Celexa®)
■ Duloxetine (Cymbalta®)
■ Escitalopram (Lexapro®)
■ Fluoxetine (Prozac®, Prozac Weekly®)
■ Fluvoxamine (Luvox®)
■ Paroxetine (Paxil®, Paxil CR®, Pexeva®)
■ Sertraline (Zoloft®)
■ Venlafaxine (Effexor®)
■ Desvenlafaxine (Pristiq®)

Self-Care for Anxiety and Depression

If you are reading this and are in the acute phase of anxiety or have moved to depression, talk to your physician about the appropriate medication to restore you to a state where you can function. You can then tackle adding the self-care tips discussed below. If your anxiety or depression is mild, allow yourself to experience the benefits of self-care for stress. The following suggestions do not require a prescription and do not cost anything—only your determination to implement the proven methods of stress control.

The "Fight" or "Flight" Stress Reaction

Where does the stress that causes anxiety that can lead to depression begin? The process begins when a new event—stressor—is perceived by a person as a threat. The stressor can be a real or imagined threat. No matter whether the stressor is real or imagined, the first and natural response of humans is to respond with a stress reaction called the "fight" or "flight" (flee or run away) reaction. This reaction makes people feel they are in danger and have to do something to protect themselves or others. High levels of anxiety caused by the event prepare the body to remove itself from danger.

If we hear a car racing as we are crossing the road, we tense and run quickly to get out of its way—it's a natural instinct for self-preservation. It can also happen when an event, such as a loud noise awakens us at night—we do not know whether it is threatening or not, until it is evaluated. This fear experience may also occur when we remember a time in our lives when a tragic event happened—simply thinking about it brings back feelings of stress and anxiety.

This stress reaction, although normal, can turn into complete physical and emotional exhaustion (depression) if it lasts too long. The secret to stopping this downward spiral is to use all available tools to manage your reactions to stress. A diagnosis of breast cancer is a real threat. It makes sense that your anxiety will be acute until you find how to regain your control and make the problem manageable—assemble your treatment and support team, get information, etc. The best advice is to avail yourself of all the support available from your treatment team and then add a program of self-care. You will find that even though your reality doesn't change, taking active steps will drastically change your thinking. With that change in thinking comes a big reduction in stress, and with reduction in stress comes an improvement in mood and increased energy.

THE STRESS RESPONSE

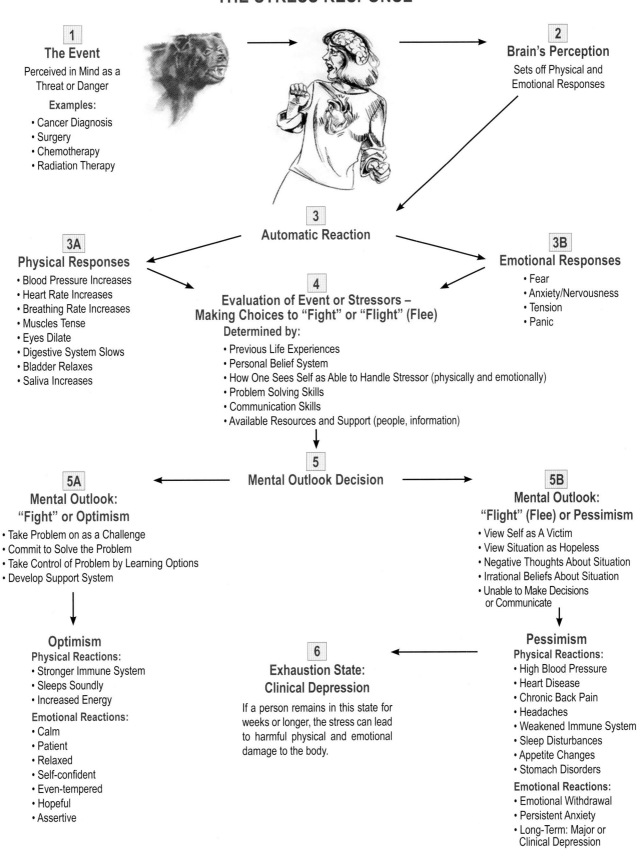

1
The Event
Perceived in Mind as a
Threat or Danger

Examples:
• Cancer Diagnosis
• Surgery
• Chemotherapy
• Radiation Therapy

2
Brain's Perception
Sets off Physical and
Emotional Responses

3
Automatic Reaction

3A
Physical Responses
• Blood Pressure Increases
• Heart Rate Increases
• Breathing Rate Increases
• Muscles Tense
• Eyes Dilate
• Digestive System Slows
• Bladder Relaxes
• Saliva Increases

3B
Emotional Responses
• Fear
• Anxiety/Nervousness
• Tension
• Panic

4
Evaluation of Event or Stressors –
Making Choices to "Fight" or "Flight" (Flee)
Determined by:
• Previous Life Experiences
• Personal Belief System
• How One Sees Self as Able to Handle Stressor (physically and emotionally)
• Problem Solving Skills
• Communication Skills
• Available Resources and Support (people, information)

5
Mental Outlook Decision

5A
Mental Outlook:
"Fight" or Optimism
• Take Problem on as a Challenge
• Commit to Solve the Problem
• Take Control of Problem by Learning Options
• Develop Support System

5B
Mental Outlook:
"Flight" (Flee) or Pessimism
• View Self as A Victim
• View Situation as Hopeless
• Negative Thoughts About Situation
• Irrational Beliefs About Situation
• Unable to Make Decisions
  or Communicate

Optimism
Physical Reactions:
• Stronger Immune System
• Sleeps Soundly
• Increased Energy

Emotional Reactions:
• Calm
• Patient
• Relaxed
• Self-confident
• Even-tempered
• Hopeful
• Assertive

6
Exhaustion State:
Clinical Depression

If a person remains in this state for
weeks or longer, the stress can lead
to harmful physical and emotional
damage to the body.

Pessimism
Physical Reactions:
• High Blood Pressure
• Heart Disease
• Chronic Back Pain
• Headaches
• Weakened Immune System
• Sleep Disturbances
• Appetite Changes
• Stomach Disorders

Emotional Reactions:
• Emotional Withdrawal
• Persistent Anxiety
• Long-Term: Major or
  Clinical Depression

115

The Stress Response

The Stress Response, also called the General Adaptation Syndrome, was first identified in the early 1900s by Hans Selye. It is a basic description of the role of stress, the way people respond to stress in their environment and how, if not relieved, stress can negatively impact health. No one can avoid stress; it is a part of life. However, we can learn to control and change some of the things that cause stress. This skill is especially important after a cancer diagnosis because cancer brings many stressors that need to be handled effectively so that the negative effects of stress will not slow your recovery.

One of the secrets to reducing the harmful effects of stress in your life is to understand the stress process and learn how you can intentionally interrupt it.

"Fight" or "Flight" (Flee) Response

When an unexpected event happens and is perceived as a threat, we naturally respond with a heightened sense of awareness. The shock can either give us a healthy surge of emotions and energy that prepares us to move from danger or it can cause us to become completely overwhelmed with fear. This is called the "fight" or "flight" (flee) response. A number of changes occur throughout the body as we prepare to "fight" or flee from this unexpected event. Sometimes the "fight" or "flight" response occurs when we merely remember or think about something that is frightening.

After years of working as a navigator, I realized how this stress response model was evident in patients. Understanding the main principles of stress could help them identify what was happening to them and how they could manage their response. The diagram on page 115 illustrates the stress process. The following numbers correspond with the diagram.

1 The Event: A Cancer Diagnosis

A cancer diagnosis comes with little warning and is perceived as a threat. It sets off the stress response spiral. Other events during cancer treatment, such as surgery, chemotherapy, radiation therapy and diagnostic tests, can also cause high levels of stress.

2 Brain's Perception

The event is interpreted in the mind as unknown or threatening and is viewed as dangerous. This is an initial and automatic response.

3 Body's Immediate Reaction

The brain releases a cascade of stress hormones, mainly cortisol and adrenaline, to prepare the body to take action. These stress hormones change every body system, preparing the person to fight or flee.

3A Physical Responses include tensed muscles, increased blood pressure, racing heart, rapid and shallow breathing, dilated eyes, slowed digestion, relaxed bladder, increased saliva and numerous other changes.

3B Emotional Responses are ones of fear, producing anxiety, nervousness, tension and panic.

4 Evaluation of Event or Stressors

After the initial stress happens and the body panics, an evaluation of what to do occurs. Does this event really require you to take action? Do you fight or flee the stressor? You'll probably decide whether to fight or flee based on your past preparation for coping, including:

- Previous life experiences (Is this something I know how to solve?)

- Personal belief system (Is it the right thing to do in this situation?)

- How capable you feel of handling the stress physically and emotionally (Can I face this and not be destroyed emotionally or physically?)

- Problem solving skills (Do I know what to do?)

- Communication skills (Can I ask for help and feel that someone will respond?)

- Available resources and people (Do I have enough information about the stressor to understand what to do? Do I have someone to help me with this problem?)

Depending on how you evaluate your ability to deal with the stressor, you'll either respond by saying, (5A) "I will fight this" (an optimistic response) or (5B) "I can't do this—I will try to flee" (a pessimistic response).

5 Mental Outlook Decision

At some point after the stress event a mental decision is made to choose either optimism or pessimism.

5A Mental Outlook: Fight or Optimism

"I am going to do all I can." This leads to seeing the event as a problem to be solved. It becomes a challenge and a commitment to take control of the situation and learn what can be done to change things. Part of this decision is reaching out to find the information you need and getting help from others to fight this new battle.

When the stressor is viewed as a challenge and a problem to be solved, the emotional and physical reactions change. Emotionally, you will notice reduced nervousness and a sense of calm because you believe that you are capable of dealing with the stressor. You will probably feel more assertive as you ask questions and begin your quest for information about what you can do. As you change your perception from victim to challenger, you reduce the stress hormones in your body. With reduced stress hormones, you'll sleep better, experience increased energy and boost your immune system. "I will fight this!" is the decision.

5B Mental Outlook: Flee (Give In) or Pessimism

The other option is to give in. The stressor seems to be too big to deal with. You might not view yourself as having the skills needed to fight the stressor. The decision (most often unconsciously) is to surrender to the stressor—"I give in." You might view yourself as a victim of the stressor and see your future as hopeless. Negative, frightening thoughts that may be irrational cause you to be unable to communicate your fears, make decisions about what could be done or ask for help. These thoughts are frightening and cause emotional withdrawal from people and activities. "My situation is hopeless and it is useless to fight; I will give in," is the decision.

Giving in keeps the body under stress and allows the stress hormones to continue to be secreted. This chronic anxiety may manifest itself with symptoms such as constant fatigue, high blood pressure, heart disease, chronic back or generalized muscle pain, chronic headaches, sleep disturbances, appetite changes and stomach and bowel disorders. The prolonged presence of stress hormones weakens the immune system, and you may notice an increase in infections, colds and viruses.

6 Exhaustion State

If the state of hopelessness with its host of symptoms is maintained for longer than a few weeks, it will lead to a condition psychologists call a state of "exhaustion" or clinical depression. Clinical depression is a condition that should be considered serious and needs treatment like any other malfunction in the body.

Stress Buster Skills

Now that you understand how the stress response works, you can learn to recognize it when it begins and take steps to manage or reduce your stress. We can never prevent events that threaten us from entering into our lives. We can, though, learn what we can do that will reduce their impact on our health.

"While we cannot direct the winds that enter our lives, we can adjust our sails."
—**Author Unknown**

Controlling Stress With Self Care

Stress control begins with identifying exactly what you are afraid of and taking steps to do what you can to make it less threatening. Dr. Herbert Benson, of Harvard Medical School, recognized as the world's leading expert on elicitation of the relaxation response, advises patients to use the following formula: **stop, breathe, reflect** and **choose.**

1. **Stop**. Recognize you are at the beginning of a stress response.

2. **Breathe.** Take several deep breaths and let them out slowly. This slows down the body's physical response and allows you to think more clearly.

3. **Reflect.** Ask yourself:
   - What am I afraid of that is causing these feelings?
   - What about this event or thought is upsetting or distressing me?
   - Am I jumping to conclusions about what happened or may happen?
   - Is this a present reality or a future worry?
   - If a present reality:
     - What can I do to change it?
     - What information can I gather?
     - With whom can I talk to understand what I need to do?
     - What is the worst thing that can happen? If that happens, can I handle it?

4. **Choose.** Take the steps of action you identified—you may still feel fearful, but addressing your fears is the way to make them manageable. Make a deliberate decision not to think about them so anxiously—remember, 90 percent of what we worry about never happens.

Stress Control by "Self-Talk"

An important part of recovery is "self-talk" or what your mind is saying to you. It is helpful to choose some encouraging phrases to say repeatedly to yourself when you begin to be fearful or worried. Sometimes "self-talk" is the quickest and easiest way to calm your nerves.

Calming "Self-Talk" Phrases Include:

- I can handle this.
- I am doing the best I can.
- I've done hard things before; I can do them again.
- I don't have to be perfect; I'd rather be happy.
- Let it go; it's not worth it.
- This, too, will pass.
- My health is more important than my need to be right.
- I have so much to be thankful for.

Using the stop, breathe, reflect and choose formula and repeating positive "self-talk" phrases allows you to reduce your stress when an event occurs. Chronic stress can also be reduced by using methods that elicit the relaxation response to calm the body. These techniques include deep breathing, meditation or imagery (focused thinking about something positive), praying or repetitive prayers, repetitive exercise, progressive muscle relaxation and yoga.

The Relaxation Response

Dr. Benson identified the relaxation response (deep breathing and repetitive phrases) as a means to manage stress when you are dealing with things you cannot control. The relaxation response has been clinically proven to reduce heart rate and blood pressure, thus relaxing the entire body and counteracting the harmful effects of chronic stress.

Learning to Elicit the Relaxation Response

To learn any new skill requires practice and perseverance. Most people have difficulty relaxing their bodies and need a way to free themselves from the stress of their environment to enter into a state of relaxation. It begins with a conscious effort.

How to Elicit the Relaxation Response

1. Find a quiet room away from interruptions and sit up straight in a chair.

2. Place your hands comfortably in your lap. Relax your muscles.

3. Close your eyes.

4. Select a focus word, phrase or prayer that gives you a sense of peace, love and safety. Some suggestions are:

   - **General:** One; Peace; Calm; Relax; Let go; Let it be; Love; My time

   - **Christian:** Come, Lord; Lord, have mercy; Our Father, who art in heaven; Lord Jesus Christ, have mercy on me; Hail Mary; The Lord is my Shepherd

   - **Jewish:** Sh'ma Yisroel ("Hear, o Israel"); Echod ("One"); Shalom ("Peace"); Hashem ("The Name")

   - **Eastern:** Om (the universal sound); Shantih ("Peace")

   - **Aramaic:** Maranatha ("Come, Lord"); Abba ("Father")

   - **Islamic:** Allah

5. Breathe slowly and naturally, and, as you do, silently repeat the phrase or word you have selected as you exhale.

6. Continue inhaling and repeating your phrase while exhaling. Do this for approximately 20 minutes.

7. When your mind wanders to another thought, refuse to entertain it and gently bring your thoughts back to your breathing and repetitive phrase.

8. Open your eyes and gradually re-orient yourself to your surroundings.

As you practice the relaxation techniques, you may find it is difficult to keep your mind focused. Admittedly, it is hard, but don't get discouraged. Fortunately, there are a number of ways to focus your mind. Mindful breathing is one of the keys.

As you practice, take a few deep breaths to help turn your attention inward, and then allow your breathing to follow its own natural rhythm. During relaxation you may feel sensations such as a tingling, a sense of floating, drifting or dropping. This indicates that your body is relaxing. It is suggested that the relaxation response be practiced twice a day to provide maximum benefit from stress.

Mini Relaxation Responses

You may find yourself in a stressful situation such as a diagnostic test or I.V. stick when you cannot leave or escape to a quiet place. Simply concentrate on breathing and repeating your phrase either silently or quietly with your eyes open, if necessary. Taking a deep breath increases the oxygen to the brain and clears the thinking. Focusing on a word or phrase during concentrated breathing interrupts the anxiety produced by the stressful situation. Many patients have said this technique has been invaluable and comforting when confronting a stressful event such as receiving chemotherapy or radiation, having an I.V. puncture, enduring a diagnostic test or a new procedure. Keep your body in a more relaxed state by practicing the mini relaxation response anytime, anywhere.

Visualization Relaxation

Another relaxation technique is to replace the repetitive phrase with a mental picture of a scene that brings a sense of peace and safety—a garden, park, seashore, etc. As you breathe slowly, mentally feel and explore the beauty of this favorite place in your mind—smell the fragrances, feel the warmth of the sun and hear the familiar sounds.

Additional Chronic Stress Busters

One of the major ways to control chronic stress is to start a program of regular exercise. You may not feel you have the energy to do anything, but any effort to increase your daily movement will bring positive benefits. Set goals for yourself to increase your daily activity. Exercise has proven to be one of the best ways to reduce stress and improve your mood. Exercise promotes the release of endorphins, chemicals in your body that naturally increase mood and decrease pain. Massage and sexual activity have also proven to increase the release of your natural endorphins, which elevate your mood.

Another way to control chronic stress is to watch what you eat. A nutritious diet and adequate hydration (water intake) promote better moods and increase energy. Mayo Clinic psychiatrist, Daniel K. Hall-Flavin, M.D., reported that some people with depression have low blood levels of eicosapentaenoic acid (EPA), a fatty acid found in fish oil. These omega-3 fatty acids have been shown to play an important role in brain function as well as normal growth and development. A good way to get more omega-3 fatty acids, including EPA, is to simply eat more fish. Try salmon, mackerel and tuna. Other dietary sources of omega-3 fatty acids include flaxseed, canola oil, soybeans, pumpkin seeds and walnuts. Increase your intake of these foods.

Conquering Anxiety and Depression

No one can avoid daily events which cause anxiety. Most often we are able to manage these everyday stressors until a crisis comes. During a crisis, we have to deal with so many threatening unknowns that we become overwhelmed with stress and experience acute anxiety. Acute anxiety is a natural response to something we find frightening and triggers the fight or flight response. We can't change what happens to us, but we can change many of our responses. We can change what we think about the event. We can get support and help understanding what we can do. We can manage stress by incorporating physical activity and eating a nutritious diet. Then, if we don't find relief, there are medications for anxiety and depression. Remember, it's hard enough to fight breast cancer physically. No one has to tough it out emotionally, dealing with anxiety or depression that robs you of your ability to function. Reaching out for help is a sign of strength and not weakness. If you need help, don't hesitate to call your healthcare team.

One patient shared her advice to other women going through treatment:

When the news is good, I don't allow myself to get too high, and when it is bad, I don't allow myself to get too low because I know that things will constantly change. My job is to manage my emotions, and the doctor's is to manage my cancer. You've got to get off of that emotional roller coaster; it will destroy you.

This is a hard change for many people to make because they feel that paying attention by worrying is necessary.

Remember

Plan to keep your friends and family involved in your life while undergoing treatments. They are a great buffer against stress. Ask for help when you need it.

Anxiety is the initial response to a new stressor and is expected. Prolonged anxiety can negatively affect your physical health.

Depression is not a sign of weakness.

Most depression is generally short-term and usually responds to counseling and/or medication.

Seeking help for anxiety or depression is a sign of strength.

Learn self-care skills to interrupt the stress response and reduce the potential for depression.

CHAPTER 15

Sexuality After Breast Cancer

"Resuming sexual relations with my husband after surgery was not easy for me. I was not comfortable with my own sexuality and wasn't sure what I wanted or expected from my husband. Fortunately, he was more comfortable with this than I was. He very tenderly and lovingly helped me come to terms with this part of our recovery."

—*Harriett Barrineau*

Breast cancer has changed many things in your life. One of the potential changes may be in the area of your return to normal sexual functioning. Women share that their sexual attractiveness to their partner was of primary concern during their recovery. Many factors are involved in successfully adjusting to the change breast cancer has brought. It is helpful if you evaluate your present status and take steps to restore any areas that may not have returned to normal.

A woman's breasts play an important part in her femininity, and any breast surgery or disease will threaten her sense of being a woman. This is a normal response. However, it is important that you take steps to incorporate these changes into a healthy perspective that allows you to return to your former state of functioning. Changes brought about by surgery are often related to your personal view of your new body image.

Focus Group Research

EduCare Inc. conducted research on sexuality after breast cancer treatment in focus groups of breast cancer survivors. The groups were convened in 11 different hospitals nationwide and consisted of women who had taken chemotherapy. We wanted to know about the impact that treatments had on their sexual functioning and quality of life. The focus groups investigated the physical changes experienced, the sexual changes, the impact on the relationship with their sexual partner, their educational needs before treatment and the women's requests for future services of pre-treatment education and support to be offered by their healthcare team and facility.

"We had to learn to navigate my new body. It was important for us to resume the intimate part of our life as it was the one thing we and we alone shared. Also, after the tremendous assault on my body, we looked upon the tenderness together as healing."

—*Anna Cluxton*

Judy C. Kneece, RN, OCN, conducted the focus groups, with patients invited by their healthcare facility. A total of 126 survivors responded to 143 questions using individual Audience Response Interactive data pads. These hand-held computer pads allowed all answers to be anonymous. Each woman was free to express her true feelings without anyone knowing how she answered. The computer automatically analyzed the data entered at each individual site and then combined the 11 sites for the final analysis. Throughout this chapter, findings from these surveys will be shared to help you understand what other women experienced.

Your Body Image

One of the hardest and most important steps is viewing the incision area and the changed or missing breast. This is indeed difficult, but it is an essential step to recovery. Your partner shares your pain and loss and, when allowed to join you in viewing the incision, will be better able to respond to your needs. Not allowing your partner to participate will build a wall of separation that will affect the sexual relationship.

Breasts add pleasure to the sexual relationship but are not essential for sexual pleasure to occur. It is not the loss of a breast that changes the relationship as much as the way you and your partner accept the loss. Facing the loss together and openly communicating about how your surgery may change your sexual relationship are the first steps in successfully adjusting. The earlier this is done, the smoother the transition to recovery.

It is helpful to plan to view the surgical scar as early as possible. The first dressing change is a good choice, if possible. However, some women find that they prefer a time more emotionally suitable for them. The goal, however, is that you allow your sexual partner to view your new body image. This is an important step to restoring normal intimacy. Delaying may make it even more difficult.

SURGICAL SCARS

Partners' viewing of scar:

- 75 percent replied that it was within days after surgery

Perception of partners' response when viewing the scar:

- 80 percent reported their partners were accepting and supportive
- 15 percent reported a neutral response
- 5 percent reported a negative response

Note: 6 percent reported that their partner had never seen their scar. These women still dress or undress behind closed doors or in the dark.

Resuming Physical Intimacy

When can you resume intercourse after breast cancer surgery? As soon as the two of you would like. If no complications arise, the incision should heal in about four weeks following surgery. However, you may resume your sexual relationship before the area is totally healed. The best time to continue is when both of you feel ready. The surgical scar area will naturally be sore or sensitive, but you can lead your partner in how to prevent pain by altering positions to avoid pressure on the surgical area.

Some women have shared that even though their partners had viewed the incision, they found it difficult to participate in sexual intimacy unclothed. This problem was solved by purchasing a lacy camisole that could be worn with or without a prosthesis. Most camisoles purchased at a cancer boutique have a pocket for a soft fiberfill or your prosthesis. For some, this helps to preserve their feelings of femininity during the sexual relationship. Examine your feelings carefully to discover what may be preventing you from resuming your sexual relationship with the one you love.

Surgical Side Effects on Sexuality

During the period surrounding your diagnosis and surgery, sexual functioning may be affected by emotional stress or physical fatigue. This is a normal interruption that will be time-limited and, when over, should not impair your former state of sexuality.

It is understandable that sexual feelings are naturally diminished during high periods of stress. However, during periods of stress the need for emotional closeness increases. Most women express that they really need and want more touching, hugging and emotional closeness during this stressful period, but they often don't know how to express this need or are afraid to ask. You may also find yourself withdrawing from your partner. Do not allow walls of silence and emotional isolation to separate you. This will diminish your physical closeness during this time because your partner is not sure how to treat you. Let your partner know you still desire to be close and to touch but that you do not feel up to sexual intercourse. Your honesty will be appreciated. Your partner, too, is having to sort through this new experience.

Radiation Therapy Impact on Sexuality

Radiation therapy to the breast area ranges from six to seven weeks of daily treatment (Monday through Friday). If the patient is not getting chemotherapy, radiation starts several weeks (3 – 6) after breast surgery or when the incision is healed. If you are having chemotherapy, radiation usually follows the chemotherapy.

During radiation treatments, you are not radioactive and sexual contact can continue. However, you may notice that you experience increased fatigue starting around three weeks after beginning treatment, resulting in diminished sexual interest. When radiation treatments are completed, you will find there is no lasting impact on the sexual relationship if you have not/are not taking chemotherapy or hormonal therapy.

Chemotherapy Impact on Sexuality

Side effects from surgery and radiation are short term. If additional treatments with chemotherapy are required, sexuality changes become more of a long-term challenge because of the impact of the drugs. Most chemotherapy teaching for patients is about the well-known side effects of fatigue, nausea, vomiting and hair loss. Very few couples are forewarned about the impact on their sexual functioning, other than the potential for infertility if the woman is pre-menopausal. The problem is that chemotherapy most often causes instant menopause in pre-menopausal women and increases menopausal symptoms for menopausal women.

Menopause caused by chemotherapy is different because it occurs suddenly, unlike normal menopause which occurs over years. The symptoms of chemically-induced menopause are more intense because the drugs diminish the hormones made in the ovaries and the adrenal glands. Natural menopause mainly impacts the ovaries during onset, causing a reduction in the ovarian hormones of estrogen, progesterone and eventually testosterone. The adrenal glands continue to supply some hormones, causing symptoms to be less severe with natural menopause.

The other important factor to understand is the production of testosterone. Testosterone is predominately a male hormone, but women also make testosterone in the ovaries and convert hormones made by the adrenal gland. Testosterone is the hormone that produces sexual desire and the ability to experience an orgasm; it also governs the intensity of the orgasm. When a woman takes chemotherapy, she has an instant reduction of all her hormones, including testosterone, from both the ovaries and adrenal glands. Side effects of the reduction of estrogen and progesterone are very apparent—hot flashes, night sweats, mood changes and vaginal dryness. However, the side effects of testosterone reduction are seldom recognized and are often ignored. Because the symptoms are experienced by the patient and impact only her and her partner, they are very rarely addressed. By understanding all of these changes, their causes and ways to reduce side effects, your sexual relationship with your partner should not suffer but thrive because you are actively seeking interventions to deal with side effects. We will briefly discuss the major side effects.

Fatigue

Obviously, after chemotherapy treatments your energy level will be low. You may not feel like doing much of anything for several days or weeks after each treatment because of lowered blood counts, which cause fatigue. Fatigue will vary with the type of drugs you receive. Ask your physician about the drugs and expected levels of fatigue.

Fatigue has a cumulative effect, increasing as treatment progresses. Plan to get additional rest by taking naps or sleeping in when possible. Reduce as many tasks of daily living as possible during your highest levels of fatigue. Take the initiative to divide household responsibilities among family members or even consider hiring help during this time. Most women are least fatigued the week before their next treatment. This is the time to plan activities requiring more energy. You may be physically and emotionally exhausted during treatment, but this will improve.

It is recommended that you strive to stay as physically active as possible, while being careful not to overdo it. Moderate exercise, such as a walking program, has been shown to increase energy and reduce fatigue and symptoms of chemotherapy. The key is balancing the two—exercise and rest. A full discussion of the challenge and guidelines for healthy movement are discussed later in this book.

Be sure that your meals are nutritionally adequate; good nutrition is required to build new cells to replace those that chemotherapy destroys. You may be too tired to prepare nutritionally balanced meals and may need help in this area.

Treatments will end, blood counts will increase and energy will return gradually. It is important to know that the return of energy does not happen in days or weeks when treatment is completed but that it requires months; some women reported a year passed before their normal levels of energy returned. Look at this as a time to take good care of yourself physically.

FATIGUE

Women participating in the sexuality study indicated their energy level at the time of diagnosis was an average of 7.6.
(1 = no energy, 10 = high energy)

When asked how chemotherapy impacted their energy levels:

- 62 percent reported a decrease from their baseline energy during treatment

- 40 percent reported a decrease six months after completion of treatment

- 22 percent reported a continued reduction at one year after completing treatment

Nausea and Vomiting

Nausea and vomiting used to be major side effects of chemotherapy, but with new drugs, they can be controlled in most cases. It is important that nausea and vomiting be controlled because they increase fatigue, decrease nutritional intake and increase the potential for electrolyte imbalances. Report any uncontrolled nausea or vomiting to your healthcare team.

Mood Swings

When women lose their estrogen, through natural or chemical menopause, one of the first things they notice is a change in their emotions. Before menopause, this is experienced the few days before their menstrual period and referred to as premenstrual syndrome (PMS). You are probably well aware that this time is emotionally different. PMS occurs when estrogen and progesterone fall to their lowest levels to allow menstruation. During these few days, increased moodiness, tearfulness, nervousness and outbursts of anger are common symptoms in many women. The same symptoms occur during reduction of female hormones from chemotherapy. A sad fact is that some women feel that their unstable emotions are caused because they are not "handling cancer" well or that they are depressed. The fact is, their bodies are thrown into the same emotional limbo as PMS, but it continues day after day because the hormones do not return to reverse the withdrawal. This emotional roller coaster is caused by the chemotherapy drugs and not your emotional weakness or inability to "handle cancer."

MOOD SWINGS

Participants in focus groups reported an increase in emotional mood swings:

- 55 percent increase in mood swings during treatment

- 42 percent increase six months after treatment ended

- 19 percent increase at one year after completing treatment

Mood changes after chemotherapy are an expected side effect and vary in degrees of intensity. It is almost a certainty that mood changes will occur during treatments. The reduction of the female hormones caused by treatment may cause wide fluctuations in your moods. You may swing from normal to sad, then to angry, then to depressed, all with no apparent cause. It is important to understand that this is not from emotional weakness on your part. The emotional battle is not a choice, but a side effect of treatments.

What can a woman do about her mood swings? She can discuss the problem with her physician and ask for a medication called an SSRI (Selected Serotonin Reuptake Inhibitor), which increases the levels of serotonin that elevate mood. The brand names are Celexa®, Paxil®, Prozac®, Effexor® and Zoloft®. The great thing about these drugs is that they have also proven successful in reducing hot flashes, nervousness and insomnia. A recent small study revealed that tamoxifen's effectiveness was reduced if taken concurrently with Paxil®, Prozac® or Zoloft®. However, Celexa®, Lexapro® and Luvox® did not have the same impact. Check with your physician if you are taking tamoxifen for the most appropriate SSRI data.

Vaginal Dryness and Painful Intercourse

Hormonal changes cause the vagina to have less lubrication, resulting in vaginal dryness. Estrogen is the hormone that causes the wall of the vagina to be soft and pliable. With the reduction in estrogen, the vagina becomes very dry. Along with the dryness, the vagina will not lubricate adequately during sexual arousal. If this problem is not understood or corrected, it can possibly result in painful intercourse, a small amount of bleeding after intercourse and a decrease in desire. Painful intercourse is not pleasant and bleeding can scare both partners.

VAGINAL DRYNESS

Vaginal dryness from chemotherapy was reported to increase:

- 123 percent during treatment

- 134 percent six months after treatment ended

- 160 percent one year after completion of treatments*

*Note: Vaginal dryness continued to increase.

Treating Vaginal Dryness

There are two over-the-counter treatments for vaginal dryness. One is a vaginal moisture-replenishing product (such as Replens® or Vagisil®) designed to maintain the moisture in the vagina. Vaginal moisturizers are applied inside the vagina on a regular basis, several times a week, to restore and hold moisture. They are like a facial moisturizer applied to keep moisture in. They are **not** designed as a lubricant before intercourse. Some women find them helpful; others do not.

The other over-the-counter intervention is a vaginal lubricant. This is applied prior to intercourse to increase lubrication. The vaginal walls are thinner after estrogen decline caused by menopause or chemotherapy-induced menopause. You should generously apply the lubricant in the vagina and on the outside on the vaginal lips. It can also be applied to the partner to increase lubrication. It is important that the lubricant be reapplied as needed during intercourse. Use it generously.

Approximately 20 percent of women have a chemical sensitivity to vaginal lubricants that causes burning and irritation when applied. If you experience burning with regular lubricants, the cause is usually glycerin or paraben in the lubricant. Look for a glycerin and paraben-free product in the personal care section of drug stores.

Recommended Lubricants:
- Astroglide® is highly recommended by patients as being the most like natural lubrication and is easily found in your local pharmacy. Astroglide® is also available in a glycerin and paraben-free formula.
- Liquid Silk® is highly recommended by healthcare professionals. It is glycerin-free and also formulated to be bio-static, which means if it is exposed to any bacteria, yeast or fungal spores it will stop them from spreading. Liquid Silk® can be ordered online.

Avoid oil-based lubricants, such as petroleum jelly (Vaseline®) or baby oil, because they may promote vaginal infections and are not recommended for use with latex condoms.

Vaginal dryness is not only uncomfortable; it can also cause itching. The dryness of the vaginal tissues can also set up an environment for irritating or painful vaginal infections that interfere with sexual pleasure. Any itching or swelling should be reported to the healthcare team for a vaginal infection evaluation.

Vaginal dryness, unlike most side effects of chemotherapy, continues long past chemotherapy administration. Most of the women in the focus groups experienced escalating vaginal dryness after treatment conclusion. The good news is that most women can manage the symptoms with over-the-counter vaginal lubricants.

It is very important for a sexual partner to know that this vaginal dryness is not from lack of desire from the patient, but from the inability of the walls of the vagina to lubricate caused by the chemical menopause. Often, partners take this reduction of vaginal lubrication as a lack of desire for them as a sexual partner and feel rejected. Some partners feel that the use of lubricant is a sign that they are not sexually stimulating to their partner. Neither is true. Lack of vaginal lubrication is caused by chemical menopause. This is something you, the patient, cannot control.

PAINFUL INTERCOURSE FROM VAGINAL DRYNESS

Painful intercourse increased:
- 137 percent six months after treatment
- 149 percent one year after treatment completion

These figures reveal that vaginal dryness with the potential to cause painful intercourse increases after treatment is completed. Therefore, couples should be prepared to deal with the lingering side effects.

Vaginal Infections

Infections may be caused by an overgrowth of bacteria that causes a thin, gray discharge that has a fishy odor. Another cause is a fungus (Candida albicans) normally found in the body can experience an overgrowth (often caused by antibiotics) causing a discharge that has thick, white (cottage cheese like) clumps that cause itching accompanied with internal and external swelling. Both of these vaginal infections can easily be treated with medications. If you experience any vaginal discharge that is irritating or has a foul odor, report this to your healthcare provider.

Vaginal Dryness Options

During natural menopause, women are offered oral or transdermal (patch applied to skin) hormone replacement therapy (estrogen) to relieve their symptoms. At this time, this is usually not an option during breast cancer treatment. However, after treatment is completed, if the vaginal dryness continues even though vaginal moisturizers and lubricants are used, discuss other options with your healthcare provider. The first option would be estrogen vaginal cream applied inside the vagina and on the external vaginal lips. Another option is a vaginal ring of estradiol (Estring®) that is inserted into the vagina and remains in place for three months, slowly releasing the drug before replacement is needed. These localized estrogens relieve vaginal dryness and decrease urinary symptoms. After several months the vagina increases in moisture and elasticity, making intercourse far more comfortable. However, only you and your healthcare provider can determine if either option is appropriate for you.

Urinary Problems

When estrogen levels are reduced, urinary symptoms are a common side effect. Estrogen receptors are found in the lining of the urinary bladder and tubes. When estrogen levels are low, the lining becomes thinner and some women experience burning during urination, urinary urgency and urinary stress incontinence (loss of urine when walking fast, running or sneezing). They find holding their urine difficult and often a source of embarrassment. The use of estrogen vaginal cream or Estring® will also greatly reduce these symptoms.

Orgasm Ability

After treatment with chemotherapy, the ability to experience an orgasm during intercourse is reduced for most women. However, a small percentage of women will not suffer this side effect. Hormonal reduction usually continues to create problems for those women who remain in a permanent menopausal state. It can cause an inability to experience an orgasm or reduce the intensity of orgasm if one is experienced. Sexual arousal is also a challenge. One woman in the focus group described her sexual desire after chemotherapy as "that of an 11-year-old girl." Diminished sexual interest, sexual thoughts, sexual arousal and orgasm are all common side effects of chemotherapy.

It is important to understand that the loss of testosterone—the hormone that causes interest, arousal and orgasm—is the basic problem. What can

Orgasm Ability Before and After Chemotherapy

ORGASM	NEVER	RARELY	OCCASIONALLY	MOST OF THE TIME	ALL OF THE TIME
Before Treatment	1%	8%	19%	55%	17%
During Treatment	24%	27%	28%	16%	5%
One Year After Treatment	10%	23%	29%	30%	9%

Before treatment, 72 percent of women would experience orgasms, varying from most to all of the time. During treatment this fell to 21 percent. Following completion of treatment, this number rose only slightly to 39 percent, translating into a 54 percent reduction in ability to experience orgasms most or all of the time, one year after treatment.

be done about these side effects? The testosterone can be brought back into normal range by a trained, experienced healthcare provider who understands the complexity of hormonal balance. Many healthcare providers are completely unaware of this intervention. Some contend that they don't know if it is safe. However, those women who have had their levels brought back into therapeutic range with testosterone creams report that this brought back the quality of sexual life they enjoyed before treatment. Ask your healthcare team if they check hormonal levels or supplement testosterone. If not, contact the International Academy of Compounding Pharmacists (1-800-927-4227) and ask for the nearest compounding pharmacy. Your local pharmacy can refer you to the providers in your area who are skilled at testing levels of existing testosterone and prescribing testosterone cream to bring levels back to normal.

SEXUAL INTEREST AND AROUSAL

Sexual thoughts prior to diagnosis:
- 88 percent of women reported having sexual thoughts and fantasies before chemotherapy
- 32 percent had sexual thoughts and fantasies during treatments
- 41 percent reported sexual thoughts and fantasies one year after treatment completion

When questioned about the need for extra time to achieve sexual arousal after chemotherapy:
- 86 percent replied that the time for sexual arousal required had increased
- 49 percent reported decreased nipple sensitivity from sexual arousal
- 80 percent reported lack of vaginal lubrication during foreplay

Wellbutrin®, an anti-depressant, has proven helpful in increasing libido and the ability to have an orgasm for some women. Some women also report weight loss while taking the medication. If you have a history of anxiety or other disorders, the medication may not be appropriate. Ask your healthcare provider if you are a candidate for this medication.

Preserving Sexual Functioning

Nerve and muscle stimulation in the genital area must be maintained to preserve normal sexual functioning. Regular episodes of sexual stimulation cause the nerves and muscles to experience increased blood flow, helping them stay healthy. Disuse leads to decreased sensitivity of the nerves, so when someone tries to become sexually aroused, they experience less response. For this reason, routine arousal, even if you do not experience orgasm, helps maintain healthy functioning of the genital tissues. When you are going through treatment, sexual arousal, understandably, is going to decline. As soon as you regain energy, however, plan to resume sexual activity to keep the vaginal nerves healthy and reclaim your normal sexual functioning.

Return of libido and ability to have an orgasm is a quality of life issue. It has nothing to do with life and death issues and for this reason may be ignored. For some, return of libido is important to quality of life. For others, this is not an issue of importance. Only you can decide what is best for your relationship. There are no right or wrong answers, only what best meets your needs. If you find that this is an important issue, keep seeking a healthcare provider who addresses your problems, offers interventions and works to improve your quality of life.

Partner's Understanding

It is essential that your sexual partner understand the potential changes that chemotherapy may bring to your sexual functioning. One of the major differences is your increased time for sexual arousal. After chemotherapy there is a need for increased foreplay. Understanding this helps both of you approach the sexual relationship with a clear understanding of problems and potential solutions.

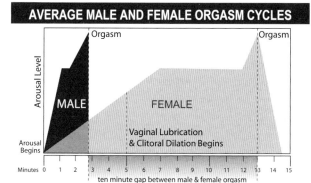

AVERAGE MALE AND FEMALE ORGASM CYCLES

Male sexual arousal time is very short compared to the time required for a woman to feel aroused, as illustrated by the chart. Many men do not understand the additional time needed for a woman to feel completely aroused for sexual intercourse. The arousal time increases after menopause and chemotherapy. Same-sex partners also need to discuss the impact of treatment on increasing arousal time. One of the first steps toward experiencing a mutually-fulfilling sexual relationship is to understand this difference and the impact that treatments may have. Full arousal makes sexual contact more comfortable and exciting. Plan to have this discussion with your partner.

The majority of women interviewed (89 percent) said they would like to have their healthcare provider explain to their partner the changes in sexuality resulting from treatment. If you feel this would be helpful to you, ask your healthcare provider to include your partner in the discussion. You can also ask your partner to read this chapter.

Talking to Your Physician

Some women feel that their physicians are only interested in saving their lives and not in their daily life functions. This is NOT true. Physicians are well aware that quality of life is one of the main components of a successful recovery. They may not ask about sexuality problems, but it does not mean that they will not discuss them with you. Don't hesitate to ask questions and report any side effects. If necessary, ask for a referral.

Breast cancer has not changed you. You and your partner may experience some new challenges after your surgery and treatment for cancer, but you are still the same loving person your partner selected. Breast cancer does not change that fact. Many couples share that the experience of cancer brought them closer together, and the meaning of the sexual relationship was enhanced because of the realization of how valuable they were to each other.

Restoring Sexual Function Self-Evaluation:

- Have I allowed my partner to see my scar? Am I still hiding in the closet to change clothes?

- Have I talked openly about my fear that our relationship will change?

- Have I expressed my desire for our sexual functioning not to be affected because of my cancer diagnosis?

- Have I shared openly about what is physically comfortable or uncomfortable during intimacy since my surgery?

- Am I honest when I am physically fatigued and would like to be held and cuddled without intercourse?

- Does my partner understand the potential side effects from chemotherapy on sexual arousal and functioning?

- Have I explained to my partner that when I do not feel up to the sexual act, I either need time to adjust or feel fatigued from treatment—I am not rejecting them?

- Have I planned a special time and saved energy for the sexual relationship to be resumed?

- Have I been honest and asked for family assistance with household duties during treatments to allow myself more time and energy for pleasurable events?

- When I have problems, such as hot flashes, dry vagina, painful intercourse or lack of sexual desire due to treatment side effects, do I talk with my healthcare team about how to manage the problems?

129

- Have I had my body image restored with a well-fitted prosthesis, reconstruction or am I planning for reconstruction?

- If interested in reconstructive surgery, have I talked to a physician and received the information needed to make a decision?

- If I am having problems adjusting to my body image or sexuality, have I asked to speak to a counselor?

- Have I asked my treatment team or called the American Cancer Society for information on sexuality after cancer?

- Have I treated myself to something to enhance my feeling of femininity after surgery, such as a lacy camisole, perfume, an item of clothing or a new haircut?

All breast cancer patients have to readjust in the area of sexual functioning. There are many things you can do. There is help from professionals to assist you in returning to your normal sexual role. Don't allow changes to occur without reaching out to your healthcare provider to ask for information and, if needed, referral to professionals in the area of sexual counseling. The earlier you address these problems, the easier they are to solve. Educational material is available, and trained counselors can help you with the transition.

Birth Control After Breast Cancer

It is necessary to discuss with your healthcare provider what type of birth control to use after your surgery. Chemotherapy usually stops your menstrual periods, and they may or may not return after the treatments are completed. If you are near menopause, they may never come back. However, if you are young, they may return. For some women, several years may go by before normal menstruation begins again. Because you may be fertile (able to conceive a child) before evidence of a menstrual period, you may want to discuss with your physician the type of birth control that is suitable for you. Do **not** take any oral contraceptives (birth control pills) without

talking to your oncologist. Alternative methods of birth control may be recommended according to the type of treatment you receive.

Note on Tamoxifen

The anti-estrogen drug tamoxifen (Nolvadex®) may increase ovulation (release of the egg from the ovary) when therapy is started. After receiving tamoxifen, women may be more fertile. Some method of birth control is recommended. Discuss with your physician what types of contraception are most suitable and the length of time your healthcare team recommends that you prevent pregnancy.

Remember

The key to preventing changes in the sexual relationship is open, honest communication with your partner and your healthcare team.

Surgery and radiation therapy may cause temporary interruption in sexual functioning due to stress and fatigue.

Chemotherapy may cause chemical menopause, impacting sexual desire, sexual arousal, ability to experience orgasm, and vaginal dryness, causing painful intercourse.

Your sexual partner needs to understand that these side effects are from treatment and not your lack of desire for them as a partner.

Ask about the need for contraception.

You are still the same loving person your partner selected. Breast cancer does not change that fact.

CHAPTER 16

The Single Woman and Future Intimacy

If you are single or divorced, a cancer diagnosis can add additional stress by impacting your view of future emotional, physical and sexual intimacy. Like many other patients, you may find it difficult to imagine how you would handle a future intimate relationship. Some women in our sexuality focus groups reported that after their cancer diagnosis and treatment, they felt as if they were "damaged goods" and that they would not be sexually attractive as a partner. This is not true! Many women have successfully developed intimate relationships after a diagnosis of breast cancer.

Single women often need help understanding the impact of diagnosis on developing future relationships. The first thing necessary is for you to rethink the subject. Cancer does not define who you are. You are still the same you! Most often a cancer diagnosis causes a person to become a stronger and more sensitive person. This life experience makes you a more attractive person. Unlike some diseases, breast cancer is treatable, and after treatment most women return to a normal state of physical and emotional health.

The first step is to make peace with yourself and take the steps needed to rebuild your self-image, whether by reconstruction, getting into shape physically or developing new skills. This is an opportunity for you to decide how you would like to change or improve.

Future Dating Reminders:

- Dating was not always successful before your diagnosis. Dating after cancer will be the same; sometimes the person is not the right one, but it has nothing to do with your cancer diagnosis.

- Most people have things they would like to change about themselves. Some are overweight, bald or are not physically "Mr. America."

- One third of Americans will have a cancer diagnosis. Ask yourself, if this person had a history of testicular or prostate cancer, would you reject him?

One of the best ways to prepare for a future relationship is to talk to other breast cancer patients about their experiences in developing intimacy after their diagnosis. Support groups are a great place to talk to other women. The Young Survival Coalition listed in the reference section of this book is a nationally recognized resource. Professional counselors are also an excellent resource to have your fears and concerns addressed and to make plans for how to deal with them in the future. You need to prepare how you will share your diagnosis when you do find a new partner. Understanding how other women have handled the issue will give you a sense of preparedness and allow you to develop your own plan.

Sharing Your Diagnosis

Sharing the details of your diagnosis with a new partner should not occur on the first date. The best time is when the relationship has passed the mutual friendship stage and is progressing. However, it is important to share before the relationship becomes serious or intimacy may occur. Only you know when this is happening. When you feel the time is right, select a time and place where you will feel comfortable discussing your diagnosis. If you should become upset, you need to be in a place where you would not feel embarrassed.

Tips for Sharing the Details:

- State that you desire respect and honesty in your relationship and you have something you need to share.

- Share the facts about your diagnosis honestly and openly: "In (year) I was diagnosed with breast cancer. This required that I have a (mastectomy/lumpectomy) that was followed by (type of treatments). I have been cancer-free for (time) or at the present I am dealing with (problems). I feel that what I went through has allowed me to become a stronger person by having to deal with a lot of hard issues. I wanted to be very honest with you before this relationship progressed. I will be happy to answer any questions you have about my diagnosis, treatment or present health."

- Do not appear as a victim; you do not want pity!

- Ask your friend what they think about what you just shared. Allow them to talk.

- If the person is hesitant to discuss your revelation, simply suggest that you know the information may have come as a shock: "Why don't you call me in the next couple of days after you have had a chance to think about this, and we will discuss your feelings?"

Remember, if this person leaves the relationship after this, this is a person who would have deserted you in the future if things did not go well. You did yourself a favor and prevented future heartaches. The nature of relationships is that some work and some don't. Your goal is to protect yourself emotionally by sharing early enough to find out if this will impact the relationship before you fall in love.

Single Woman's Goals

As a single woman, you need to be prepared to discuss your diagnosis confidently with future partners. Surround yourself with understanding peers as you work through the process of preparing what you will say in the future. Cancer has not "damaged" you; it has been a tool for expanding your ability to love and appreciate life.

Remember

Being diagnosed with cancer does not change who you are.

A cancer diagnosis can serve to make a person stronger and more sensitive.

You are not "damaged goods." You are a person who has expanded her ability to love and appreciate life.

CHAPTER 17

Future Fertility

One of the issues least thought about during a cancer diagnosis is the impact of cancer treatments from chemotherapy and hormonal therapy on future fertility. Most thoughts naturally focus on the patient and getting the most appropriate treatment for control of the cancer. However, one of the most important issues for younger couples who have not started or completed having their family is taking the time to discuss the potential impact on their future fertility. It is essential for couples to ask questions to protect their fertility or plan for future alternative fertility methods before treatment begins.

For women, infertility is the inability to start or maintain a pregnancy. Infertility can occur because of the inability of the ovaries to produce mature eggs (oocytes) for ovulation. It can also occur from the inability of the body to successfully allow implantation of a fertilized egg into the uterine wall or to maintain growth after implantation.

Women and the Fertility Cycle

When a woman is born, she has all of the eggs (approximately 200,000 immature eggs) she will ever have and does not produce more. When the female hormones gear up at puberty, she experiences the development of secondary sex characteristics such as breasts, pubic hair and menstruation. Eventually, the menstrual cycles are accompanied by the release of a mature egg at mid-cycle (ovulation, around day 14) ready for fertilization by the male sperm. If conception does not occur, or if the fertilized egg does not successfully implant into the uterine wall, the prepared uterine wall sloughs off, evidenced by the menstrual flow. The entire process begins again for another monthly cycle. Each full cycle averages from 28 to 32 days.

"We were newlyweds when I was diagnosed. This raised a lot of questions about our future for becoming parents. Would chemotherapy rob us of the anticipated joy of one day having our own children?"

—Anna Cluxton

Each ovulation reduces the number of stored eggs. It is estimated that approximately 500 eggs reach maturity and are released over the fertile period of a woman's life. Eventually, as hormonal levels decrease, the supply of eggs that mature is reduced, ovulation ceases, hormones decrease to pre-menstrual levels and eventually the menstrual periods stop. This cessation of ovarian function with the loss of fertility is called menopause. With menopause comes not only infertility, but also hot flashes, vaginal dryness, changes in moods, urinary changes and other side effects.

Fertility Threatened by Chemotherapy

Surgery has no effect on fertility, other than creating stress that causes change in the hormonal balance that may temporarily alter ovulation and possibly menstruation. This usually resolves itself in several months. Radiation therapy to the breast alone has only temporary effects, similar to surgery, because of stress and fatigue temporarily altering hormonal functioning. The major cause of infertility comes from chemotherapy.

Chemotherapy drugs work to treat cancer by killing rapidly dividing cells throughout the body. Chemotherapy drugs are cytotoxic (cyto=cell, toxic=poison). These drugs kill cancer cells, but in the process kill healthy, rapidly dividing cells as well. Shortly after chemotherapy administration, women notice hormonal changes in their body. The large majority of women suffer irregular or complete cessation of periods during treatment. Factors that determine the extent of side effects and impact on future infertility are the patient's age, the type of drug or the drug combinations that may create a compounding effect of toxicity on the body. It is very difficult for an oncologist to accurately predict who will suffer side effects with their hormonal functioning. Some women have their fertility return after the drugs are discontinued, but for others, infertility may be permanent.

Factors That Help Predict Future Fertility

1. The nearer a patient is to menopause, the less likely she is to have hormonal function (menstruation and ovulation) return. The younger the woman, the more likely hormonal functioning will return.

2. A class of drugs, called alkylating agents, has an especially destructive effect on hormonal functioning. The most common one used in breast cancer treatment is cyclophosphamide (Cytoxan®). Other drugs that increase infertility in this category are melphalan (Alkeran®) and busulfan (Myleran®). Cisplatin (Platinol®) is usually considered an alkylating agent and also impacts fertility even though it works differently than the others in this category.

Addressing Issues of Fertility

Since physicians cannot predict with absolute certainty whose fertility will be permanently affected, there are steps to take to preserve your future ability to have children.

1. The most essential step is telling your healthcare team **before** treatments that having children in the future is a top priority in making treatment decisions.

2. Ask your healthcare team to discuss treatment recommendations and their potential for causing infertility.

3. Ask for written information on the subject of chemotherapy and fertility.

4. Ask for a referral to a fertility specialist if you still have questions or concerns.

5. Ask for treatment protocols that reduce potential for infertility.

6. Explore alternative fertility preservation options.

Fertility Preservation Options

Embryo Freezing

Hormones (like tamoxifen, proven safe to use in breast cancer patients) are used to stimulate egg production. Mature eggs are removed by a physician in a minor surgical procedure, fertilized in vitro (in a glass test tube) with sperm, frozen for future use and then stored. This procedure is called in-vitro fertilization (IVF). Pregnancy rates average 10 to 25 percent with each frozen embryo.

Egg (Oocyte) Freezing

Hormones (like tamoxifen) are used to stimulate egg production. Mature eggs are retrieved by the physician, frozen for future use and then stored (not fertilized). This method is new and at present has an estimated three percent pregnancy success rate.

Ovarian Retrieval and Transplantation (Research in Progress)

Ovaries are surgically removed by a laparoscope (instrument that allows surgery to be performed through a small incision in the abdomen), divided into small strips, frozen and later transplanted back into the body when fertility is desired. Drugs are given to stimulate ovulation. Some researchers call the process ovarian grafting. This method is experimental but appears to have potential for women who will have chemotherapy that will damage their ovaries. The first successful birth after chemotherapy with ovarian retrieval and transplantation occurred recently. Check with your healthcare team on the continued progress of research.

Expense and Time Requirements

The procedures for fertility preservation are expensive and usually require several months for egg retrieval, which may delay treatments. At this time, most of the cost is not covered by insurance. During treatment decisions, this adds another difficult choice for some couples who still desire to have a family of their own, but this is an important consideration if future fertility is desired.

It is important to know that some cancers require immediate attention. One of these is inflammatory carcinoma, a cancer that is already systemic because of the involvement of the lymphatic system and requires that treatment start within days of diagnosis. Discuss with your physician if any type of delay would reduce your chances for survival.

Optional Parenthood Choices

Some couples find that their priority during the diagnostic period is optimal cancer treatment and that preserving fertility is not the most important issue for them.

Options for Couples Who Wish to Become Parents:

- Use donor eggs if fertility does not return
- Use a surrogate mother
- Adoption

Pregnancy After Breast Cancer Facts:

- Pregnancy does not reduce patient survival or trigger recurrence.

- Women who have had systemic chemotherapy have been able to conceive and deliver healthy, normal children with the chance of birth defects near that of the normal, untreated population.

- Developing eggs exposed to chemotherapy may suffer genetic damage. Some physicians suggest waiting six months after regular menstrual periods return before pregnancy is attempted. However, the time recommendation varies according to many other variables and will need to be given by your own healthcare team.

Questions to Ask Before Chemotherapy:

- What is the predicted impact of the drugs on fertility?

- What percentage of women who take these drugs experience permanent infertility?

- Are there drugs with less potential for infertility that can be used?

- What options do I have to preserve my fertility?

- Do you make referrals to physicians specializing in fertility preservation, if I desire?

- If I decide to pursue embryo freezing as an option, will the time required to collect the eggs impact my survival outcomes by delaying treatment for several months?

- If my fertility returns, how long do you suggest I wait before becoming pregnant?

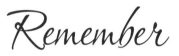

Future fertility is an issue that may not be discussed by your healthcare team unless you bring up the subject.

If future fertility is important to you, ask for information and referrals to a fertility specialist to discuss options best suited for you and your partner.

The Young Survival Coalition

www.youngsurvival.org

1-877-972-1011

CHAPTER 18

Care of the Surgical Arm

After surgery for breast cancer, it is important to begin your journey to recovery by restoring the normal function of your surgical arm through an exercise program and learning to protect and care for your arm in the future. In this text, we will refer to the "surgical arm" as the arm on the side of your surgery, and the "non-surgical arm" as the opposite arm.

Surgical Arm Changes

After your surgery, sensation in the area of your incision will be diminished, and your arm may feel numb or tingly. The area under the arm (if the lymph nodes are removed) contains nerves that, if injured or cut, can cause different types of sensations. The most common are numbness and a tingling sensation. The area under your arm and the back of your arm is where the numbness usually occurs. If the nerve is stretched or injured during surgery, these sensations may improve in a few months. If the nerve is cut, the numbness will be permanent; however, this will not affect the use of your arm.

The surgical arm will feel very tight when you attempt to stretch it up over your head. Removing your lymph nodes also requires the removal of an area of fat around the lymph nodes. This causes the area to feel pulled and tight after surgery, but the feeling is temporary and will improve as you begin your exercise program and gradually stretch this area.

After surgery, your surgical arm needs to be exercised to restore your normal range of motion. However, do not begin any exercises until your surgeon gives you permission. Most physicians prefer that all drains and sutures or staples be removed before you attempt an exercise routine. Ask your physician when to begin range of motion exercises. Additional instructions as to types of exercises may be provided by your physician.

"I give a great deal of credit to my Reach to Recovery visitor for my physical recovery. She provided me with a wealth of information. For the first time, I had something I could read and re-read. I was discovering fast the necessity of education in this new and strange world."

—Harriett Barrineau

"Doing my exercises gave me an immediate sense of control. I could feel my body getting stronger each day."

—Anna Cluxton

"Working in medical records, I had problems with this side of my body (surgical arm), lifting up charts. It was so painful just to reach up, but I had to do it."

—Earnestine Brown

137

Arm Exercise Program

When you begin the exercise program, you will find that you may tire easily and that there will be some discomfort as you attempt to perform the movements. However, you should continue to perform them to the point of slight discomfort but not until it becomes painful. It may take several weeks before you are able to complete some of the exercises. Work at your own pace. Your progress will be gradual. Some women find the routine is less uncomfortable when they take their pain medication, aspirin, Advil® or Tylenol® an hour before starting, or if they take a warm shower just prior to beginning the exercises.

Exercises should be performed on a regular basis—preferably two or more sessions a day, 10 to 15 minutes each session. Persistence is the key to regaining complete range of motion. Do the exercises slowly and hold the position when you get to the end of the range. This helps stretch and strengthen the muscles. Some exercises require a small rubber ball to squeeze and a broom handle or yardstick to hold in your hand. Many of the exercises may be performed either standing or sitting down.

If you are having difficulty performing the exercises and feel you are not making progress, tell your surgeon. Some women need the assistance of a physical therapist to regain complete range of motion, or they may need the motivation of an exercise group led by a professional.

After breast surgery, it is not uncommon for some women to favor the use of their non-surgical arm and become "one armed" as they resume their daily activities. Weakness in the surgical arm, which most women experience to some degree, will cause this to happen. However, it is helpful if you remember that normal use of the surgical arm will gradually increase strength and range of motion.

Remember: The "surgical arm" is the arm on the side of your surgery, and the "non-surgical arm" is the opposite arm.

SURGICAL ARM LIFTS

- Lift your surgical arm away from your side toward the ceiling with your palm turned forward.
- Raise your arm as high as possible and hold it there for a few seconds.
- Repeat six times.

SURGICAL ARM RAISES

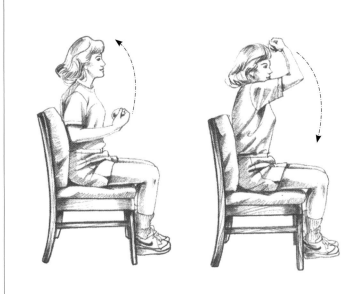

- Clench a rubber ball in your surgical hand with your elbow bent.
- Slowly lift your arm toward your head, keeping your elbow away from your body.
- When you reach your head, hold this position for a few seconds.
- Repeat six times.

SURGICAL ARM REACH

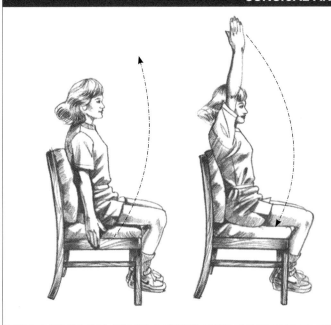

- Hold your surgical arm straight beside your body.
- Slowly raise your arm as high as possible over your head while keeping your elbow straight.
- Hold the position for a few seconds.
- Repeat six times.

SURGICAL ARM SWINGS

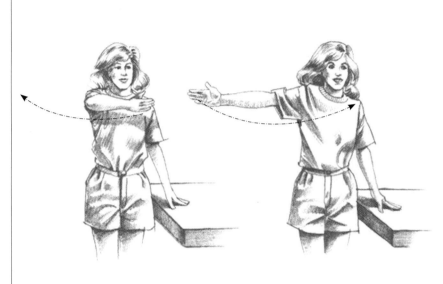

- Place your non-surgical arm on a table to support your body.

- Put your surgical arm across your chest, placing your hand on the opposite shoulder.

- Move the surgical arm slowly away from your body until it is extended straight out.

- Keep your arm at shoulder level as you perform the exercise.

- Repeat six times.

LATERAL RANGE OF MOTION

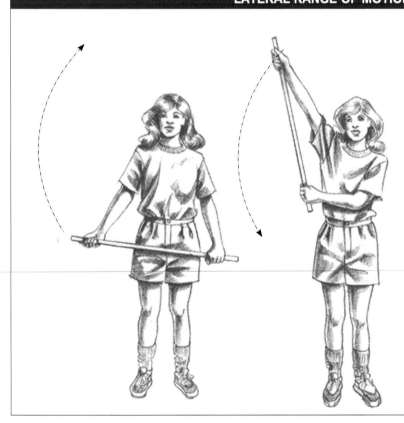

- Hold a stick with your surgical hand palm up and your non-surgical arm palm down.

- Push your surgical arm directly out from your side toward the ceiling until you feel a stretch.

- Hold this position for several seconds.

- Repeat six times.

SURGICAL ARM CIRCLES

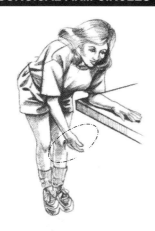

- Lean on a table with your non-surgical arm.
- Move your surgical arm in a circle clockwise and then counter-clockwise.
- Repeat six times.

SURGICAL ARM SWINGS

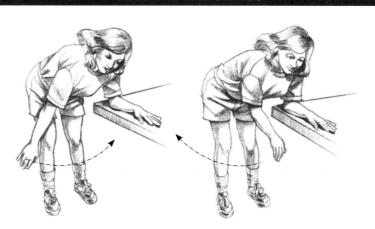

- Lean on a table with your non-surgical arm.
- Swing your surgical arm up until you feel a stretch.
- When you feel the stretch, hold the position for a few seconds.
- Repeat six times.

OVERHEAD RANGE OF MOTION

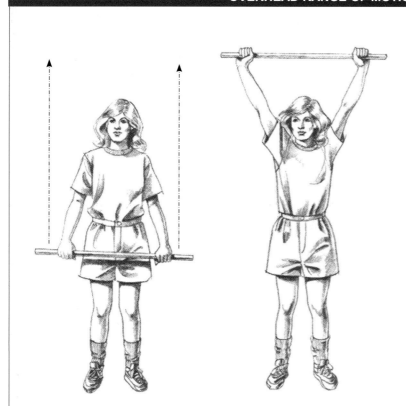

- Hold a stick with both hands palm down.
- Without bending your elbows, bring the stick directly over your head, leading with the non-surgical arm.
- Reach back over your head until you feel a stretch.
- Hold the position for a few seconds.
- Repeat six times.

Assessing Range of Motion

After having performed your exercises for several months following your surgery, ask these questions to determine whether you have regained adequate range of motion in your arm.

If You Could Perform the Following Prior to Surgery, Can You Now Easily:

- Brush and comb your hair?
- Pull a tee shirt or sweater over your head?
- Close a back-fastening bra?
- Completely zip up a dress that has a long back zipper?
- Wash the upper part of your back in the shoulder blade area of the opposite side of surgery?
- Reach over your head into a cabinet to remove an object?
- Make a double bed?

When you master the full range of motion exercise described below, congratulate yourself on the hard work required to stick with your dull, routine exercise program to accomplish this task. If you cannot perform your full range of motion approximately eight weeks after surgery, ask your surgeon to refer you to a physical therapist for help. It is advantageous to your recovery that you regain your range of motion early in your recovery.

Lymphedema

Removal of the lymph nodes under your surgical arm or radiation therapy to the underarm area may cause a swelling called lymphedema (lymph, from lymphatic fluid; edema, swelling from fluid accumulation). Having only sentinel nodes removed will greatly reduce this potential. However, radiation therapy may cause fibrosis (the excessive development of scar-like connective tissue) in some women, increasing the potential for lymphedema.

FULL RANGE OF MOTION EXERCISE

- With both of your arms straight by your side, raise both hands above your head and hold the position for several seconds.

- Repeat six times.

This exercise will be one of the last to master and will be proof that your surgical arm has regained full range of motion.

Lymphatic fluid is high in proteins. These proteins leak from vessels into surrounding tissues when vessels are obstructed. The protein then draws water into the tissues. This condition results in swelling from the slower flow and removal of lymph fluid and accumulation of protein and water in the tissues of your arm. Only a small percentage of women experience lymphedema after surgery, but all women need to know of the potential risks and available treatments if it should occur. It can occur anytime from shortly after surgery to years later. It is suggested that you measure or have someone measure your arm three inches above and below the elbow prior to surgery so you can monitor with more accuracy whether you develop any swelling.

Arm lymphedema can produce pain, restricted movement of the shoulder and arm and increased susceptibility to an infection called cellulitis. Medications and treatments are often limited in their effectiveness; therefore, the best strategy is to prevent the problem before it occurs. Lymphedema management starts with understanding the causes, knowing how to prevent it, recognizing symptoms if they occur, understanding the need for early reporting of swelling and being familiar with the signs of cellulitis. In the management of lymphedema, you gain nothing and risk a lot by waiting to address the problem.

Causes of Lymphedema:

- Surgical removal of lymph nodes
- Poor range of motion in your surgical arm
- Infection
- Obesity
- Radiation therapy to the breast and underarm area
- Constriction caused by clothing or jewelry
- Long periods of positioning the arm below the level of the heart
- Repetitious tasks using the surgical arm

The first line of defense against lymphedema is regaining the full range of motion of your arm by using the exercises suggested in this book or by your physician. While these exercises may seem dull and unnecessary, they serve to facilitate the flow of the lymphatic fluid from the arm area. Do not begin an exercise program until your physician gives you permission.

Lymphedema Prevention:

- For several weeks after surgery, when lying down, prop your arm up on a pillow above the level of your heart to help drain the fluid. Elevation of the arm helps reduce swelling and prevents additional accumulation of fluid.
- Avoid using your arm and hand in a dependent position (below the level of the heart) for long periods of time. If you need to perform a task of this sort, periodically hold your arms above your head to promote drainage.
- Make a fist or squeeze a small rubber ball in your hand repetitively for two to three minutes several times a day to assist the accumulated fluid in returning to general circulation.

Injury and Infection Prevention:

- Do not allow the surgical arm to be used for blood pressure checks, blood samples or injections. Ask your nurse for a pink wristband or ribbon to be placed on the wrist of your surgical arm as a reminder to all your healthcare givers.
- Do not wear anything tight on the surgical arm or hand, such as rings, watches, bracelets or tight elastic in sleeves.
- Do not hold a cigarette in this hand.
- Do not cut your cuticles; keep hands soft by using hand lotion regularly. Avoid nail salons that use rotary files that could injure your cuticles.
- Do not carry heavy packages or purses on the side of your surgery.
- Wear protective gloves when working in the garden, washing dishes or using any irritating chemicals, such as hair dye or cleaning products.

- Avoid burns and cuts when cooking.

- Wash all cuts or injuries with antibacterial soap, apply an antibiotic medication and cover the area with sterile gauze or a Band-Aid® until the wound heals.

- Avoid sunburn. Wear long sleeves or sunscreen at all times when in direct sunlight for a period of time.

- Use a thimble when sewing.

- Avoid insect bites by wearing insect repellent.

- Be careful with animals. Avoid scratches.

- Use an electric razor under your arm.

When to Notify Your Physician

If you have persistent swelling several weeks after your surgery, the first treatment is simply to elevate the arm. Raising the arm above the level of the heart by propping it on a pillow for 45 minutes several times a day will usually reduce most lymphedema. Sleeping with the arm elevated on a pillow is helpful. If the swelling persists after several days of elevation, notify your physician.

When accumulated lymph fluid becomes infected with bacteria and inflames the surrounding tissue, it is a condition called cellulitis.

Signs and Symptoms of Cellulitis Include Any of the Following:

- Localized pain, redness, swelling and tenderness in arm or breast

- Skin that resembles an orange peel (peau d'orange)

- Pitting of skin with pressure

- Red streaks may appear on skin

- Fever, chills, fatigue

Antibiotics are necessary to treat the infection. Early intervention is essential to prevent the spread of infection to other parts of your body. If you have any symptoms of cellulitis, your healthcare provider needs to be notified as soon as possible. Cellulitis is a problem that needs immediate attention. If it occurs outside of office hours, call or page your healthcare provider.

Lymphedema Treatments

Elastic Sleeve for Lymphedema

A special elastic sleeve, designed to reduce swelling, may be ordered by the physician. The sleeve looks a lot like support hose and can be worn under long-sleeved clothing. A professional fitter will measure the arm and order a customized sleeve to fit your measurements.

Elastic Sleeve Tips:

- Get your physician to write a prescription for insurance reimbursement.

- Purchase two sleeves so that you can wash one while wearing the other one.

- Wash in lukewarm water and allow sleeve to air dry thoroughly. Do not wring out while wet. Do not put it in the dryer.

- Do not wear a sleeve that does not fit well. This causes skin irritation and can increase your swelling after wearing.

- If you have a problem with the top of the sleeve rolling down on the arm, ask for a water-soluble adhesive lotion to apply under the top of the sleeve. This adhesive washes off easily with soap and water when the sleeve is removed.

- Have the fitter re-measure your arm periodically to see if the sleeve is still the appropriate size. To be effective in reducing swelling, sleeves must fit properly.

- Replace your sleeve about every six months because it will stretch and lose elasticity from repeated use. Contact your insurance provider and ask how often they will pay for a sleeve replacement.

- It is suggested that you purchase and wear an elastic sleeve for long airline flights. Pressure changes can cause an increase in lymphedema.

Lymphedema Massage
A gentle, specialized massage technique, Manual Lymph Drainage (MLD), also known as complex decongestive physiotherapy, is performed by some trained physical therapists and massage therapists to remove swelling from the arm. This method stimulates the skin and underlying lymphatic vessels by a special technique that is different from traditional massage therapy. Traditional massage may increase, rather than decrease, swelling because it is so vigorous. MLD therapists are trained to delicately move their hands over the surface of the skin slowly in circular or pumping motions to move fluid toward the shoulder. These sessions last approximately an hour. At the conclusion of the massage, the arm is wrapped in a special bandage to prevent re-accumulation of fluid in the arm. Instructions are given on how to massage the arm with the bandage in place. This method of massage and bandaging is performed several times a week for several weeks or until swelling has been reduced to a manageable level. Patients and family members are often instructed in the massage and bandaging techniques so that treatment may be continued at home.

When seeking treatment for lymphedema, always ask if the therapist is trained in or has certification in manual lymph drainage for breast cancer. If your physician does not have a recommended therapist, you can find a list of specialists on the National Lymphedema Network online (www.lymphnet.org).

Compression Pumps for Lymphedema
Your physician may order a sleeve hooked to a compression pump. This is a special sleeve connected to an air pump that compresses your arm. A compression pump requires several hours of time a day to manually remove the accumulated fluid. There are two types of compression pumps. One is a gradient pressure pump that has the air pressure greatest at the area of the hand with less pressure at the top of the sleeve. Another type is a sequential pressure pump that exerts pressure that starts at the hand and gradually moves up the arm to the shoulder in a milking-like fashion. Pumps are expensive, and their progress is often not monitored by a trained therapist but rather by a salesperson for the company. It is recommended that you use a pump only with a physician's order and that a trained professional monitor your progress throughout use of the pump. Overuse or too much pressure may increase swelling.

Diuretics for Lymphedema
Medications called diuretics that remove excess water from your entire body are **not** generally recommended for treating lymphedema. Swelling is caused by leakage of protein from the vessels in the arm. Diuretics cannot remove the protein that has seeped out into the arm. They may remove some of the water temporarily, but once you stop taking the diuretics, swelling returns because the excess protein in the arm pulls the fluid back.

Remember, lymphedema usually has nothing to do with cancer. This condition occurs because lymph nodes and vessels in the breast have been removed during surgery, scar tissue has formed after surgery, or radiation therapy has caused changes in the area. These conditions slow down the removal of the lymphatic fluid that accumulates in the breast and arm area, resulting in swelling of the arm and hand.

Lymphedema and Weight Lifting
A new study from the University of Pennsylvania School of Medicine was conducted with breast cancer patients who had pre-existing lymphedema. The study concluded that patients who participated in progressive weight-lifting exercises for 13 weeks had a reduction in symptoms, compared to women who did not lift weights during that time. Previously, it has been recommended that women with lymphedema avoid weight-lifting. However, this new study showed that participating in a safe, structured weight-lifting routine, supervised by a certified

fitness professional can help women with lymphedema take control of their symptoms and reap the benefits of resistance training, including increased bone density and weight control.

It is recommended that a well-fitting, elastic compression sleeve be worn during workouts and that a trained professional supervise correct techniques for weight-lifting. Consult your healthcare team for their advice.

Surgical Scar Massage

During the first four weeks after surgery, your surgical incision will heal and will eventually turn into a scar. Scars form fibrous (thickened) tissues that are firm and do not stretch or move easily. The goal of surgical scar massage is to soften and restore pliability (movement) to the scar area. This is especially important if you are having reconstructive surgery.

Instructions for Scar Massage:

- Start four weeks after surgery.
- Lubricate your scar with vitamin E, sesame, almond or any other natural oil.
- Use your index (pointer) and middle fingers to gently rub across the scar making small, round circles.
- Do not rub along the length of the scar.
- Massage the area for several minutes each day.
- Continue until the scar is soft and moves easily.

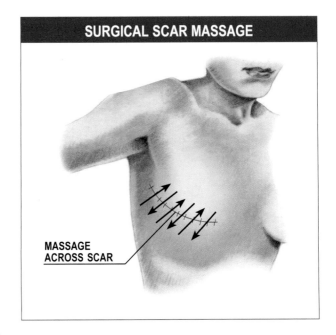

SURGICAL SCAR MASSAGE

MASSAGE ACROSS SCAR

Remember

Exercise is essential to restore normal use of your surgical arm.

Exercise to the point of some discomfort but not pain.

Protect your surgical arm from injury.

Treat lymphedema by elevating your surgical arm. If this is not successful, call your physician.

The best treatment for lymphedema is prevention of swelling.

Immediately report any sign of infection in your surgical arm.

CHAPTER 19

Health Insurance
and Employment Issues

"Nothing prepared me for the magnitude of the responsibility I would have in seeing to it that I received the insurance benefits to which I was entitled. I was overwhelmed by the number of bills I received following surgery. Good record keeping was essential."

—Harriett Barrineau

When you are diagnosed with breast cancer, inform your insurance provider and ask for guidelines for filing or payment of claims. The following questions may need to be clarified. Some of the answers may be found in your insurance policy manuals.

- Do I need a second opinion for procedures?
- Do I need pre-approval for diagnostic tests, scans or hospital admissions?
- How do I file claims?
- What is the name of a person at the company who can answer questions about my case?
- What is the amount of the deductible, if any, required before claims are paid?
- Are there any limits imposed on the amount paid for surgery, chemotherapy, radiation therapy or reconstruction?
- What is the policy regarding coverage for new treatments or treatments considered "experimental" (new medications or treatments)? Are there limits on what amounts will be paid?
- What is the policy regarding coverage for a permanent prosthesis? If delayed reconstruction is considered, will insurance pay for both, or does one exclude payment for the other?
- What is the policy for reconstruction? Does this cover surgical repair of the other breast?

"So much to do—so little time. I made the effort to write down the name, time and date every time I spoke with someone regarding my benefits. Don't take no for an answer. Keep everything!"

—Anna Cluxton

"My co-pay was fifty dollars for every specialist visit, and sometimes I'd see three or four specialists a week. I hit my insurance maximums and ended up owing $14,000 out of pocket. I pay what I can."

—Earnestine Brown

Reimbursement Record Keeping

After breast cancer, it is very important that you take steps to receive payment for services covered under your insurance. Many women find this task overwhelming. Often, a partner or a friend will volunteer to perform this job for you. Ask for assistance in this area. Keeping accurate records will make the task much easier.

Record Keeping Tips:

- Keep calendar records of all appointments (a pocket calendar is helpful).

- Write on the calendar the physician you visited, procedures performed and medications purchased.

- Provide physicians with appropriate information for filing claims.

- Ask for copies of all charges at the time of service or ask to have copies mailed to you.

- Keep copies of **all** charges from appointments or services **in one place** (a box, a notebook or file folder).

- Periodically check to see if appropriate payment is made to medical providers.

- If problems arise, ask your healthcare facility or provider to help you understand or assist you in providing information for adequate repayment.

- Call your insurance providers and talk with a claims representative. Offer additional records or assistance for getting information from your medical providers. Always write down the date of contact and the person's name.

- Keep all premiums current; **do not allow your insurance to lapse.**

Insurance After Diagnosis

After any major illness, insurance is more difficult to obtain. For this reason, keep all premium payments current. If you decide to change jobs, be sure that you will be covered under the new employer's insurance program before making a decision. If you have private insurance or coverage through your employment, be very alert to these areas before making major decisions.

COBRA Health Insurance

In 1986 Congress passed the Consolidated Omnibus Budget Reconciliation Act (COBRA) health benefit provision. This law allows certain former employees, retirees, spouses, former spouses and dependent children the right to temporary continuation of health coverage at group rates. This coverage, however, is only available when coverage is lost due to certain specific events. Group health coverage for COBRA participants is usually more expensive than health coverage for active employees, since the employer usually pays a part of the premium for active employees while COBRA participants generally pay the entire premium themselves. It is ordinarily less expensive, though, than individual health coverage. If you or your spouse is leaving a company with group insurance coverage, talk to the company's benefits officer to see if you qualify for continuing your insurance by converting to a COBRA policy.

Financial Assistance

If your illness is going to be a financial burden to you, ask to speak to the social worker in the cancer treatment center. Social workers are trained to help you with the social issues of your illness, including helping you secure financial help for needed medical services. There are various services available, but you will need to apply for them. The earlier you can make this need known, the more effective the social work team can be in helping you file the forms. People often feel embarrassed to ask for help and postpone the issue. Many people find that an unexpected illness drains their financial reserves. You are not alone. Ask for help early.

Financial Tips:

- If your insurance requires a copayment (usually $10.00-$50.00) with each office visit, pay it at the time of each visit if possible. These charges accumulate quickly and can seem overwhelming if not kept current.

- If you have an insurance deductible or annual "co-insurance" requirements, speak with the business office at the cancer treatment center about a monthly payment plan. Make sure the payment is reasonable and something that you can afford to pay each month. Begin making these payments before you receive your first bill. The treatment center will reimburse you if you overpay.

- If you are on a payment plan with the hospital or cancer treatment center and you cannot make your payment one month due to unexpected bills—or if you have a change in your monthly budget—contact the business office to discuss the problem.

- Check with your hospital about patient assistance for your surgery or other treatments. Most hospitals are obligated by law to provide some patient assistance. Their funds tend to run low by the end of the year, so check as soon as you think you need help.

Employment Issues During Treatment

Breast cancer surgery and treatment will require some time away from your job. Most employers are very understanding and offer their support during this time. You will need to give notice of your absence and expected time away from your job.

Occasionally, however, a breast cancer patient will be discriminated against because of illness. If you have reasons to believe that your employer has treated you unfairly because of your illness, there are laws to protect you. There are federal laws and varying state laws that offer protection against discrimination or unfair practices. Listed in the reference section of this book are names and telephone numbers you can call to receive information on how to best manage your situation.

Family and Medical Leave Act

In 1993, the Family and Medical Leave Act (FMLA) granted certain employees up to 12 weeks of unpaid, job-protected leave per year. It also requires that the employee's group health benefits be maintained during the leave. As a cancer patient, your illness meets the requirements if you are employed by a public agency, a public or private elementary/secondary school or a company with 50 or more employees.

You Are Eligible for Leave if You:

- Have worked for your employer at least 12 months.

- Have worked at least 1,250 hours over the past 12 months.

- Work at a location where the company employs 50 or more employees within 75 miles (some states have additional laws; check with your own state).

Documentation of Illness

You will be required to provide a note or form signed and dated by a doctor.

Necessary Information:

- You have a cancer diagnosis

- When the illness started

- Whether absences are expected to be continuous or in short blocks of time

- When you may be expected to return to work

- Whether further treatment will be required after the absence

To learn more about FMLA provisions and rules, read the FMLA Fact Sheet posted on the United States government's Department of Labor Web site at: www.dol.gov (enter FMLA in the search box), or call the Wage and Hour Division's referral and information line at the Department of Labor at 1-866-4 US WAGE (1-866-487-9243). They can give you other helpful information and tell you how to reach the Department of Labor division office nearest you.

What Do You Tell Your Co-Workers?

It is necessary for you to decide how much to tell your employer, fellow employees and friends about the details of your illness. Some women are very open about their illness and treatments. Others feel that this is a private matter and would rather not share the details with everyone. Decide what you wish for others to know. It is helpful if you inform your support partner or family members so that your wishes can be carried out when people call or drop by.

You do not have to constantly share your "illness story" with others if this makes you uncomfortable. The simple reply, "I appreciate your concern, but right now I am not up to talking about it. Thank you for understanding," allows you the right not to share. You need to communicate, but you do not need to feel that you have to talk with everyone who asks about your illness. It may be helpful to allow family members to answer the phone and screen your calls if you would rather not talk. Plan to do what best suits your particular personality.

When Co-Workers Don't Call or Come

Often women find that their co-workers or friends don't call or come to see them after their diagnosis. This can be emotionally painful because these are people that you saw and worked with every day. Why does this happen?

- They don't know what to say.
- They don't know what to do.
- It hurts them to see you in emotional pain when they can't do anything about it.
- It hurts them to see you in physical pain.
- Your diagnosis serves as a reminder that they, too, could be diagnosed with cancer. It becomes easier for them to avoid you than to face their own vulnerabilities.

Breaking the Silence:

- Call your friends and co-workers. Let them know that you are handling your diagnosis as well as you can and that you miss them.
- When they ask if they can help, be specific: pick up the children, take me to lunch, pick up a prescription, drive me to the doctor, etc. They want to know that they will not add to your burdens but can truly help you during this time.
- Invite them over for a cup of coffee or tea.
- Ask them to go for a walk.
- Be sure that you have not sent out unspoken messages that you want your illness to be a private affair.

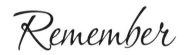

Remember

Simple record keeping will help take the hassle out of insurance filing.

Recruit someone to help with record keeping.

Keep your insurance premiums current.

Do not change jobs unless you know you will be covered by the new insurance.

If you experience discrimination on the job, seek assistance from professionals.

Decide how your friends can best help you during this time.

Don't be afraid to reach out to your friends.

CHAPTER 20

Monitoring Your Health After Breast Cancer

After your surgery, you will see your oncologist every three to six months for the first three years. If no problems arise, you will then progress to office visits every six months for several years and then to once a year thereafter. It is very important that you keep these visits with your doctor, even when you are feeling great. Other physicians involved in your care may require return visits for their area of specialty. Some women are referred back to their primary care provider.

Your physician will monitor your general health and order routine exams and screening tests when deemed necessary to detect any recurrence or new problem. A complete update of your physical history since your previous exam and a physical exam of the surgical area will take place on each visit. Bone scans, chest X-rays and other staging exams are ordered when needed to provide additional information. Ask about your physician's schedule for follow-up tests. Continue to have pap smears, mammograms and bone density scans on a regular basis.

Follow-up Care Questions:

- How often will I need to return for a checkup?
- Do I call and make the appointment, or will your office call me?
- What symptoms should I be aware of that might indicate a possible recurrence?
- What can I expect as normal, long-lasting side effects of my treatment?
- What should my arm and breast area look and feel like (painful, numb, tingling)?
- What changes might occur that I should consider dangerous and worthy of alerting you?
- Are there any special things that I should do or that I should avoid (particular activities, medications, food)?

Healthcare Team Communication

Some women report that one of their most difficult tasks during treatment is communicating with their healthcare team or physician. This is a challenge, because for most, cancer is a new experience. There are so many questions, so many unfamiliar terms and so many different physicians that it is an overwhelming task to sort it all out.

Communication Methods

Ask your doctor about the preferred method of patient communication concerning emergency and non-emergency needs. Ask if you can communicate your non-emergency questions by email. Some physicians have email services that allow them to communicate with their patients through secure transfer of information online.

Keep These Things in Mind:

- Know that you deserve to have your questions answered by your healthcare team. This is not unreasonable; getting answers to your questions is an important part of your recovery.

- Do not be embarrassed to ask any question. There are no silly or stupid questions, and there are many other people who have asked those same questions. Ask if you do not know.

- Realize that physicians and other members of the healthcare team are on a working schedule that allows a certain amount of time for each patient. If they appear rushed, it is not that they do not care or want to take the time; in today's healthcare economy they have to see a certain number of patients to maintain the financial viability of a medical practice.

- Understand that calling and asking to speak to a physician at the time of the call is difficult because of other scheduled patients. For questions and non-emergency situations, call and give the question to an assistant or nurse and ask to have someone call you with the answer. This may be a trained educator or physician's assistant. If you have a series of questions, call and schedule an appointment just for questions.

- Prepare to communicate effectively with your healthcare providers by reading about your disease and learning some of the new terms involved, or have a family member do this and go with you to the appointments.

- Make the most of your allotted appointment time. Forget the small talk and be sure that you are using your time to get the information you need.

- Specific questions for each type of physician you will be visiting are located in the tear-out worksheets at the back of this book. Reviewing these before the visit will prepare you to ask questions that are in the area of the physician's expertise. One physician is not able to specifically answer all questions regarding your treatment.

- When going to an appointment with your healthcare provider, it is essential to prepare a list of what you need to discuss in order for your physical and mental recovery to progress as smoothly as possible. Often, patients think they will remember what to report or ask during the appointment, but they leave with important questions unanswered. As you are well aware, appointment times are short and many things have to be checked by your provider. It is normal for healthcare providers to concentrate on your physical disease and treatment; however, your questions about quality of life and side effects deserve to be brought to their attention as well. Part of being an active participant in your healthcare is being prepared to relay your physical and psychological concerns during this time in the most effective manner possible.

- If you do not understand a term or instructions, say so. Simply say, "I'm sorry, but I am having trouble understanding what you just said. Would you please explain it again?"

- Ask if they have written information on the subjects discussed.

Appointment Preparation

Keep a written list of questions that arise between visits to ask during the appointment. If the list is long, it may be helpful to inform the nurse or give her the list of questions prior to seeing the physician. Ask if you need to make a return visit to have your questions answered.

Symptoms to Report Early in the Visit:

- Bleeding from anywhere in the body: when, amount, how long it bled and how it was stopped
- Fever: date experienced and temperature elevation and how long it lasted
- Dizziness or fainting: dates and any other event that happened during the same time
- Persistent headaches
- Persistent cough
- Painful or frequent urination
- Chest or arm pain: description, intensity and date of pain
- Vision changes: type and date of change
- Constipation: frequency
- Abdominal pain
- Diarrhea: frequency, including number of loose stools in a 24-hour period and number of days
- Vomiting: when, frequency and number of episodes during a 24-hour period
- Swelling or new lump in any part of the body
- New pain in any part of the body
- Changes in surgical scar, nipple discharge or rash on breast or chest wall
- Shortness of breath or difficulty breathing

Quality of Life Issues

Other areas that you should bring to a healthcare provider's attention are in the area of quality of life. Simply, these are issues that impact your ability to enjoy day-to-day activities; they are not life-threatening, but they are important just the same and need to be presented in quantified terms.

- **Physical energy:** Report level in understandable terms, like "unable to stay up over three hours without rest" or "unable to work."
- **Depression or feeling "blue" most of the time:** "I feel too depressed to participate in everyday activities with my family." "I find myself crying frequently."
- **Anxiety or nervousness:** "I feel anxious and shaky most of the day and it interferes with my ability to concentrate and interact with my family. Can you help me with this?"
- **Pain:** Report on a scale from 0 (no pain) to 10 (severe pain): "I am having pain in my (area) that averages a (number you give your pain) most of the day, and this interferes with my ability to rest and participate in daily activities. Can you help me find a way to reduce my pain to a manageable level?"
- **Nausea:** Report any nausea or vomiting between checkups by telling your healthcare team when and how long you were nauseated or how often you vomited.
- **Appetite:** Report a reduced appetite or inability to eat.
- **Sleep:** Report inability to go to sleep or stay asleep and how long you are able to sleep uninterrupted: "I have problems going to sleep and sleep only (amount in hours) before I wake up. I then find it difficult to return to sleep. I wake up the next morning exhausted and feel sleepy during the day; can you help me with this problem?"
- **Hot flashes or night sweats:** Report the approximate number you are having daily and if they awaken you at night. "I am having at least (number) hot flashes a day, and they awaken me at least (number of times) at night. Can you help me with this problem?"

- **Dry vagina or painful intercourse:** "I am having a problem with vaginal dryness that is causing painful intercourse. Can you help me with this problem?"
- **Information needs:** Keep a written list of information or referrals needed.

At the conclusion of the appointment ask when you will need to return, if there are any normal changes you should expect before your next visit and for any changes in recommendations for your care or medications.

As a patient, you can maximize your checkup time with your healthcare providers by being prepared with your own information and by reporting anything new that has occurred since the last visit. Remember, this needs to be done early in the appointment to allow the physician time to consider if any action is needed. This makes you an active partner in your healthcare. This is the patient that every physician dreams of having—one who comes prepared to report physical status and needs, is educated on the basics of her cancer and understands the time constraints in a medical practice.

Remember

Recovery is a partnership between you and your healthcare team.

Take an active role in preparing for your appointment.

Maximize your appointment time by reporting any changes in your health and asking any questions you may have.

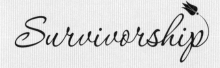

Survivorship

Courage is an act of your will. No one can give it to you. No one can sell it to you. No one can give it in a treatment or a pill. You have to decide that this is the mental approach you will take. It is a decision of the mind, often not felt in the heart, at the time of the decision. However, the heart follows quickly and verifies that the peace gained from having courage is far greater than cowering in fear.

Courage is the best of all medicines for the mind and the body. Take it in big doses during recovery. Then share it with other women who cross your path.

—Judy Kneece

CHAPTER 21

Diet and Exercise

"As soon as possible, I got out of the house to get into the fresh air and sunshine. I asked how soon I could start doing arm exercises, and then I did them every day. I was training to get back into life."

—*Anna Cluxton*

A breast cancer diagnosis can provide the perfect opportunity to slow down and reevaluate your life. It can also allow you to take care of yourself without feeling guilty. It is more important than ever that you fuel your body with good food and keep moving physically.

As you recover, it is helpful to keep in mind that chemotherapy and radiation treatments kill cancerous cells and, in the process, destroy normal, healthy cells that have to be replaced. New cells are rebuilt from what you eat and drink. Therefore, it is important you have the nutrients necessary to rebuild healthy cells for recovery to occur. What you eat and drink is important.

Maintaining as much energy as possible is also vital. New research shows that physical movement during treatment and recovery can contribute to a sense of well-being and can increase energy.

This chapter on diet and exercise is not about restrictive diets and workouts at a gym but about suggestions that are flexible and easily incorporated into your normal lifestyle. I encourage you to consider your diet and exercise as a vital part of your recovery. You alone can make these decisions. This is a gift only you can give yourself.

Diet

Your goal during treatment should be to eat a nutritious, balanced diet, which maintains your body weight while not making you feel hungry or deprived. This is not the time for fad diets, which often cut out food groups. You should not attempt any diet that causes extreme hunger or is highly restrictive. Restrictive diets do not promote recovery; they only increase stress, which is definitely not good for you. The focus in this chapter is to provide tips that will help you eat nutritionally and make better choices without the stress of a restrictive diet. Remember that every time you make a food selection, you have the opportunity to give your body the fuel needed to rebuild healthy cells.

Weight Gain During Treatment

Some women undergoing chemotherapy for breast cancer experience weight gain and some do not. Like other side effects, weight gain is usually time-limited.

Weight Gain May Be Caused By:

- Hormonal changes caused by chemotherapy or hormonal medications

- Fluid retention from chemotherapy medications

- Keeping food in the stomach to relieve nausea
- Increased eating caused by stress
- Decreased activity during treatments

If you find that you gain weight during treatment, do not panic and go on a restrictive diet which could impact your recovery. Don't allow the numbers on a scale to determine how you feel. Avoid daily weighing during this time because medications can cause wide fluctuations in weight. Think of this time of treatment as temporary—your body will undergo changes you don't like, but they are time-limited.

Dietary Tips During Breast Cancer

While going through treatment, it is helpful to evaluate your dietary habits to ensure that you are eating nutritious foods from all food groups and that you are not adding empty calories that could add to weight gain. The following tips offer simple changes that can easily be adapted to your lifestyle. The goal is to incorporate as many of the dietary tips as possible to maintain your energy and prevent unwanted weight gain.

Hunger Control

It takes fewer calories to prevent hunger than it does to deal with it once it occurs.

Tips:

- Eat three balanced meals a day and plan to include nutritious snacks between meals to keep hunger at bay.
- Reduce portions at meals and eat throughout the day to help curb hunger. Try eating five to six times a day. Going without food for several hours can lead to hypoglycemia (low blood sugar) which causes fatigue, increases potential for nausea and slows your metabolism.

Stay Hydrated

Drink lots of water! Water (fluid intake) is crucial to your health. Water makes up about 60 percent of your body weight, and every system in your

body depends on water to function properly. Lack of water can lead to dehydration, a condition that occurs when you don't have enough water in your body for your cells to carry on normal functions. Even mild dehydration can sap your energy and make you tired. That is why it is important to report to your physician any nausea, vomiting or diarrhea that you cannot control within 12 – 24 hours. It is essential that you are able to drink and retain adequate amounts of fluid to maintain your energy.

Early Signs and Symptoms of Dehydration:

- Thirst
- Fatigue
- Headache
- Dry mouth
- Muscle weakness
- Little or no urination
- Dizziness or lightheadedness

How Much Water Do You Need?

There are different recommendations for water intake. The National Institute of Health recommends that women drink about 2.2 liters (9 cups) a day to maintain water balance. The average recommendation is eight 8-ounce glasses per day. This amount increases when activities cause excessive sweating.

When You Don't Like Water

Some people find drinking plain water difficult. The goal is to drink fluids that are not calorie dense and loaded with sugar. Sugary drinks do not rebuild cells but can add weight.

Tips for Making Water More Tasteful:

- Squeeze lemon into water.
- Add whole strawberries or slices of cucumber, orange or lime to a pitcher of water and allow flavor to permeate.
- Add products like Emergen-C® (found in discount or health food stores) which come in

individual packages in many flavors and can easily be added to a bottle or glass of water to provide a healthy, energizing drink containing extra vitamin C, B vitamins and electrolytes.

Eliminate Empty Liquid Calories:

- Strive to avoid all sugary drinks when possible—soft drinks, sweetened tea, sweetened coffee drinks or sports drinks. These drinks are all full of calories and cause a quick rise in blood sugar. We may get a rush of energy, but the down side is that our blood sugar drops quickly afterwards, leaving us fatigued.

- Avoid diet drinks as well; they have been associated with weight gain in some people and add no nutritional value to your diet.

- Monitor the amount of fruit juice you drink because it is also high in calories. Choosing to eat the whole fruit with fiber is a better choice when possible. Eat an orange at breakfast rather than drinking a glass of orange juice.

- Select 100 percent vegetable or tomato juice, one percent or skim milk, soy milk, tea or coffee for lower-calorie choices.

Understanding Carbohydrates in Your Diet

Carbohydrates (carbs) are foods that when eaten and digested break down into glucose (sugar), which gives you energy. In the past few years, some of the fads in dieting have promoted low-carb diets for weight control. The goal during cancer treatment is to avoid fad diets and eat foods from all food groups, including carbohydrates. However, some carbohydrates are healthier choices than others for maintaining energy and weight control. They are identified through the glycemic index (GI).

The glycemic index is a measure of how quickly a carbohydrate will raise your blood sugar (glucose) level. The glycemic index ranks carbohydrate foods by how much and how quickly they raise the levels, which is called the "glycemic response." Foods that raise glucose levels quickly have a higher glycemic

index rating than foods that cause a slower rise. The lower the rating, the better the carbohydrate is to help control your appetite and your risk of diabetes. Lower-rated carbs are healthier choices, because they are usually lower in calories and higher in fiber, nutrients and antioxidants. Choosing low glycemic index foods may help you control your appetite because they tend to keep you feeling full longer, along with other health benefits.

LOW GLYCEMIC INDEX FOOD BENEFITS

- Control your blood glucose levels by maintaining a more constant level of energy
- Control your appetite by maintaining your blood sugar level
- Lower your risk of getting heart disease by helping control your cholesterol levels
- Lower your risk of getting type 2 (adult-onset) diabetes by keeping blood sugar levels lower

Glycemic Index Rating

Carbohydrates on the glycemic index are rated as low (55 or less), medium (56 – 69) or high (70 and up). Your goal is to select lower glycemic foods.

Low Glycemic Foods (55 or Less):

- Skim milk
- Plain yogurt
- Soy beverage
- Apples/plums/oranges
- Sweet potato
- Oat bran bread
- Oatmeal (slow-cook oats)
- Bran cereal
- Converted or parboiled rice
- Pumpernickel bread
- Pasta
- Lentils (beans)
- Honey

Medium Glycemic Foods (56 – 69):
- Bananas, pineapples, raisins
- Popcorn
- Brown rice
- Shredded wheat cereal
- Whole wheat bread
- Rye bread

High Glycemic Foods (over 70):
- Dried dates, watermelon
- Instant mashed potatoes
- Baked white potato
- Instant rice
- Corn Flakes®; Rice Krispies®; Cheerios®
- Bagel, white
- Soda crackers
- Jelly beans; candies
- French fries
- Ice cream
- Cookies
- Table sugar

Maximize Good Carbohydrates
Good carbs are lower on the glycemic index and include beans and grains. The fiber content will fill you up while promoting healthy blood sugar levels.

Beans
- Beans are also filled with nutrients and phytochemicals (plant chemicals) that have been shown to be active in prevention of diseases.
- Beans are inexpensive, easy to prepare and last for several days when refrigerated. They can be eaten alone, over brown rice or added to soups, salads or stews. Aim for one half cup serving or more of beans each day.
- Good choices are soybeans, lentils, kidney beans, chickpeas (garbanzo), butter beans, navy beans, black beans, white beans or split peas.

Grains
- Do not deprive yourself of breads and cereals; just make sure that you choose 100 percent whole gains—whole wheat, whole oats, brown rice, rye, barley, etc.
- When buying grain products look for the word "whole" in front of "grain."

Vegetables and Fruits
- Vegetables are low in calories and high in fiber. Vegetables are natural appetite suppressants because they are very filling and are packed with vitamins, minerals and phytochemicals.
- Best choices include cabbage, kale, broccoli, cauliflower, brussel sprouts, collards, carrots, garlic, onions, leeks, tomatoes, asparagus, spinach, dark varieties of lettuce, red or orange bell peppers.
- Try to limit or avoid the high glycemic index or starchy vegetables such as corn, white potatoes, parsnips and rutabagas, which raise your blood sugar quickly.
- Fruits are highly nutritious. Strive to include two servings a day.
- The best fruits if you are watching your weight are berries (any variety), cherries, plums, any whole citrus, cantaloupe, grapes, peaches, apples, pears, dried or fresh apricots.
- Limit amount of the higher glycemic fruits such as bananas, mangoes, papaya, pineapple, raisins and dates.

Healthy Proteins
- Proteins provide a steady, prolonged blood glucose level with minimal insulin response and will keep you feeling satisfied longer between meals.
- Healthy proteins are fish (oily varieties such as salmon, tuna, mackerel, sardines, herring and trout), shellfish, skinless poultry, nuts, seeds, soy, wild game, lean dairy products (cottage cheese and yogurt), beans/legumes and eggs.

- Limit other protein sources such as red meat or pork to two servings a week.

- Eating protein at breakfast is especially important for energy and weight control.

Fats

Newer dietary studies have shown the important role of dietary fat. During and after chemotherapy, the body requires fat to repair cells. It is important to eat good sources of dietary fat.

- Dietary fat makes food taste better, satisfies your appetite and reduces hunger.

- Many of the good fats are found in the sources of protein listed above. Additional sources include extra virgin olive oil, canola oil, nuts, seeds and avocados.

- Avoid trans fats. These are vegetable oils that have been processed, such as margarines and shortenings.

- Minimize saturated fats found in fatty cuts of beef, pork, lamb, whole dairy products (whole milk, cream, ice cream and cheese) and palm or coconut oil.

- Green salads with olive oil dressing are an excellent way to get a healthy serving of fat.

Nuts

- Unsalted, unprocessed nuts are a great source of protein, make an easy, healthy snack and can aid in weight loss.

- Walnuts, almonds, cashews, pistachios, hazelnuts, Brazil nuts, pecan and pine nuts are good choices.

- Include one to 1½ ounces of nuts in your daily diet. Buy raw nuts in bulk and divide into smaller packages to carry as a handy snack.

Portion Control

When eating a meal, limit portion sizes at any one sitting to no more than the equivalent of your hands cupped together. The exception to this rule is non-starchy vegetables which can be consumed in unlimited amounts.

Healthy Eating Preparation

Eating right requires being prepared. When you are hungry, or when your energy is low from treatments, it is easy to eat the most convenient food.

- Purchase and have healthy foods, snacks and drinks available.

- Stock your pantry and freezer with an assortment of healthy foods before you begin chemotherapy. Use the week before your next treatment to replenish your supplies.

- Cook several meals and freeze them for the days when you don't feel up to cooking.

- Buy large packages of nuts and whole grain crackers and divide them into small plastic bags.

- Keep small amounts of food in your stomach to help prevent nausea and to prevent fatigue caused by low blood sugar.

- Carry water and a healthy snack of nuts, fruit or whole wheat crackers with you to avoid getting hungry when away from home. Don't get caught without something nutritious to eat.

Nutrition During Chemotherapy Tips

If you take chemotherapy drugs, you may experience numerous side effects that alter your dietary intake. Taste changes, nausea, vomiting, diarrhea or constipation may all change how, when and what you eat. Some people find that they need to adjust their diets to maintain their calorie intake during therapy.

- Make every spoonful and every drink you take count nutritionally. Your body is building healthy new cells to replace those damaged by chemotherapy.

- Eat five to six small meals rather than three large ones. Small meals are better tolerated.

- Because your body is building new cells, it is essential to get adequate protein. You need more protein when you may least feel like eating. Good choices are whole wheat bread or crackers combined with peanut butter, almond butter (tastes like peanut butter and is highly nutritious), hard-boiled eggs, yogurt, liquid yogurt or cottage cheese.

- Limit amount of fluid you drink with meals to avoid getting full too quickly. Drink between meals instead. Adequate fluid intake and staying hydrated are essential. Monitor your intake to be sure you are getting enough fluids. Filling a bottle with your daily intake at the beginning of the day will help you monitor how much you are drinking.

- Make your own high-protein smoothies in a blender out of yogurt, fresh fruit or peanut or almond butter. This is a smart way to get calories and lots of protein while avoiding the hassle of food preparation.

Nausea or Vomiting Nutrition Tips:

- If nausea is a problem, take your nausea medication 30 – 60 minutes before smelling food or trying to eat. Studies now show that ginger (fresh ginger or capsules, not flavoring) can decrease nausea when taken 30 minutes before a meal.

- Cold food is better tolerated because it has fewer aromas. Ask your family to allow your meal to reach room temperature to reduce odors before bringing it to you. Try eating chicken or turkey cold instead of hot.

- Avoid foods high in fat; they may cause nausea to increase. Bland white foods such as Cream of Wheat®, mashed potatoes, rice and cottage cheese have been found to be easily tolerated.

- If you have been vomiting, take your medication with a small sip of fluid and wait 30 – 60 minutes. Then, try several spoonfuls of food and wait 10 – 15 minutes before attempting to eat a full meal. Don't try to eat your favorite foods; you may create an aversion to them later. Starting out with dry toast, salty crackers or clear soups, such as chicken broth, is often helpful.

Constipation or Diarrhea Tips:

- Some cancer medications and pain medications cause constipation. This increases your discomfort. After nausea passes, be sure that your diet contains high-fiber content. Ask your physician or nurse about recommendations for a fiber supplement or stool softener if you are constipated. Constipation should not be ignored.

- If diarrhea occurs, be sure to drink adequate amounts of fluids to prevent dehydration. Try eating bananas, rice, applesauce and dry toast during episodes.

Remember, chemotherapy is time-limited, and problems affecting your eating and nutrition will come to an end. Additional information is available from the American Cancer Society.

Staying Physically Fit

Recovery from breast cancer is also a time to consider an exercise program as part of your personal fitness plan. Your hospital or clinic may offer or recommend exercise classes for breast cancer patients with a focus on regaining the range of motion of the surgical arm. These programs are very beneficial. I encourage you to join if there is one available. If not, refer to Chapter 18 and perform the arm exercises shown there until the full range of motion is restored to your surgical arm. In addition, take a serious look at how physical exercise can increase your physical stamina, reduce treatment side effects and shorten your recovery time.

Why Should I Exercise When I'm Already So Tired?

Most people who have not participated in regular exercise think of exercise as an additional activity that will decrease their available energy. The opposite is true. Physical exercise has proven to restore energy and reduce many side effects during cancer treatment and recovery.

Normal fatigue is expected after surgery, radiation therapy and chemotherapy. The traditional recommendation in the past was "you need to rest," and many patients reverted to bed rest to manage their fatigue. It was believed that the more you rested, the quicker you would recover. However, newer studies have shown that bed rest can actually promote physiological changes that increase, rather than decrease, fatigue.

Studies by Greenleaf and Kozlowski revealed, "Maintenance of optimal health in a person requires a proper balance between exercise, rest, and sleep, as well as time in an upright position."

Bed Rest Versus Activity Study Revealed:
- Too **much** rest promotes fatigue (imbalance).
- Too **little** activity promotes fatigue (imbalance).
- A dynamic **balance** between rest and activity decreases fatigue.

Their conclusion was that patients need to remain as active as possible during periods of physical recovery. There has to be a balance of activity and rest for maximum energy to be maintained.

Clinical Study of 100 Cancer Patients Reveals Benefits of Exercise:
- Exercise functioned as a stress relief mechanism in coping
- Patients maintained a feeling of control over their lives
- Increase in measurable functional energy using peak oxygen uptake as an indicator of functional capacity
- Increase in internal control (ability to make decisions based on Levinson Locus of Control)
- Increase in mood elevation (Profile of Mood States tool)
- Decrease in tension and anxiety
- No harmful or debilitating effects reported
- 40 percent gain in functional capacity at end of 10 weeks
- Decrease in complaints of nausea and vomiting

Another interesting outcome involved those who did not participate in regular exercise. Unlike those who exercised, those who did **not** participate reported a worsening of mood states as treatment progressed.

It is important that you understand the newer concepts of energy building, especially after a cancer diagnosis. The older recommendations for bed rest have to be replaced with the new facts.

- Too much rest can decrease available energy.
- Exercise can build energy.
- Decreased movement may make a person feel worse.
- Excessive bed rest and inactivity are enemies of recovery.
- Too much rest can cause increased fatigue.
- Activity and rest must be balanced to maintain or build energy.
- Maintaining or starting a moderate exercise program based on your present ability can speed recovery and reduce symptoms of treatment; it will **not** harm you.
- Exercise activities can reduce the need for pain and nausea medications that have side effects of fatigue.

With the new information available, this is your opportunity to make recovery a time of balance between appropriate rest and appropriate exercise. If you did not participate in an exercise program prior to your cancer diagnosis, now is the time to build energy by adopting moderate physical movement as a part of your complete recovery plan.

Whatever exercise you select and consistently do will raise your energy levels and speed your psychological recovery from breast cancer by decreasing depression. In addition, exercise reduces pain by promoting the release of natural painkillers referred to as "endorphins" or "natural morphine" into the body.

Exercise Programs During Cancer Treatments

Before beginning any exercise program, ask your physician if you have limitations. While it is important to maintain physical activity, it is also necessary that you understand that your tolerated level of activity may change during treatment. Strive to maintain your activity at a level that allows you to exercise regularly without exhaustion. Enjoy the activity and look at this as a special time set aside to take care of your own needs. The rewards will be increased physical stamina and psychological well-being.

What Type of Exercise Program Is Best?

Some women prefer group/peer exercise groups, and others prefer to exercise alone or with a family member or friend. The goal is for you to decide what type of physical activity is suitable for you and take steps to start. The right exercise for you is something you can physically do, you have the time to do, is convenient for you and you enjoy. You do not need to join a gym or health club. Walking programs, Pilates, yoga, biking, swimming or gardening are all good choices.

Walking Program

Starting a regular walking program is a good choice because you can do it anytime you choose, it does not cost anything and it can be adapted to your present physical condition. A walking program can be easily modified to meet your changing needs during treatment; it can be started, suspended, decreased or accelerated according to your physical energy.

Recommendations for a Walking Program:

Frequency: Four times a week minimum, six times a week maximum; try not to skip more than one day in a row if your health allows.

Goal: Gradually increase and maintain your heart rate at 100 to 120 beats per minute during your walk.

Duration: Brisk walking at your own rate; start at 10 minutes per session and increase gradually to 30 minutes per session, as tolerated.

Place: Preferably outdoors, when weather permits; indoor mall or treadmill.

Attire: Comfortable shoes designed for walking and layered, loose, cotton clothing to absorb perspiration. Investigate purchasing a pedometer that measures the distance you walk and monitors your heart rate.

Evaluation: Use the "talk test" to determine if the activity is too strenuous. During your exercise you should be able to talk in sentences without feeling out of breath. If you cannot say a sentence, you should reduce your exercise level. Stop any exercise if it causes or increases pain.

Walking Routine

1. Five minutes of slow walking to warm up.

2. Increase walking to a brisk pace to increase heart rate to 100 to 120 beats per minute (take your pulse for 6 seconds and multiply by 10 to check your heart rate).

3. Gradually increase the time your pulse remains at your target heart rate by extending your walk as tolerated. Walking should increase your energy after your heart rate returns to normal, without causing fatigue. Do not exercise to a point of causing fatigue; this is not healthy or recommended.

4. For the last five minutes, reduce your pace to allow your heart rate to return to normal gradually.

Walking Tips:

- Walk with a partner, if possible.

- Carry personal identification with you.

- Listen to inspirational tapes or your favorite music if you walk alone.

- Keep an exercise log or diary to monitor your progress.

- Exercise at the same time of day, if possible, to make walking routine.

- Drink a full glass of water before and after you walk.

- Walk in a safe area, away from traffic.

Exercise Evaluation

The ultimate test to evaluate whether you are overdoing your exercise is to wait one hour after completion and then ask yourself, "Do I have more energy and feel more relaxed?" If the answer is yes, you are exercising in a range that is building energy. If the answer is no, you are over-taxing your body's physical reserves, and you need to reduce the intensity or duration of your exercise.

Do Not Exercise if You Have:

- Fever

- Nausea or vomiting

- Muscle or joint pain with swelling

- Bleeding from any source

- Irregular heart beat

- Dizziness or fainting

- Chest, arm or jaw pain

- Intravenous chemotherapy administration on the same day

- Blood drawing on the same day—may exercise afterwards, but prior exercise may alter counts

- Any restrictions placed on exercise activities by a physician

Exercise Precautions During Treatment

If you are receiving chemotherapy, your nurse or physician will alert you if your counts are in a range where exercise is not advised. Ask your nurse when you have your blood drawn if your counts are still in a safe range.

Do Not Exercise When:

- White blood count less than 3,000 mcL

- Absolute granulocyte count less than 2,500 mm^3

- Hemoglobin/hematocrit less than 10 gm/dL

- Platelet count less than 25,000 mcL

Diet and Exercise

What you eat and how you move your body are predictors of how you will feel during treatment and recovery. Eating nutritious food and getting regular exercise are keys to increasing your energy and improving your mood. When your body has nutrients from food available and the ability to transport oxygen to all its cells, it increases its capacity to heal, increases available energy, elevates mood, decreases pain, lowers anxiety, decreases depression and boosts immunity.

Plan to select changes that will enhance your recovery and that can easily fit into your lifestyle. These are changes that no one can make for you. Food and exercise are habits. The good news is that bad habits can be broken and new habits can be implemented. If you recognize that there are changes that may benefit you, now is the time to plan what you need to change and when to get started. If you find change hard to stick with, enlist a friend or support partner to join you or be your cheerleader. Share commitment. You will never regret these positive changes. This is a gift that you can give yourself.

My support person for change:

_____

Changes I plan to make in my diet:

_____

Exercise I plan to start:

_____

Date I plan to start:

_____

Remember

Exercise can elevate your mood and increase physical endurance.

Walking is one of the best forms of exercise.

Ask someone to join you; this will increase the likelihood that you will continue the program.

Do not select a diet to lose weight; instead, select a diet to create health.

Diets that limit the amount of food eaten and create hunger are psychologically stressful and should always be avoided.

Do not allow three numbers on a bathroom scale to dictate how you feel about yourself.

Concentrate on choosing foods that will give your body the nutrients needed to rebuild healthy cells.

CHAPTER 22

Monitoring Your Breasts After Surgery

"My husband is proud to say that he is as much an expert on the landscape of my breasts as I am! After all, we were newlyweds when I was diagnosed!"

—*Anna Cluxton*

After breast cancer surgery, there is an increased risk that you may have cancer in the remaining breast or a recurrence in the surgical breast. Therefore, breast self-exams are an important part of monitoring your health. Monthly self-exams combined with mammography and regular clinical exams by your healthcare provider will provide the best surveillance of your breast health. It is important to remember that women find most suspicious lumps themselves and that finding them early increases the chances for successful treatment. Early detection is the best weapon we have against breast cancer.

Many women report that it is difficult to perform a breast self-exam after having surgery for cancer. If you find it difficult, make an appointment with your healthcare provider for a clinical breast exam and ask your healthcare provider to explain what is felt in your breast tissue. This routine exam can help you begin your breast self-exams knowing that what you feel in your breast is normal breast tissue and not suspicious.

Normal Nodularity

Your goal for breast self-exam is to carefully check your breast(s) to learn what is normal for you. Hormones produced by the body cause women's breasts to feel different at different times of the month. Often the breast will feel lumpy because of hormonal stimulation of the breast tissues, referred to as **normal nodularity.** After checking your breast(s) regularly, you will discover a normal nodularity pattern. During breast self-exam, you will be feeling for unique changes in your tissue, especially new lumps or areas of thickening. Report any changes to your healthcare provider.

When to Check Your Breasts

Check your breast(s) when they are least filled with fluid.

- **Menstruating women** should check their breast(s) the last day of the menstrual period or several days past.

- **Menopausal or pregnant women** should select the same date each month.

■ **Women receiving treatment,** who are not having a regular menstrual period, need to select the same date each month.

Self-Exam After Surgery:

■ **Mastectomy patients** should begin their exam of the surgical area after complete healing of the incision, usually two to three months after surgery.

■ **Lumpectomy patients** should begin exams of their surgical area after complete healing, usually in two to three months, or at the completion of radiation therapy.

■ **Reconstructive surgery** patients should begin exams when their incision is completely healed, from two to three months after surgery.

Normal Changes After Surgery

Soon after surgery, you need to become familiar with how your incision area feels. It will feel different from surrounding tissue; the scar will feel firm to your touch. Occasionally an area in the incision will be slightly firmer. This is scar tissue formation. Areas where drains were placed may also feel firm. This firmness is normal. Breast cancer occurring in the scar area the first few months after surgery is very rare. Knowing what your normal scar feels like will help you recognize suspicious changes should they ever occur.

A sporadic pain, like a shooting sensation in the area of the incision, is not uncommon during the healing process. This sensation can occur for months, especially in breast conserving surgery.

Normal Radiated Breast Changes:

■ Color change, generalized darkening of the skin

■ Swelling (edema) of breast tissues for up to a year

■ Gradual decrease in swelling and a firmness of the radiated tissues, which will feel lumpy to the touch

■ Skin thickening, greatest in the area of the nipple and areola

■ Slight decrease in the size of the radiated breast when edema subsides

Monthly exams of the radiated breast allow you to become familiar with normal changes and prevent misinterpretations of post-radiation changes. You will notice most of the changes within the first six months, but changes may continue to occur eighteen months past treatment.

MammaCare® Method of Self-Exam

The exam described below has been taken from the MammaCare® method. This method was developed from research at the University of Florida and is considered the state-of-the-art breast self-exam technique.

Area to Be Examined

The breast tissue extends beyond the breast mound. It covers a large portion of the chest wall. Examine the area from the middle notch of your collarbone, following under the collarbone until you reach mid-underarm, then straight down until you reach your bra line. Follow the bra line to the middle of the breastbone and then back up to the notch. Fifty percent of cancers occur in the upper, outer quadrant of the breast and eighteen percent under the nipple. Examine these areas carefully.

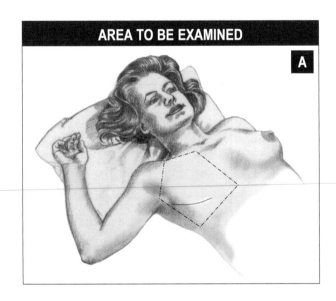

AREA TO BE EXAMINED

A

Finger Positions

Use the flat pads of your three middle fingers, from the first joint down to the tips. Place flat pads of fingers in a bowing position on the breast tissue.

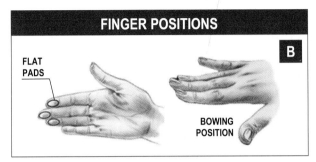

Three Levels of Pressure

Using three levels of pressure allows you to carefully examine the full thickness of the breast and not displace small lumps into fibrous tissues or into your rib area. Pressures do not injure your breast tissue.

1. Position your fingers on the first spot to be examined.
2. Use your fingers to make dime-sized circles using light pressure (barely moving the top layer of skin).
3. Without lifting your fingers, repeat the circles using medium pressure (go halfway through the thickness of the breast).
4. Again, without lifting your fingers, repeat the circles using deep pressure (go to the base of the breast next to the ribs).
5. Lift your fingers. Move to the next position and repeat the process.

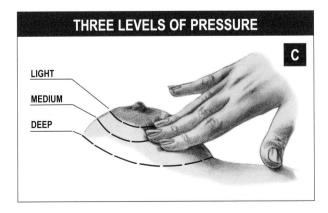

Remember: Do not lift your hand or release the pressure from your breast until you have completed the three circles in each area.

Performing Your Exam

Step One: Side-Lying Position

Use the following techniques to examine the lumpectomy breast or the mastectomy site:

- Lie down on the bed, roll onto your left side to examine your right breast (D).

- Pull your knees up slightly, rotate your right shoulder to the flat of the bed.

- Place your right hand, palm up, on your forehead. Your nipple should point directly toward the ceiling. Use your left hand to examine your right breast. You may place a small pillow under the arch of the back to increase comfort.

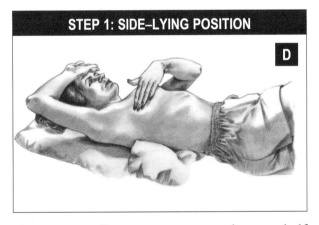

This position allows you to examine the outer half of the breast by spreading out the tissue. Fifty percent of all cancers occur in the area of the breast which extends from the nipple to underneath the arm. The side-lying position prevents breast tissue from falling into the underarm area.

Step Two: Side-Lying Exam

- Using the flat pads of your three middle fingers in the bowing position (B), begin your exam under the arm. Make dime-sized circles using the three levels of pressure in each spot (C), following the up and down pattern of search (E). Do not release the pressure as you spiral downward. Ten to sixteen vertical strips will be needed. Continue the pattern of search until you reach your nipple area.

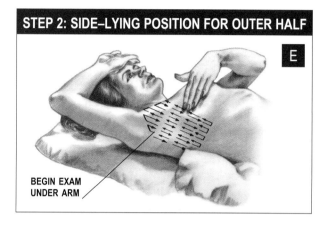

STEP 2: SIDE–LYING POSITION FOR OUTER HALF

E

BEGIN EXAM
UNDER ARM

Step Three: Back-Lying Exam

▪ When you reach your nipple area, roll onto your back; remove your hand from your forehead and place this arm alongside your body on the bed (F).

▪ Continue the exam of the nipple area using the same pressures (C). Do not squeeze the nipple.

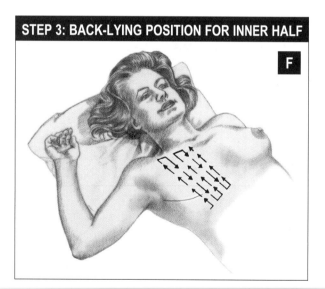

STEP 3: BACK-LYING POSITION FOR INNER HALF

F

Report any discharge from your nipple not associated with the onset of a menstrual period, hormonal medications, sexual stimulation or excessive manipulation of the breasts. A bloody discharge or a discharge from only one breast needs to be reported promptly.

▪ Examine the remaining breast tissue with the same pressures and pattern of search until you reach the breastbone.

Repeat steps 1 – 3, examining the opposite breast.

Step Four: Lymph Node Exam

▪ Make a row of circles above and below your collarbone on each side (G).

▪ While standing, check the depressed area near your neck by rolling your shoulders upward and turning your face toward the side you are examining. With the opposite hand, place your fingers in the formed depression and check carefully.

▪ Feel under each arm for axillary lymph node enlargement.

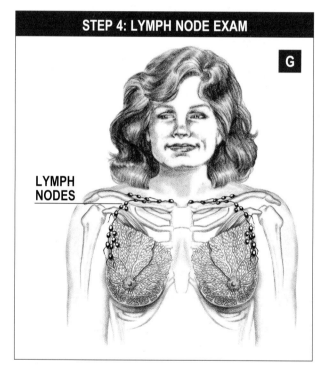

STEP 4: LYMPH NODE EXAM

G

LYMPH
NODES

Lymph nodes are soft to hard, pea-like areas in the lymphatic system. They may become enlarged from cancer or infection. Enlarged lymph nodes do not always indicate cancer, but you should report any lymph node enlargement to your healthcare provider.

Step Five: Visual Exam

A visual inspection of your breast(s) is important. Some cancers do **not** form a hard lump. The first indication of cancer may be one you can see and not feel. Looking into a mirror, closely examine your breast(s) in these four positions:

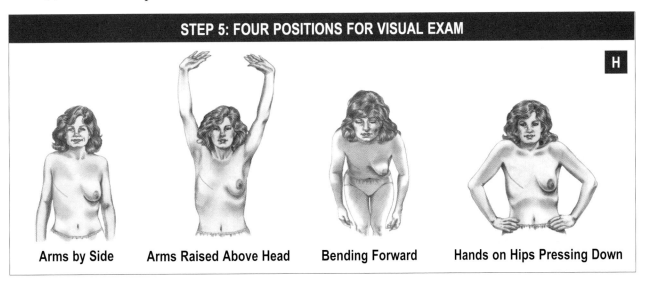

STEP 5: FOUR POSITIONS FOR VISUAL EXAM

| Arms by Side | Arms Raised Above Head | Bending Forward | Hands on Hips Pressing Down |

Carefully observe your incision. It is normal for it to be raised and red in the beginning. The color will gradually begin to fade to a light pink and the scar area will flatten out. A lumpectomy scar area may have a depression or sinking in of the tissues.

Look for the Following Changes Surrounding Your Scar and the Non-Surgical Breast:

- Skin texture that resembles an orange peel (1)
- Color changes in breast tissues
- Swelling or decreased size of the non-radiated breast
- Dimpling, bulging or pulling in of the skin (2)
- Inverted nipple (not normally inverted) (3)
- Crusty material or irritation around nipple
- Open sore or bump; red rash
- Difference in vein pattern over one breast (4)

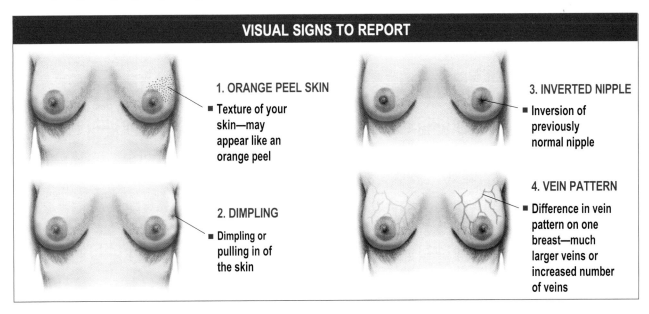

VISUAL SIGNS TO REPORT

1. ORANGE PEEL SKIN
- Texture of your skin—may appear like an orange peel

2. DIMPLING
- Dimpling or pulling in of the skin

3. INVERTED NIPPLE
- Inversion of previously normal nipple

4. VEIN PATTERN
- Difference in vein pattern on one breast—much larger veins or increased number of veins

What Cancer Feels Like

Ninety percent of cancers form a very hard lump, feel anchored in the surrounding tissues, are usually painless and do **not** change in degree of hardness during a menstrual cycle. Ten percent of cancers do **not** form a lump but may cause visual changes in the breast. Therefore, both a manual exam and a visual exam are needed each month to ensure your best surveillance of your breast health.

Self-Exam After Surgery

When you complete your monthly exam, congratulate yourself for taking an active part in guarding your health. Then forget about it until the next month.

Mammograms After Surgery

Mammograms, on a regular schedule, are an important part of monitoring your breast(s). After a diagnosis of breast cancer, it is very important that the lumpectomy breast and remaining breast be monitored with mammography. If you had bilateral mastectomies, a prophylactic mastectomy or reconstruction, ask your physician for recommendations concerning regular mammograms. Some physicians may require more frequent mammograms for lumpectomy and mastectomy patients the first several years. Other physicians feel yearly mammography is adequate surveillance. Your physician will tell you what schedule you will follow. Remember, even if you are under age 35, your doctor may now want you to go for your mammograms on a yearly basis. Remind your doctor if your annual checkup does not include a mammogram.

When Going for Your Mammogram:

- Schedule your mammogram at the end of your period when your breast(s) are least filled with fluid.
- Do not wear deodorant, perfume or powders to the exam. They may show up as debris on the film.
- If a past mammogram was uncomfortable, stop caffeine intake several weeks prior to exam to reduce discomfort. You may also take ibuprofen several days prior to your exam.
- If you change facilities for your mammogram, obtain your old film for comparison prior to your scheduled exam. Your previous images are an important part of your health record, and it is necessary for a new physician to have the old images to compare with your new films.

Remember

Breast self-exam is a valuable tool for monitoring for local recurrence.

When you complete your monthly exam, congratulate yourself for taking an active part in guarding your health. Then forget about it until next month.

Have a mammogram as often as recommended by your physician.

Practice breast self-exam monthly. Remember, do not to look for cancer but rather for changes to report to your physician.

Have a healthcare provider perform a clinical exam at least yearly—or more often, if necessary.

Using these three methods will help ensure that a vigilant watch is being kept over your continued good health. You need to practice all three methods of detection.

Chapter 23

Monitoring Your Future Health for Recurrence

"They found more calcifications (thankfully benign) in my breast during follow-up, so I had to have another biopsy. Before cancer I would have rushed back to work. Now I'm learning to take care of myself. People take time off to go to the beach, time off to do whatever. This is my health. I can take time off to take care of me."

—Earnestine Brown

Breast cancer recurrence is often hard for healthcare providers to discuss. When patients are ending treatments and there is no evidence of cancer, it's a happy time for patients and healthcare providers alike. Somehow, we think that if we don't talk about the potential for recurrence, a patient won't worry about it. However, the opposite is true. Survivors report that their number one fear after breast cancer treatment is the possibility of recurrence. One patient said:

Fear of recurrence is like a black cloud in my blue sky. Some days it is right over my head causing everything to appear dark and gloomy. Some days it is far away, and my day is sunny. But I'm always aware it is there.

Not talking about recurrence is like seeing a pink elephant standing in the middle of the room and having everyone ignore it—everyone sees it, but they're afraid to mention it. Failing to mention it only creates more anxiety for everyone involved. Talking about the potential for breast cancer recurrence and telling you how you can take appropriate steps is a better solution. Having worked with breast cancer patients for over twenty years, I can tell you that most patients overestimate their recurrence potential. Talk to your doctor and find out about your particular situation. Then remember that you are an individual, not a statistic. My goal in this chapter is to talk about the "pink elephant" and empower you to face this common fear.

"Being so involved in the cancer community, I am acutely aware of the potential for recurrence. To protect my future, I keep up with my appointments and keep a list of questions to discuss with my doctors."

—Anna Cluxton

Breast Cancer Recurrence

The majority of breast cancer recurrences occur within the first five years, with an estimate of 60 to 80 percent occurring in the first three years after treatment. Therefore, it is very important that you keep your appointments with your physician for close monitoring of your health. Recurrence is highly unpredictable—no one can say absolutely if and when. Your physicians have given you the best protection against recurrence through recommended treatments. The next step is a partnership with your physician for monitoring your future health for any signs of recurrence.

Breast Cancer Recurrence Types

After a breast cancer diagnosis, there are three categories of potential breast cancer recurrences. If breast cancer recurs, your cancer will be re-staged.

1. **Local recurrence** is cancer that returns to the local area of removal. This type of recurrence is considered failure of primary treatment and not a sign of a more aggressive cancer. This happens because it is impossible to destroy every cancer cell during surgery and radiation. A local recurrence does not change the stage of your cancer.

2. **Regional recurrence** is when cancer spreads outside the breast and underarm lymph nodes. This spread may be to the chest muscles, internal mammary nodes underneath the breastbone or in the nodes above the collarbone.

3. **Distant recurrence** is when the cancer is found in a distant site such as the bones, lungs, liver, brain or other sites in the body.

Monitoring Your Future Health

The American Society of Clinical Oncology (ASCO) recommends follow-up guidelines for the management of a breast cancer patient and a follow-up schedule for physician visits.

Recommended Surveillance Guidelines:

- Physician physical examination including complete patient history
- Patient education about signs and symptoms to report on a scheduled basis
- Breast self-exam
- Mammography
- Pelvic examination
- Diagnostic/surveillance testing when a patient has symptoms that indicate a need

Recommended Physician Visit Schedule:

- 1 – 3 years past treatment, every 3 – 6 months
- 4 – 5 years past treatment, every 6 – 12 months
- 6 years or more past treatment, every 12 months

Returning to your physician for a physical exam and update of your history is the most important thing you can do to monitor for recurrence. It has been proven that a physician's exam and review of your recent physical changes is the number one way that most recurrences are detected. Make the most of your appointment by preparing to report any changes you have experienced since your last visit. Write down any changes before you go to the exam so you don't forget. Report these changes early in the visit so that the physician will have the time to further evaluate the change.

During your physical exam, your doctor will look for any physical changes that relate to your general health and/or any symptoms that may suggest your cancer has recurred locally or spread to another part of your body (systemic disease). In addition to performing a careful breast exam, your doctor will closely examine your entire chest wall and check for lymph node enlargement in other areas of your body. Your heart and lungs will be listened to, and your abdomen, liver, spleen, neck and other areas will be checked for swelling or tenderness. Your doctor will also check for any changes in your neurological (nerve) functioning that may be associated with recurrence.

Signs and Symptoms to Report for Potential Local Recurrence:

- Change in size, shape or contour of the lumpectomy breast
- Nipple discharge that is clear or bloody
- Nipple inversion
- New onset of breast pain
- A new lump that may feel like a small pea
- Thickening in breast tissues or on chest wall after mastectomy
- Changes in the skin: dimpling (pulling in of skin), scaly appearance, rash, redness or any discoloration on breast or chest wall
- A lump or thickening in the underarm area

Monitoring for Potential Regional or Distant Recurrence:

- New lump or thickening in area above the collarbone
- Chronic bone pain or tenderness in an area
- Chest pain with shortness of breath
- Chronic cough
- Persistent abdominal pain or abdominal swelling
- Headaches, dizziness, fainting or rapid changes in vision
- Increasing fatigue unrelated to treatments
- Inability to control urine or bowels
- Persistent nausea or loss of appetite
- Changes in weight, especially weight loss

Do not hesitate to report any other changes that you observe in your health to your physician. The most common way recurrence is discovered is when a patient reports symptoms or changes she has experienced in her health. Don't ignore any change as being unimportant. Instead, let your physician or nurse make the decision. What may seem unimportant to you may be important to your healthcare team.

Additional diagnostic tests will be recommended after the physician's assessment and physical exam if the tests would be helpful to further explore or clarify any changes. With this open partnership, any recurrence should be detected early.

Potential Diagnostic Tests

Your physician may supplement your physical exam with additional diagnostic tests if your reported symptoms warrant the need for more diagnostic information. Diagnostic tests may include: MRI or dedicated breast MRI, PET scan, computed tomography (CAT scan), chest X-rays, bone scans, liver ultrasound or tests for breast cancer tumor markers such as CA 15-3, CA27.29 or CEA.

Monitoring Your Health

- **Breast Self-Exam:** Perform a breast self-exam each month. This includes a careful check of your breast(s) or surgical site for any new lumps, redness or swelling. This is particularly important if you have had breast surgery of any kind (lumpectomy or mastectomy, with or without reconstruction or implant). If you do not feel competent performing a self-exam, your healthcare provider can instruct you on how to do a correct exam. You will then be able to tell the difference between a lump, normal breast tissue, normal scar tissue, changes in a radiated breast and implant material. It is recommended that you perform a breast self-exam each month. This self-exam does not replace mammography as a screening tool, but it provides additional monitoring between your scheduled mammograms. This interval monitoring may detect changes that need to be reported before the next scheduled mammogram or physician's exam.

■ **Mammography After Breast Surgery:** Have a yearly mammogram. If you had breast-conserving therapy (lumpectomy), you should have your first post-treatment mammogram six months after completion of radiation therapy, then annually or as indicated by your doctor. (Some physicians keep the six-month schedule for lumpectomy patients for several years.) If you have had a mastectomy, you still need to have a mammogram of the other breast. Some physicians may also prescribe a mammogram of the tissue remaining at the site of the mastectomy, and some may order a mammogram if you have an implant(s). Ask your physician about your recommended schedule.

■ **Pelvic Exam:** Every woman should have a pelvic exam at regular intervals. For most women, this will be yearly. If you have had a total abdominal hysterectomy and oophorectomy (removal of your ovaries), the exam may be done less often. Your periodic pelvic exam should include a Pap test as well as a rectal exam. If you take or have taken tamoxifen, you could be at increased risk for endometrial (uterine) cancer and, therefore, your physician will ask you specifically about vaginal discharge or bleeding. There is no need for routine endometrial biopsies as was once recommended.

■ **Bone Density Scan:** Treatment with chemotherapy for breast cancer accelerates the loss of bone density during the first year after treatment. Decreased bone density puts survivors at higher risk for osteoporosis, a bone thinning disease that can increase the risk for bone fractures. The most common sites for fractures are the hips, spine and wrists. However, osteoporosis causes progressive bone loss throughout the skeleton, causing fractures in any site. Osteoporosis can be difficult to fight because it is a silent disease. It is often missed until a person suffers a fracture.

Bone density testing is a safe, non-invasive radiological procedure that helps determine if individuals have a bone density level that puts them at risk for osteoporosis or strongly suggests that they have osteoporosis. The recommended standard today is the dual energy X-ray absorptiometry (DEXA) measurement of the spine and hip. It is suggested that all women over the age of 50 and all women completing breast cancer treatment have a DEXA to measure their bone density. Bone density tests of other sites of the body such as the wrist and heel are less accurate because they are screening tests, not diagnostic procedures like DEXA. If a screening test indicates low bone mass, a DEXA should be ordered to determine true bone loss. Screening tests should never be used as a follow-up to measure improvement in bone density. A score of minus 1 to minus 2 indicates osteopenia (some bone loss), a condition that can lead to osteoporosis. A value of minus 2 (some use minus 2.5) or greater shows osteoporosis.

Osteoporosis has no cure, but women diagnosed with the condition can usually prevent further loss by following their healthcare providers' treatment plan.

Treatment for Osteoporosis:

■ Diet adequate in calcium (1,200 mg daily) and Vitamin D (400 – 800 IU daily)

■ Appropriate physical activity, including weight-bearing

■ Review of any medications you are taking that can cause bone loss

■ Regular visits for counseling and check-ups

■ Medications to prevent or slow additional bone loss (Fosamax®, Miacalcin®, Evista®, Actonel®, Boniva® and Reclast®)

■ Estrogen replacement therapy may be used if your tumor was estrogen negative

Your Future Health

This chapter is a guide to how you can protect your future health in partnership with your healthcare team. It is very important to remember that after breast cancer you will still experience the same illnesses, aches and pains that all people experience. Not every symptom is a sign of recurrence. Don't be over-vigilant, automatically fearing that every ache and pain is a sign of cancer. A good guideline is that if a symptom lasts more than two weeks, you should give your nurse or healthcare team a call and simply report the change. Their experience in cancer nursing can provide guidance about whether you need to have additional evaluation of the symptom. Your responsibility is not to tolerate a symptom that is lingering without informing your healthcare team. Monitoring for recurrence is a partnership with your healthcare team.

Dr. David Spiegel addresses the subject of patient anxiety about aches and pains experienced after cancer. These aches cause patients much concern about potential recurrence, but people wrestle with whether they should call the doctor or ignore it. In *Living Beyond Limits,* he writes:

> My rule of thumb is, if it is on your mind, do something about it. You treat anxiety by doing something. Even if you are just humoring yourself, you are still reducing your anxiety and that in and of itself is worthwhile. If your doctor thinks you are worrying about nothing, he or she can tell you so. Doctors count on their patients to be good reporters of what they feel in their bodies.

Remember

Remember to write down any questions to ask your physician before your follow-up visit.

Your understanding of what to report and when to report it is an essential part of monitoring your health.

You are still human and will have aches and pains.

Don't ignore persistent symptoms. Report them to your healthcare providers and let them determine their significance.

Keep your scheduled appointments.

Communicate openly with your healthcare team.

Survivorship

It is a fact that there is no way to rewrite our past. What happened has happened. Acceptance is the only way to make peace with our past and move on after a cancer diagnosis.

Our goal should be to become designers of our future life. We need to add to our life things or events that make us smile, inspire us to keep going and let us experience a deep, inner sense of peace. What do you plan to add to your life in the future?

A major sign of emotional recovery is when we reach out to help others in need. It is in serving others that we rediscover our worth as a human being and recapture the best we can be.

Helping other people is a powerful secret for healing ourselves.

—*Judy Kneece*

CHAPTER 24

Facing the Future After Breast Cancer

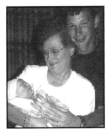

HARRIETT BARRINEAU

"I consider myself a survivor, not a victim. I think about recurrence, but it no longer consumes me. I do not fear death, nor do I fear life after having had breast cancer. My life will never be the same as before, but any negatives breast cancer has brought have been matched by positives."

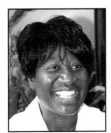

EARNESTINE BROWN

"The most important thing about cancer is learning you can say 'no' to others. I couldn't before. I couldn't say 'no' to my kids, I couldn't say 'no' to my mother, but I can say 'no' now. It's a very important thing to be able to do."

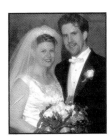

ANNA CLUXTON

"I remember that while I was still in the hospital I said to my mother-in-law that I needed to find out why this had happened to me. I know she thought I was looking to place blame. But I was really looking for meaning. Somehow, after struggling with all the normal emotions and asking 'why,' I finally arrived at the inner feeling that I had been given the gift of being diagnosed with breast cancer—yes, a gift! But I had to do something to make this a reality. So I changed careers, got involved in local breast cancer causes, and joined the Young Survival Coalition. Now I am 'fighting for our future' and working to ensure the quality and quantity of the lives of young women affected by breast cancer. Every day, I am on the front lines seeing that others have the tools they need to negotiate their own diagnosis. My life is extremely fulfilling and emotionally rewarding."

What about my future after breast cancer treatment is over? What do I need to do to get back on track with my life? How do I plan? What can I do? These are all legitimate questions about your future. How do you take what has happened and rebuild your life?

Eileen Crusan said in *Coping* Magazine:

To me, cancer was like a tornado. There is no warning before a tornado strikes. There is very little time to prepare for the destruction it leaves in its path. It's hard to find a safe place to hide. It sucks you into its terrible motion and tosses you about like a toy. When the storm has run its course, some things are left standing and others are totally flattened. The landscape is significantly changed.

No woman would ever choose to have breast cancer. Breast cancer changes your life, and there are some things that will never be the same after your diagnosis. Many women have shared, though, that their breast cancer experience added a new dimension to their lives—one that allowed them to enjoy life even more than before. If you are reading this chapter shortly after your diagnosis, you may find this unbelievable. However, as time passes and side effects subside, many women find that their diagnosis presents an opportunity to reevaluate their lives and make positive changes that they had postponed because they were waiting for the right time.

If you are like many women and your life has centered on doing for others, take it from other patients who have survived. Now is the right time to look at your life closely and plan to incorporate things you always wanted to do but didn't because you were too busy putting others first. Not to plan, means that you leave decisions up to others or to chance. To plan, means that you chart your own course and take steps to build the life that you would like. This is not being selfish; it is becoming the best version of yourself.

Survivorship Attitudes

I began my work twenty years ago as a Breast Health Navigator in a hospital working with women throughout the entire breast cancer experience. There I learned that women facing a challenge are strong and resilient if they are given information about what they need to know and what they can do to make a difference in their own lives. From those women I observed the coping skills and survivorship attitudes that can help build an even richer life after a breast cancer diagnosis. These skills and attitudes are not new. There are no secrets revealed here. Sometimes, though, in the midst of a crisis it can be helpful if someone reminds you of what has worked for others who have encountered a similar experience.

Survivorship attitudes and coping skills lead to happiness in spite of the event that paid an unexpected visit to your life. Survivorship attitudes do not deny the loss and pain you've endured, but rather encompass the loss as a learning and motivating experience. Breast cancer survivors have used these lessons to make changes in their lives, including taking care of themselves emotionally and physically. Survivorship is mostly attitude—the attitude that "I CAN." Become the best survivor ever!

As you read through this list, think of how these attitudes may help to add a sense of control and joy back to your life. This is what this final chapter is all about, how to maneuver the ups and downs of treatments and recovery to emerge a stronger, happier person.

Cancer Recovery Tips
Recovery Timetable

Recovery from breast cancer is a gradual process for the mind, just as it is for the body. Physical healing usually comes long before psychological healing. Your treatment team will focus on your physical healing; you must manage your psychological recovery on your own timetable. Some women are eager to put the experience behind them, while others need time to absorb the impact of the changes that cancer brings. Only you can decide what is best for you. Just as your treatment team has plans for you to recover physically, you need to chart a mental recovery plan.

Understand Your Cancer and Treatment

- Demystify cancer. Learn the facts about cancer. Correct your misconceptions. Cancer is a scary word and experience. However, because each person's cancer experience is unique, you have to learn the details of your own cancer and treatment plan to correct misconceptions and move forward with correct facts.

- Participate in your treatment decisions. Get answers to your questions before you agree to surgery or treatments. This is your life and your breast(s), and you will feel much more in control when you express your needs regarding treatment decisions. Remember to ask yourself, "How do I want to look a year from now?" Rushing to get things over is not the best longterm decision. Evaluate treatment decisions carefully. Refer to the tear-out worksheets to find questions for each physician involved in your care. Ask the questions you choose. Answering your questions about treatment is part of a physician's responsibility. Participating in decisions about your body is the beginning of your own recovery.

- Form a partnership with your treatment team to battle the disease. Learn how you can best participate for maximum response during treatment. Communicate openly and honestly with your treatment team. They need your input. Remember, you are the only one who knows what is really happening to your body and what tools you need to recover.

Dealing With Emotions and Fears

- Some people get emotionally stuck trying to figure out "why." In the field of breast cancer, we don't know why most women have breast cancer. Concentrate instead on what you can do now that it has happened. Do not concentrate on the "what ifs." Thinking about what you could or could not have done differently will not change anything. The past is the past, and yesterday cannot be changed.

- Do not suppress your emotions. Strong emotions are expected after a cancer diagnosis. Cry when you need to, and talk about your experience. Grieve over your loss. Grief is not a sign of emotional weakness; it is a normal response to a loss in life. Talk to someone you can trust about your feelings and fears. It may be necessary to find this person outside of the family unit—a professional counselor or peer.

- Identify your fears. Write them down and take action to disarm them. Fear is a paralyzing factor. Our fears rob us of peace in the moment and torment us about decisions in the future. Fear can only be mastered by naming the fear and facing it with action.

- Acknowledge that there are going to be days when things don't go well and you won't feel well physically or psychologically. Remember to reach out, ask for help if you need it, and know that this, too, will pass. Don't try to be a superwoman. Prepare yourself for emotionally trying days (of treatment, medical tests or anniversary dates) with a stress-free schedule as often as possible. Recruit a friend to share this time or plan a special treat to soften the experience. Be proactive in planning for your own mental health.

- If your emotions turn into continuous anxiety or clinical depression, ask your physician about counseling or medication. Do not suffer emotionally without seeking help; delaying only slows down your physical recovery. If you had diabetes, you would seek help. Clinical depression and chronic anxiety can be helped as well. Remember, you have to reach out to your treatment team to get emotional help. It is available, but you have to ask.

Stress Management Tips

Planning is the first step to eliminating unnecessary stress in life. The second step is to be realistic and expect certain things to be stressful. Determine to accept the things you can't change, and work to change the things you can.

- Plan a schedule for daily living. The body performs better when it sleeps the same hours. Schedules help you avoid a lot of unknowns.

- Plan what you want to accomplish daily. List in order of importance. Do one thing at a time. You don't have to do everything for everyone. There are no rewards for over-commitment!

- Spend some time meditating or having a devotional period before you begin your day. Prepare your mind for the day by reviewing your reasons to be grateful, even in your present circumstances. Get mentally dressed before tackling your day.

- Reduce the noise in your environment. Use voice mail to control a constantly ringing phone. This lets you talk when you feel you are physically or emotionally up to it.

- Take mini breaks. Take a series of deep breaths when you feel yourself getting stressed. It sends oxygen to the brain, reduces tension in your body and elevates your mood. Plan time for a walk. Exercise is good medicine for the mind and body.

- Avoid people who are "stress carriers" or those who are "negaholics." Say "no" to the things you don't want to do or that cause you stress. Saying "no" to others is saying "yes" to yourself. One patient said, "I finally realized that I can say 'no' and feel guilty for thirty minutes or I can say 'yes' and feel resentful for thirty days." Plan something new or good for yourself every day. Remember, no one else can do this for you.

- Monitor your "self-talk," the internal conversation you have with yourself daily. Is it positive or negative? Remember, you can't prevent negative thoughts coming your way, but you can stop

them from camping out. Refuse to entertain them. Replace them with positive affirmations, scriptures or meditations.

- When you feel like your last nerve has been used, put a big smile on your face and hold it. (You may need to leave the room to try this.) A smile can reduce stress. Try being angry with a smile on your face—it won't work!

- Avoid being a "TVaholic." The majority of shows are depressing. Spend some of your time reading, writing a journal, taking up a new hobby, volunteering at your local nursing home or healthcare facility or doing things that bring you pleasure and satisfaction.

- Learn to express your needs and to communicate your feelings. Use "I feel" or "I need" statements. Don't make others guess what you need. Ask. Unmet needs create stress.

- Shy away from criticizing, condemning, blaming, pouting and getting even. These are all energy drainers and accomplish little except to increase your stress. Practice letting it go. Choose to be happy and at peace rather than fighting to be right.

- When something happens that begins to cause you stress, examine the event and determine what you can do to reduce or stop it. Practice saying, "I refuse to let something like this bother me." "This is not worth my getting upset." "What difference will it make in a month anyway?" "I don't have to win to be happy." "Some people are just naturally unhappy and negative, but I refuse to participate in their pity party."

- Laugh every chance you get. Rent old movies. Watch old comedy TV shows. Laughter is as good as medicine for elevating the spirit.

- Look for beauty in the small things that come your way daily—the people, the smells, the colors and the sounds. Savor the moment.

- Set up your own personal reward system. After getting chemotherapy or completing radiation therapy, go out to eat, see a movie, do some shopping or visit with a friend. Plan to celebrate the milestones in life. It helps when you have something to look forward to.

- Share your own "oil of kindness" with others who cross your path. Speak, smile and say, "I appreciate you." "I love you." "You are such a wonderful help." "You do such a good job." "I always enjoy seeing you." "You certainly did a good job." "I hope you have a blessed day." Recognize their value as a person. When we give the "oil of kindness" away, it automatically spills onto us in the process. We feel better.

- Plan special times for you and those special to you. Enjoy life together whenever possible.

- End each day remembering the reasons you have to be grateful. Our happiness in life is more dependent on what we think about our life than on our circumstances. Keep the reasons for your gratefulness in the forefront of your mind.

Places to Find Encouragement
- Participate in a support group. Find a group that provides education as well as support. Women who attend support groups tend to adjust better than those who do not reach out.

- Use your spiritual faith as a source of strength and a place to find answers and give meaning to the hard questions of life.

- Allow your family and friends to participate in your recovery by helping you. Tell them what is helpful. It is therapeutic for them to feel needed. Stop long enough to say "thank you" or "I appreciate you" to your caregivers, whether they are the healthcare staff, family or friends. Like you, they need to know they are appreciated and valued. Being a caregiver is not always easy, and most people forget to share what they feel.

- Find outside support resources for your family, such as written materials and support groups, to help them understand and adjust to your

diagnosis. Encourage them to reach out for their own sources of support.

Diet and Exercise
- Eat healthy foods, exercise regularly, rest when needed and get enough sleep. These are the foundations for physical and emotional health.

- Don't resort to covering your anxiety with alcohol or recreational drugs. This only postpones your psychological recovery and can lead to depression.

Monitoring Your Health
- Follow your physician's guide for medical monitoring after cancer. Keep your appointments, perform breast self-exams monthly and get your mammograms, pap smears and bone density scans, but don't make a "career" out of cancer. Don't let it dominate your thoughts and actions. If a lingering symptom is bothersome, call your nurse and ask if it should be evaluated.

- It is vital to remember that you are not a breast cancer statistic. You are an individual. Do not look at your future purely through statistics. If only one person has ever beaten the odds, you have the right to become the second.

Charting Your Future
- Look at the breast cancer experience as a "caution light" in your life that allows you to slow down and examine your real needs and wishes for the future.

- Take time to do the things that make you feel good, whatever they may be. Plan your own fun times. Don't wait for happiness to come. Go and find it!

- Decide that you are going to make this a time of intensive personal growth. Start a journal and list the things you have always wanted to do and never gotten around to doing. Writing your goals down is essential. This list will serve as your road map for personal recovery. Chart new courses for yourself—take a class or go back to school, change careers, read a long book, take a trip, plant a flower garden, get physically fit or do whatever you have always wanted to do "when I have time." Beginning a new project will give you new energy and facilitate recovery. Cancer can be the reason you decide that your goals and dreams are important. Remember that you, and you alone, can start making your heart's desires a reality. Today is the day!

- Surround yourself with things you love and that cause your spirit to soar … music, books, pets, hobbies, whatever makes you smile. You deserve it.

Tear-out Worksheet
Personal Plan for Recovery - Page W • 27

Remember

"There comes a time after you grieve your losses that you have to choose if you want to live your life as a memorial service around the event or learn from the horrible things sent your way and build a new and even better life."

—Brenda Harmon

Dear Survivor

Breast cancer is an unwelcome visitor in any woman's life. You have found yourself forced to embrace an enemy. Yet, even in the midst of this frightening and often lonely experience, you **do** have the capacity to find new strength as you work through this challenge.

Recovery is not a "one-size-fits-all" journey. It is an individual journey. Only you can decide what you need to master the challenge of living well with breast cancer. It takes time. Be patient. Becoming a triumphant survivor is achieved by taking life one day at a time and learning to live with the uncertainty cancer brings—it is a gradual process, not an event.

As I said on the first page of the book, "There may be scars on your chest, but there need not be scars on your heart." It takes longer to heal the heart; but, like thousands of other women, you, too, can turn this unexpected crisis into a time of personal growth and emerge stronger, emotionally and physically.

It has been my privlege to share this part of your journey with you. I hope you have found needed information to make decisions. But, most importantly, I hope you have found the encouragement you needed to make your journey with breast cancer a little easier.

My love and best wishes for a happy and healthy future,

Judy

APPENDIX A

Understanding Diagnostic Tests

BLOOD COUNTS

Your doctor will monitor your blood counts by drawing blood from your finger, arm or implanted vascular port on a regular basis. This blood test evaluates how you respond to the effects of chemotherapy, monitors for infections and detects changes in your blood chemistry.

Main Counts Monitored Will Be:

- Red blood cells (RBCs)—carry oxygen to all parts of your body

- White blood cells (WBCs)—combat infection and provide immunity

- Platelets—determine how your blood will clot

- Electrolytes (potassium, magnesium, calcium, sodium, chloride, glucose and carbon dioxide)

- Hemoglobin (iron)—the portion of the red blood cells (RBCs) that attaches to oxygen

Remind the technician drawing the sample not to use your surgical arm. If you had bilateral mastectomies, the technician will need to use sterile procedures to reduce the potential for infection.

BONE SCAN

Your physician may order a nuclear medicine test called a bone scan after your diagnosis to see if cancer has spread to your bones.

How the Bone Scan Is Performed

On the day of your scan, a radioactive substance is injected into a vein, usually in the hand or arm. Approximately three to four hours later, when the injected substance has traveled throughout your bloodstream, you will have your scan. The scanning part of the test will last about one hour.

The images taken during your scan will show how evenly the radioactive material has been distributed throughout the bones in your body. Normal distribution areas appear uniform and gray with no areas of increased or decreased distribution. Increased areas of the radioactive material are called "hot spots" and may indicate an abnormality that the physician will evaluate for evidence of cancer in the bones.

What to Expect When Having a Bone Scan:

- There is no preparation prior to the scan. You can eat, drink or take any medications the day of the exam.

- You will be asked to sign an informed consent.

- An I.V. injection of a radioactive substance is given into a vein three to four hours prior to the test.

- Bring something to read if you are planning to wait in the same facility.

- Prior to the test, you must remove jewelry and other metal objects. You may be asked to wear a hospital gown.

- Plan to use the restroom prior to the exam.

- A technologist will instruct you to change positions during the exam while the machine moves above your body taking images from head to toe.

- There is no discomfort from the exam unless you have difficulty lying still. If you think this may cause discomfort, ask your physician for medication prior to the exam. If the medication ordered is sedating, you will need someone to drive you home; otherwise, you will be able to drive yourself.

- The radioactive substance given is of insufficient radioactivity to necessitate taking any special radiation precautions. The radioactive material will be excreted through the urine within 24 hours. You are not a risk to your family members during this time.

- The physician who ordered the bone scan will receive the report from the exam and give you the results.

BREAST CANCER GENETIC TESTING

In the mid 1990s, scientists discovered two genes that, when mutated (altered or changed), greatly increase the risk of a person developing breast and/or ovarian cancer. The genes are known as BRCA1 and BRCA2 (BR=breast; CA=cancer). The normal function of these genes prevents cells from becoming cancer by helping to repair mutations (changes) that occur in other genes—making them "tumor suppressor genes." But an inherited mutation within either the BRCA1 or BRCA2 gene greatly increases the probability of malignant transformation and cancer. When a mutation in either gene exists, there is a high risk of developing breast or ovarian cancer. It is estimated that approximately 7 to 10 percent of diagnosed breast and ovarian cancers are caused by one of these altered genes.

Understanding Hereditary Breast Cancer

Everyone is born with two copies of approximately 25,000 genes. One copy comes from your mother, and one copy comes from your father. With regard to breast and ovarian cancer, when a woman inherits a mutated BRCA1 or BRCA2 gene from either parent, her risk for developing breast and ovarian cancer is increased. It was once believed that risk for hereditary breast and ovarian cancer came only from the mother's side of the family. We now know that people are just as likely to inherit BRCA mutations from their fathers' families. A father's family history is as important as a mother's. Men in the family may be the gene carrier.

A man or a woman may inherit and thus "carry" a BRCA mutation without ever developing cancer. This may cause the disease to look as though it has skipped a generation. In smaller families or families with more men, it may be harder to "see" the hereditary cancer risk because there are fewer women to develop cancer. It was once thought that the number of relatives with cancer was the highest predictor of a hereditary syndrome. We now know that other important factors, such as young age at diagnosis, a history of more than one cancer in the same person or male breast cancer in the family, are also strong clues that may indicate the presence of a mutation existing in a family.

Certain ethnic groups have a greater likelihood of carrying a BRCA mutation. For instance, 1 in 40 Jewish persons of Northern and Central European descent (Ashkenazi) may be carriers of a mutation. Specific testing of three common mutations in this population can be ordered at a lower cost than the more extensive test generally needed for non-Ashkenazi Jews.

What Are the Risks?

Women who inherit a BRCA mutation have a 56 to 87 percent risk of developing breast cancer by age 70. They also have a 27 to 44 percent risk of developing ovarian cancer. Women also face increased risk of developing a second breast cancer if they carry a mutation. These risks vary depending on which gene has the mutation. Increased risks for other cancers exist but are much lower than the risk of developing breast or ovarian cancer.

Hereditary Breast and Ovarian Cancer Syndrome Testing

After a breast cancer diagnosis, your treatment team will look at your family cancer history and at the characteristics of your diagnosis and decide if you need to pursue genetic testing. Genetic testing requires that a small sample of your blood be drawn and sent to a specific laboratory to determine the presence of a BRCA mutation. If your test results show that you have a mutation in either the BRCA1 or BRCA2 gene, this may significantly change your surgical treatment options.

Genetic Testing May Be Recommended if You:

- Were diagnosed with either breast cancer before age 50 or ovarian cancer at any age
- Have a family history of male breast cancer

- Have one first* or second degree** blood relative younger than 50 who was diagnosed with breast and/or ovarian cancer

    *first degree relative: mother, father, sister, brother, daughter, son

    **second degree relative: aunt, uncle, grandparents, grandchildren, niece, nephew, half-brother or half-sister

- Have two or more first or second degree blood relatives (on one side of the family) with breast or ovarian cancer
- Were diagnosed with bilateral (both sides) breast cancer or have multiple primary sites of cancer
- Have a blood relative who is documented as being a BRCA mutation carrier

Do not hesitate to remind your treatment team of any characteristics you see in your history that may qualify you for genetic testing. If there are any questions that cause you or your treatment team doubt, seek the advice of a genetic counselor or professional. A genetics professional uses a tool called a three-generation pedigree to record the family history. This helps determine the pattern of cancers in the family and whether genetic testing may be appropriate.

Potential Outcomes of Genetic Testing:

- A negative test result will allow you to move forward with breast conservation, if recommended. Other treatments may be recommended by your treatment team.

- A positive test for either a BRCA1 or BRCA2 gene will limit your surgical options. At the present time, breast conservation followed by radiation therapy is not a recommended option. Instead, bilateral mastectomy and high risk ovarian surveillance (transvaginal ultrasound exam and CA-125 testing) or oophorectomy (ovary removal) are often recommended treatments.

Positive Gene Impact on Your Children:

If you are diagnosed with a positive mutation in either BRCA gene, you can pass the mutated gene equally to either your sons or daughters. This places your children at increased risk for developing breast, ovarian and, to a much lesser extent, prostate, colon and pancreatic cancer. Each child has a 50 percent risk of inheriting the mutation from a carrier parent. Knowing if you are a carrier allows you to tell your children so that they can pursue genetic testing (after age 18) to see if they inherited the gene from you. If they are identified as carriers, your daughters can take steps of "high risk" surveillance.

High Risk Surveillance Recommendations:

- Perform monthly breast self-exams and have an annual clinical exam beginning at age 25
- Start having screening mammograms or breast MRIs between ages 25 – 35
- Start transvaginal ultrasound exams and CA-125 testing between ages 25 – 35

Chemoprevention Recommendations:

- Drugs such as tamoxifen or Evista® be taken
- Oral contraceptives be taken for ovarian protection

Prophylactic Surgery Considerations:

- Prophylactic mastectomy (after breast-feeding desired children) to prevent occurrence
- Prophylactic ovary removal (after age 35 or having desired children) to prevent occurrence

BREAST MRI

Breast MRI may be used to more closely evaluate breast abnormalities first seen on a mammogram. Mammography uses low dose X-rays to image the breast while MRI uses powerful magnetic fields. MRI may be used to study the extent of the breast cancer after a diagnosis. Breast cancer can be multi-focal (in more than one area of the breast) but difficult to see on a mammogram; therefore, a physician may want to evaluate both breasts carefully before lumpectomy surgery.

MRI is useful in helping to determine whether breast cancer has spread into the chest wall. If there is evidence of breast cancer in the chest wall, the patient may undergo chemotherapy before surgery. Physicians can also use MRI to detect recurrences in women who have already been treated for breast cancer with lumpectomy.

Breast MRI is also used to examine implants to see if they are intact or leaking and to further evaluate whether the cancer has spread within the breast or to surrounding areas. It allows physicians to easily visualize the muscle and chest wall in the vicinity of the breast along with the breast tissue. Recently, researchers have studied MRI as a screening tool for women who are at high risk for breast cancer, are young or have dense breasts.

Benefits of Breast MRI:

- Highly sensitive to small lesions
- Effective in visualizing dense breasts
- Evaluation of inverted nipples for evidence of cancer
- Evaluation of the extent of breast cancer
- Visualization of breast implants and ruptures
- Detection of breast cancer recurrence (return) after breast conserving therapy
- Characterization or identification of small lesions missed by mammography

- May be useful in screening women at high risk for breast cancer

What to Expect During an MRI Breast Exam:

- The patient lies face down on a special padded table with the breasts falling through openings in the table (no compression is used). The table contains special MRI coils (antenna) that receive the imaging data during the exam.

- A series of images will be taken while the patient lies still.

- A tapping sound is heard coming from the machine during the MRI exam.

- The exam typically takes between 30 and 60 minutes.

Preparation for Exam:

- Inform your physician if you think you will have difficulty lying still on your abdomen.

- There is no pain or compression during the exam.

COMPUTED TOMOGRAPHY (CT) SCAN

The CT scan (also called a CAT scan) is an imaging exam that uses X-rays to create cross-sectional pictures of the body.

How a CT Scan Is Performed

During a CT scan, you will be asked to lie on a narrow table that slides into the center of the CT scanner. The area of your body being scanned will determine if you lie on your stomach, back or side. When the table is inside the scanner, the machine's X-ray beam rotates around you, creating images. These images can be stored, viewed on a monitor or printed on film. During your time in the scanner, you will be able to talk to the technologist. You must lie still during the exam, because movement causes blurred images. Your technologist may ask to hold your breath for short periods of time.

Contrast Agents

Certain CT exams require a special dye, called a "contrast agent," to be delivered into the body before the scan starts. Contrast agents are given to highlight specific areas inside the body to help create clearer images. There is a potential for some people to have an allergic reaction to I.V. contrast agents. The most common type of contrast given into a vein contains iodine. If a person with an iodine allergy is given this type of contrast, nausea, sneezing, vomiting, itching or hives may occur. Medications, such as an antihistamine like Benadryl®, may need to be taken before the contrast agent is given. Inform your physician if you have ever experienced an allergic reaction to iodine or seafood.

The type of CT ordered determines if you need a contrast agent. If contrast is used, you may also be asked not to eat or drink anything for 4 – 6 hours before the test.

Contrast Can Be Administered:

- Through a vein (I.V.) in your hand or forearm.

- Through the rectum using an enema.

- By drinking the contrast agent before your scan.

What to Expect During a CT Scan:

- Your physician will tell you before your exam if you will receive a contrast agent and if you can eat, drink or take medications on the day of your scan.

- If a contrast agent is given by I.V. you may experience a slight burning sensation in the vein during administration along with a warm flushing sensation in your body, especially in the perineal area (between vaginal opening and anus), followed by a metallic taste in the mouth.

- CT scan is painless.

- Plan to use the restroom prior to the exam.

- You will be asked to lie still on a table as it enters into the scanner. Some people have difficulty lying on the hard table.

- If you have problems feeling claustrophobic in small places, ask your physician prior to the exam about medication to relax you.

- A built-in communications system enables a two-way conversation between you and the technologist at all times while in the scanner.

- If you require medication to relax during the scan, you will need someone to drive you home; otherwise, you can drive yourself.

- Results of your scan will be made available to the physician who ordered the scan.

If you are given a contrast agent, it will naturally leave your body within 24 hours. You should increase the amount of water you drink to help get rid of the agent from your body through your kidneys. CT scans give off no more radiation than a series of regular X-ray studies, and you will not be radioactive. This is a painless procedure.

LIVER SCAN

Your physician may order a liver scan after your diagnosis to evaluate liver functions and to see if cancer has spread to your liver.

What to Expect When Having a Liver Scan:
- There is no preparation prior to the scan. You can eat, drink or take any medications the day of the exam unless otherwise instructed by your physician.

- You will be asked to sign an informed consent.

- An I.V. injection of a radioactive substance will be given prior to your exam usually into a vein in the hand or arm.

- Prior to being scanned, you must remove jewelry and other metal objects. You will be asked to wear a hospital gown.

- Plan to use the restroom prior to the exam.

- A technologist will instruct you to change positions during the exam while the machine moves above your body taking images of the liver.

- There is no discomfort from the exam unless you have difficulty lying still or turning when requested. If you think this could cause discomfort, ask your physician for medication prior to the exam.

- The level of radiation during a liver scan is minimal and is not considered significant enough to cause harm.

- The physician who ordered the liver scan will receive the report from the exam and give you the results.

MAGNETIC RESONANCE IMAGING (MRI)

Magnetic resonance imaging is a noninvasive test that uses powerful magnets and radio waves to take pictures of your body. No radiation is used in an MRI. The MRI scanner contains a powerful magnet that causes the hydrogen atoms in the body to line up in a certain way, similar to the way the needle on a compass works. When the radio waves are sent to these lined-up atoms, they bounce back and a computer records the signals made. Different types of body tissue send back different signals. Each signal sent back is called a "slice." The images can be stored on a computer or printed onto film for your physician to interpret.

Because an MRI works with a magnet, please report any metal implants in the body before scheduling because they may disqualify you from the exam. A physician would need to evaluate if the implant would interfere with the exam.

Report a History Of:
- Inner ear (cochlear) implants
- Brain aneurysm clips
- Certain heart valves (physician will decide if you are a candidate)
- Older vascular stents (physician will decide if you are a candidate)
- Artificial joints (physician will decide if you are a candidate)

Patients with a pacemaker are not candidates for an MRI.

What to Expect When Having an MRI:

- Your physician will inform you if you need to fast before your exam.

- You will be asked to wear a hospital gown or come to the exam wearing clothing that does not have any metal fasteners. Many people wear sweat pants and a tee shirt.

- You will be asked to remove any metal items such as jewelry, hearing aids, eyeglasses or dentures.

- If your physician has ordered it, prior to the exam you may receive a contrast agent in a vein in your hand or forearm. A contrast agent provides more information about blood vessels in the body.

- You will be placed on a narrow table that slides into the MRI machine. If you are claustrophobic, inform your physician prior to the exam so that you may receive a mild sedative to relax you. Some MRI machines are "open" and the scanner is not close to your body. Ask your physician about the machine that will be used for your exam.

- There is no pain from the exam, unless lying still causes you pain. It is important that you remain completely still because movement will blur the images being taken.

- You will hear the machine making humming and thumping sounds as it moves over your body.

- The person taking your exam will watch from outside of the room. A two-way communication system allows you to talk during your exam.

- Time in the MRI scanner varies according to the area being scanned.

- After the exam you are free to return to normal activities. If you have received a sedative, you will need someone to drive you home.

- The physician who ordered the test will give you the results of the exam.

MRI BREAST BIOPSY

Your physician may recommend a Magnetic Resonance Breast Imaging (MRI) biopsy of an abnormality found in your breast. MRI locates the abnormality by creating images using a large, powerful magnet instead of X-ray.

Preparation for the Exam:

- Inform your physician if you have problems lying on your stomach.

- Inform your physician if you have any allergies.

- Tell your physician about any prescription or over-the-counter medications you are taking to evaluate the potential to increase bleeding.

- Inform your physician if you are claustrophobic (fear small places).

Day of Your Exam:

- You will be asked to sign an informed consent for the exam.

- You will have an I.V. inserted into your arm.

- You will lie face down on a table. The breasts are allowed to fall through a cushioned opening where they are visualized by a special coil that encircles the breast.

- The breast being biopsied will be placed in a compression device which has grid-like small openings.

- You will enter a cylinder-shaped machine where you will hear tapping sounds caused by the images being taken.

- You will then receive a contrast material (Gadolinium DTPA) through your I.V. site to improve quality of contrast between the tissues, highlighting the abnormity for the physician.

- Your images will be reviewed to determine the entrance site and lesion depth for placement of the biopsy needle.

- The skin is cleansed with an antiseptic at the site for the needle entrance.

- The area is then numbed with an injection.

- The biopsy needle guide is then inserted through the grid on the compression device in the area of the breast abnormality. After the correct positioning is confirmed, the biopsy needle is inserted, and samples of the lesion are taken to be sent to a pathology laboratory for evaluation. A small biopsy marker is placed in the area for future identification during imaging.

- When the biopsy is completed, you will have compression of the area (like an ace bandage) along with an ice pack to reduce potential for bleeding.

- No pain is involved other than the needle stick for the I.V. and the injection of the anesthesia to numb the breast. You will feel slight compression of the breast from the compression device to stabilize the breast and some pressure as the biopsy needle enters.

- When the anesthesia wears off, you may have local discomfort, and there may be discoloration of the breast from the procedure.

- The biopsy procedure usually takes less than an hour, unless there are complications.

Report to Your Physician Following Your Biopsy:
- Any pain that is sudden or severe
- Bleeding that soaks through your bandage
- Appearance of a hard lump at the biopsy area (caused from internal bleeding)
- Signs of infection at biopsy site, such as fever over 100.5°F, redness of biopsy area or a colored drainage (infection is rare)

PET SCAN (POSITRON EMISSION TOMOGRAPHY)

A PET scan is a nuclear medicine diagnostic imaging test based on detection of positrons, which are tiny particles of a radioactive sugar substance injected into the patient prior to the exam. During the scan, the machine creates images based on how the positrons collect in the body. PET scans are used to detect cancer, determine the stage of cancer and evaluate the effectiveness of cancer treatment such as chemotherapy or radiation therapy.

The PET machine looks like a large doughnut because it has a hole in the middle of the machine. Inside the machine are multiple rings of detectors that detect the positrons and show the images on a computer outside the room.

Preparation for a PET Scan:
- Wear comfortable, loose-fitting clothes.
- Do not eat for four hours before the scan.
- You will be encouraged to drink lots of water.
- Your physician will instruct you on taking any regular medication before the procedure (ask specifically about insulin, pain, blood pressure or heart medications).

Before Your Exam:
- You will be given a radioactive substance (I.V.) that is attached to a natural substance like glucose (sugar).
- You will wait approximately 30 – 60 minutes for the substance to travel throughout your body and be absorbed by the tissue that is being studied.
- You will be asked to rest during this time, avoiding any significant movement and talking.

During the Exam:
- The PET scan will be started and requires approximately 30 – 45 minutes of lying on a table in the open area of the machine.

- The images of a PET scan reflect the accumulation of the substance in different colors. For example, a glucose substance may be attracted to organs that use a lot of glucose. Because cancer requires a lot of glucose to divide and grow, these areas will show up with brighter colors. The images will be shown on a computer outside the room.

- The testing physician may compare previous CT or MRI scans with the PET images.

After the Exam:

- Drink plenty of fluid to flush the radioactive substance from your body.

- There are no restrictions on daily routines after an exam is completed.

- The testing physician will send a report to your physician.

ULTRASOUND

Ultrasound imaging, called sonography, involves using sound waves to produce pictures of the inside of the body without using radiation like X-rays. The test utilizes high-frequency sound waves that are sent out from a transducer, a microphone-like instrument that moves across your body transmitting the waves back to a sensor within the machine that produces a picture on a monitor. Ultrasound images are captured on the monitor in real-time so that you can see the structure and movement of the internal organ. Doppler ultrasound is a procedure used to assess blood supply and blood flow.

Ultrasound may be used after mammography to further evaluate a lump or abnormality. Ultrasound is not recommended by the American College of Radiology as the best method of screening for breast cancer, but rather as an ancillary procedure. It is especially helpful in determining if a lump is solid or fluid-filled. Ultrasound is safe when a woman is pregnant. Ultrasound is also used to provide a physician real-time guidance when

performing a fine needle aspiration (FNA), a hand-held core biopsy or a vacuum-assisted biopsy. Using ultrasound allows the physician to see the movement of the biopsy instrument and fluid movement in the breast in real-time on the screen and to capture still pictures when needed to document the procedure.

What to Expect During an Ultrasound:

- There is no advance preparation for the exam. The exam is painless.

- You will lie on a table and the examiner will apply a gel that allows the transducer to move smoothly over your breast, evaluating the area of concern.

- There is no discomfort unless lying on your back is difficult.

- Your referring physician will inform you of the ultrasound finding.

What to Expect During an Ultrasound Breast Biopsy:

- You will lie flat on your back with your arm raised.

- The physician will apply the gel and move the transducer across the suspicious area.

- When the area is located, a local medication is given to numb the area.

- A small surgical nick is made in the skin where the biopsy needle is to be inserted.

- The needle is inserted and advanced to the location of the abnormality using ultrasound guidance as the physician watches on the screen.

- Tissue samples are then removed using one of two methods. The core procedure collects cores of tissues—usually three to six. With a vacuum-assisted device, vacuum pressure is used to pull tissue from the breast through the needle into the sampling chamber. Without being withdrawn and reinserted, the biopsy device rotates positions and collects additional samples. Eight to ten samples of tissue are usually collected from the area with one biopsy needle insertion.

- A small marker may be placed at the site before the biopsy device is removed from the breast so that the biopsy site can be easily identified on mammography in the future.

- The needle is removed, and pressure with a cold compress is applied to stop any bleeding. The biopsy site is covered with a dressing. No sutures are needed.

- The procedure takes approximately one hour. Avoid strenuous activities for 24 hours. You can then return to normal activities. If you receive medications to relax you for the procedure, you will need to have someone drive you home.

- Bruising and some swelling are normal and expected after the biopsy. If you experience discomfort in the area, apply a cold pack for about 20 – 30 minutes at a time and take an over-the-counter pain reliever.

- Your referring physician will receive the biopsy pathology report and give you the results.

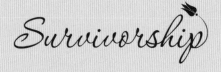

Survivorship

If I Had My Life to Live Over

I would dare to make more
    mistakes next time.
I would relax.
I would limber up.
I would be sillier than I have been
    this trip.
I would take fewer things seriously.
I would take more chances.
I would take more trips.
I would climb more mountains
    and swim more rivers.
I would eat more ice cream
    and less beans …

—Nadine Stair, age 85

APPENDIX B

Understanding Chemotherapy Drugs

There are many drugs used to treat breast cancer. The drugs listed below are the most common. Your physician and nursing staff will provide you with the names and side effects of the drugs you will receive.

Chemotherapy drugs are often given in combination. There are many combinations used to treat breast cancer. Often your treatment team will refer to the combination of drugs by the initials of each drug.

Most Common Drug Combinations:
- CMF (Cytoxan®, Methotrexate®, 5-FU®)
- CAF (Cytoxan®, Adriamycin®, 5-FU®)
- CMFVP (Cytoxan®, Methotrexate®, 5-FU®, Vincristine®, Prednisone®)
- CFP (Cytoxan®, 5-FU®, Prednisone®)
- FAC (5-FU®, Adriamycin®, Cytoxan®)
- AC (Adriamycin®, Cytoxan®)
- ACT (Adriamycin®, Cytoxan®, Taxol® or Taxotere®)
- FEC or CEF (5-FU®, Epirubicin®, Cytoxan®)
- EC (Epirubicin®, Cytoxan®)
- AT (Adriamycin®, Taxol® or Taxotere®)
- GT (Gemzar®, Taxol®)

Initials Used for Drug Administration:
- P.O. (Per Orally); given by mouth.
- I.M. (Intramuscular); given by injection into a muscle.
- I.V. (Intravenous); given by a needle into a vein.
- S.Q. or S.C. (Subcutaneous); given by injection into the fatty tissues of the body.

S.Q. Injection Instructions
Your healthcare provider will give specific storage instructions for the prescribed medication. If the medication is refrigerated, remove from the refrigerator and allow it to sit at room temperature for approximately 30 minutes before using.

Preparing the Dose:
- A disposable or pre-filled syringe should only be used one time.
- Gather supplies: syringe with medication, alcohol wipes, cotton ball and syringe disposal container.
- Recheck expiration date of medication.
- Wash your hands with soap and water before preparing medication.
- Open the package and remove the syringe.
- Hold the syringe with needle pointing up and remove the needle cover.

- Hold the syringe with the needle pointing upward and check for air bubbles in a pre-filled syringe. If there are air bubbles, gently tap the syringe with your finger until the air bubbles rise to the top of the syringe.

- Slowly push the plunger up to force the air bubbles out of the syringe.

- Continue to slowly push the plunger up to the line that matches the dose your healthcare provider has prescribed. Lay the syringe down on your work surface without allowing the needle to touch anything.

Subcutaneous (Fatty Tissue) Administration:

- Areas that may be used: outer area of upper arms; abdomen (except for 2 inch area around navel); front of the middle thighs.

- Clean the area selected with alcohol wipe. Do not touch the skin after cleaning.

- Pick up the syringe with the hand you will use to inject the medication. Hold the syringe like you would hold a pencil.

- Use your other hand to pinch up the skin that you have cleaned.

- Inject the needle using a quick, dart-like motion either straight up and down (90 degrees) or at a slight angle (45 degrees).

- Push the plunger all the way down to inject the medication.

- Pull the needle out, press a cotton ball over the injection site and hold it for several seconds.

- Place the syringe with needle (do not recap) into the disposal container.

Disposal Container

Your healthcare provider will tell you how to dispose of your container. Follow instructions for disposal. DO NOT place in household trash.

Dose-Dense Chemotherapy

Dose-dense chemotherapy is a term used for giving the same amount (dose) of chemotherapy drugs over a shorter period of time. Traditionally, administration time required a three-week schedule because blood counts needed to return to their near-normal level before the next dose. Dose-dense therapy combines special drugs to promote blood cell recovery when needed so that the administration schedule can be shortened to every two weeks.

CHEMOTHERAPY DRUGS

ABRAXANE (ALBUMIN-BOUND PACLITAXEL)

Method Administered: I.V.

Brand Name: Abraxane®

Side Effects: Lowered white (WBC) and red (RBC) blood counts; fatigue; nausea and vomiting; diarrhea; tingling in hands and feet; muscle aches starting 2 – 3 days after administration

Notify Physician of These Side Effects: Fever over 100.5°F; chills with or without fever; shortness of breath; tingling or numbness in hands or feet; nausea and vomiting not controlled with medication

Precautions: Tell your doctor of any over-the-counter medication you are taking.

CAPECITABINE

Brand Name: Xeloda®

Method Administered: P.O.

Report to Physician: If pregnant; taking a blood thinner such as warfarin (Coumadin®); taking Dilantin®; taking the vitamin folic acid; if you have a history of kidney or liver problems

Side Effects: Diarrhea; nausea; vomiting; stomach pain; constipation; weakness; tiredness; dizziness; headache; sleeplessness; dry or itching skin; dehydration

Notify Physician of These Side Effects: Severe diarrhea; loss of appetite; severe vomiting; tingling; numbness; pain; redness or swelling of the hands or feet; sores or pain in the mouth or throat; fever or infection; chills; sore throat; chest pain; rash

Precautions: Take drug within 30 minutes of a meal. Use barrier-type (condom) method of birth control. Do not breastfeed while taking capecitabine.

CARBOPLATIN

Brand Name: Paraplatin®

Method Administered: I.V.

Side Effects: Low platelet count; low white blood count; low hemoglobin; nausea; vomiting; numbness of hands and feet; hearing changes

Notify Physician of These Side Effects: Fever; chills; signs of infection; unusual bleeding or bruising; nausea not controlled with medication within 24 hours; tingling or loss of feeling in hands or feet; changes in hearing

CISPLATIN

Brand Name: Platinol-AQ®

Method Administered: I.V.

Side Effects: Decreased red blood count; nausea; vomiting; low white blood counts; decreased platelet count; potential kidney damage; potential hearing loss; diarrhea

Notify Physician of These Side Effects: Fever; chills; signs of infection; unusual bleeding or bruising; dizziness or fainting; diarrhea not controlled with medication; blood in urine or stools; decreased urine output; changes in hearing

CYCLOPHOSPHAMIDE

Brand Names: Cytoxan® and Neosar®

Methods Administered: P.O., I.V.

Side Effects: Lowered blood counts (WBCs, Platelets, RBCs); nausea; vomiting; loss of appetite; hair loss; stopping of menstrual periods; darkening of skin

Notify Physician of These Side Effects: Blood in urine; fever; chills; painful urination; unusual bleeding or bruising

Precautions: Drink lots of fluids while taking medication. One to two quarts a day is recommended during the 24-hour period following administration. If the drug is given by mouth, take in the morning and follow with adequate fluids during the day.

DOCETAXEL

Brand Name: Taxotere®

Method Administered: I.V.

Side Effects: Temporary hair loss; rare reports of permanent hair loss; decreased white blood cell count with increased risk of infection; decreased platelet count with increased risk of bleeding; hair thinning or loss; diarrhea; loss of appetite; nausea; vomiting; rash; numbness and tingling in hands or feet

Notify Physician of These Side Effects: Redness; swelling and pain in hands or feet; swelling in the ankles; shortness of breath; weight gain; if your clothes feel too tight at the waist

Precautions: Some drugs increase toxicity. Consult your physician or pharmacist. Take dexamethasone (Decadron®) medication, as ordered by your physician, prior to chemotherapy.

DOXORUBICIN

Brand Names: Adriamycin PFS®, Adriamycin RDF®, ADR®

Method Administered: I.V.

Side Effects: Hair loss; sore mouth; nausea; vomiting; lowered blood counts (WBCs, Platelets); changes in heart rhythm; darkening of nail beds; red urine; painful urination; flu-like symptoms; sensitivity to sun; inflammation of eyes

Notify Physician of These Side Effects: Fast or irregular heartbeat; fever; chills; redness or pain at injection site; shortness of breath; swelling of feet and lower legs; diarrhea for over 24 hours; unusual bleeding or bruising; wheezing; joint pain; side or stomach pain; skin rash or itching; sores in mouth

Precautions: When the drug is being administered, if burning or pain occurs at I.V. site or in nearby veins, notify your nurse immediately. If drug leaks into tissues, necrosis (cell damage) will occur in area of infiltration. Causes urine to turn reddish in color hours after administration, which may stain clothing. This is not blood and will last for one to two days after administration.

EPIRUBICIN

Brand Names: Ellence®, Pharmorubicin PFS®

Method Administered: I.V.

Side Effects: Lack of menstrual periods; nausea and vomiting; diarrhea; hot flashes; darkening of soles, palms or nails; loss of appetite or weight loss; low white blood counts; hair loss; red urine; sore mouth

Notify Physician of These Side Effects: Severe vomiting; dehydration; fever; evidence of infection; shortness of breath; injection site pain; fast or irregular heartbeat; chills; swelling of feet and lower legs; diarrhea for over 24 hours; unusual bleeding or bruising; wheezing; joint pain; side or stomach pain; skin rash or itching; sores in mouth

Precautions: When the drug is being administered, if burning or pain occurs at I.V. site or in nearby veins, notify your nurse immediately. If drug leaks into tissues, necrosis (cell damage) will occur in area of infiltration. Tell your physician if you are taking cimetidine (Tagamet®).

ETOPOSIDE (VP-16)

Brand Name: Vepesid®

Method Administered: P.O.

Side Effects: Decreased white blood count; decreased platelet counts; nausea; vomiting; hair loss; sore mouth and throat

Notify Physician of These Side Effects: Fever; chills; signs of infection; excessive bleeding or bruising; nausea not controlled in 24 hours with medications; difficulty eating or swallowing because of irritation

Precautions: Medication should be stored in refrigerator.

FLUOROURACIL

Brand Names: Adrucil® and 5-FU®

Method Administered: I.V.

Side Effects: Lowered blood counts (WBCs, Platelets); sore mouth; nausea; vomiting; diarrhea; loss of appetite; some hair loss; sore throat; sensitivity to sunlight; darkening of skin; nail changes; dermatitis or rash; dark veins where drug was administered

Notify Physician of These Side Effects: Chest pain; cough; difficulty with balance; shortness of breath; black tarry stools; diarrhea over 24 hours in duration; fever; chills; sores in mouth; stomach cramps; unusual bleeding or bruising

Precautions: Avoid people with colds and infections. Avoid prolonged exposure to sunlight.

GEMCITABINE

Brand Name: Gemzar®

Method Administered: I.V.

Side Effects: Nausea; vomiting; fatigue; diarrhea; sores in mouth or on lips; flu-like symptoms with first treatment; skin rash; swelling in hands, ankles or face; thinning hair; itching

Precautions: Do not take aspirin or medicines containing aspirin.

IXABEPILONE

Brand Name: Ixempra®

Method Administered: I.V.

Side Effects: Decreased white blood counts; allergic reactions to medication; numbness in hands and feet; loss of appetite; changes in taste; nausea; vomiting; sore mouth and throat; diarrhea; constipation; abdominal pain; hair loss; nail changes; skin rash; redness, pain and peeling of hands and feet

Notify Physician of These Side Effects: Fever; chills; signs of infection; redness, tingling, pain or numbness in hands and feet; nausea or diarrhea not controlled with medication within 24 hours

LAPATINIB

Brand Name: Tykerb®

Method Administered: P.O.

Side Effects: Nausea; vomiting; diarrhea; red, painful peeling of hands and feet; skin rash; mouth sores; loss of appetite; indigestion

Notify Physician of These Side Effects: Vomiting or diarrhea not controlled in 24 hours with medication; red or painful hands or feet; mouth sores

Precautions: Take with food or within 30 minutes of eating. If you miss a dose, do not double the dose the next day.

METHOTREXATE

Brand Name: Folex PFS®

Methods Administered: P.O., I.M. Injection, I.V.

Side Effects: Sore mouth; nausea; vomiting; loss of appetite; diarrhea; hair loss; taste alterations; blurred vision; dizziness; fatigue; infertility; itching; sensitivity to sun

Notify Physician of These Side Effects: Black tarry stools; bloody vomit; diarrhea over 24 hours in duration; fever; chills; sore throat; sores in mouth; stomach pain or unusual bleeding or bruising

Precautions: Do not drink alcohol while receiving the drug. Avoid too much sun exposure, use of sun lamps or tanning beds. Do not take aspirin or ibuprofen without first checking with your physician.

PACLITAXEL

Brand Name: Taxol®

Method Administered: I.V.

Side Effects: Decreased white blood cell, platelet and red blood cell count; allergic reaction during administration; numbness in hands and feet; low blood pressure; body aches; nausea; vomiting; diarrhea; sore mouth and throat; hair loss

Notify Physician of These Side Effects: Fever; chills; signs of infection; excessive bleeding or bruising; shortness of breath during drug infusion; tingling or numbness in feet or hands; body aches unrelieved by prescribed medication; nausea or vomiting not controlled in 24 hours with medication; inability to eat or swallow

TRASTUZUMAB

Brand Name: Herceptin®

Method Administered: I.V.

Side Effects: Chills; pain at tumor site or in abdomen or back; shortness of breath; muscle weakness or stiffness; rash; headache

Notify Physician of These Side Effects: Difficulty breathing; nausea; vomiting; diarrhea; loss of appetite; sleeplessness; unusual bruising or bleeding; swelling of the feet or ankles; rapid heartbeat; upper respiratory tract infection; excessive coughing; fever

VINCRISTINE

Brand Names: Oncovin® and Vincasar PFS®

Method Administered: I.V.

Side Effects: Hair loss; numbness in limbs; nausea; vomiting; lowered blood counts (WBCs and platelets); ovary suppression; constipation

Notify Physician of These Side Effects: Fever; chills; unusual bleeding or bruising; blurred or double vision; confusion; constipation; difficulty walking; tingling in fingers and toes; sores in mouth; pain in stomach

Precautions: This medication can cause severe constipation. Eat lots of fiber, drink lots of water and ask your physician about using a stool softener or laxative.

VINORELBINE

Brand Name: Navelbine®

Method Administered: I.V.

Side Effects: Redness and tenderness at site of injection; darkening of vein used; hair loss; nausea; vomiting

Notify Physician of These Side Effects: Difficulty walking; cramping in legs; redness and pain at site of I.V.; unusual bleeding or bruising; black tarry stools; lower back or side pain; fever; chills; painful or difficult urination

Precautions: Avoid people with infections.

HORMONAL DRUGS

ANASTRAZOLE

Brand Name: Arimidex®

Method Administered: P.O.

Side Effects: Weakness; fatigue; headache; nausea; mild diarrhea; increased or decreased appetite; sweating; hot flashes; vaginal dryness

Notify Physician of These Side Effects: Pain in lower leg; redness or swelling of your arm or leg; shortness of breath; chest pain

EXEMESTANE

Brand Name: Aromasin®

Method Administered: P.O.

Side Effects: Fatigue; hot flashes; pain at tumor site; nausea; depression; difficulty sleeping; increased appetite; weight gain; increased sweating

Notify Physician of These Side Effects: Severe hot flashes; difficulty sleeping; depression

Precautions: Keep taking the drug even though you are feeling well. Take drug after eating.

FULVESTRANT

Brand Name: Faslodex®

Method Administered: I.M. Injection

Side Effects: Nausea; feeling listless or tired; vomiting; constipation; diarrhea; abdominal pain; headache; back pain; hot flashes; sore throat; pain at injection site; flu-like symptoms; pain in chest or pelvis

Notify Physician of These Side Effects: Bloating or swelling of face, hands, legs and feet; tingling in hands or feet; unusual weight gain or loss

Precautions: Notify physician if taking blood thinners such as Coumadin®.

GOSERELIN

Brand Name: Zoladex®

Method Administered: S.Q. Injection

Side Effects: Light, irregular vaginal bleeding; stopping of menstrual periods; hot flashes; headaches

Notify Physician of These Side Effects: Pelvic pain; burning, itching or dryness of vagina; anxiety; deepening of voice; increased hair growth; mental depression; mood changes; nervousness; fast or irregular heartbeat

Precautions: When taking goserelin, your menstrual period may become irregular or cease altogether. You still need to use non-hormonal birth control methods, like condoms or spermicides, if you are sexually active. Drinking alcohol while on goserelin increases risk of osteoporosis.

LETROZOLE

Brand Name: Femara®

Method Administered: P.O.

Side Effects: Back, bone, joint or muscle pain; hot flashes; loss of hair; weight loss; decreased appetite; sleepiness; anxiety; constipation; diarrhea; stomach pain; weakness

Notify Physician of These Side Effects: Shortness of breath; chest pain; increased sweating; severe nervousness; cough; light-headedness; sudden headache; slurred speech; sudden loss of coordination; swelling of hands or feet; vaginal bleeding

LEUPROLIDE

Brand Names: Lupron®, Lupron Depot®, Viadur®, Leuprorelin®

Method Administered: I.M. Injection

Side Effects: Light, irregular vaginal bleeding; stopping of menstrual periods; hot flashes; blurred vision; headache; nausea or vomiting; swelling of hands or feet; swelling and tenderness of breasts; trouble sleeping; weight gain; bleeding, bruising, burning or itching of injection site

Notify Physician of These Side Effects: Fast or irregular heartbeat; trouble breathing; sudden, severe drop in blood pressure; swelling around the eyes; rash, hives or itching; numbness or tingling in hands or feet; anxiety; deepening of voice; increased hair growth; mental depression; mood changes; nervousness

Precautions: When taking leuprolide, your menstrual period may become irregular or cease altogether. You still need to use non-hormonal birth control methods, like condoms or spermicides, if you are sexually active.

TAMOXIFEN

Brand Names: Nolvadex®, TAM®

Method of Administration: P.O.

Side Effects: Hot flashes; nausea when first begun; fluid retention; vaginal discharge; menstrual irregularities; vaginal dryness; may have flare of bone pain when drug is first started (first few weeks of treatment); increase in fertility

Notify Physician of These Side Effects: Excessive vaginal dryness; vaginal infection; changes in vision; continued bone pain

Precautions: Take medication with food. Ask your physician about the need for birth control. A yearly gynecological exam is recommended. Some SSRI antidepressants may reduce the effectiveness of tamoxifen.

TOREMIFENE

Brand Name: Fareston®

Method Administered: P.O.

Side Effects: Nausea or vomiting; hot flashes; bone pain; dizziness; dry eyes

Notify Physician of These Side Effects: Blurred vision or changes in vision; change in vaginal discharge; confusion; increased urination; loss of appetite; pelvic pressure or pain; unusual tiredness; vaginal bleeding

Precautions: Taking a thiazide diuretic will increase side effects of drug. Taking Coumadin® increases risk of bleeding while on toremifene.

MISCELLANEOUS DRUGS

BEVACIZUMAB

Brand Name: Avastin®

Method Administered: I.V.

Side Effects: Abdominal pain; diarrhea; gastrointestinal perforations; decreased wound healing; hemorrhage; blood clots; high blood pressure; congestive heart failure; kidney problems

Notify Physician of These Side Effects: Fever; chills; signs of infection; abdominal pain; unusual bleeding or bruising; dizziness or fainting; shortness of breath; pain in chest or legs; diarrhea not controlled with medication; blood in stools; headaches

DARBEPOETIN ALFA

Brand Name: Aranesp®

Method Administered: S.Q. Injection

Side Effects: Pain at injection site; elevated or lowered blood pressure; headache

Notify Physician of These Side Effects: Headache; dizziness; fainting

DEXAMETHASONE

Brand Names: Decadron®, Dexasone®, Dexone®, Hexadrol®

Methods Administered: P.O., I.M. Injection, I.V.

Side Effects: Euphoria; restlessness; insomnia; stomach irritation; increased appetite

Notify Physician of These Side Effects: Dizziness; fainting; shortness of breath; fever; wounds that don't heal; swelling of feet or legs

Precautions: Take medication with food. Do not take more medication than prescribed. Do not stop taking medication without informing your physician.

DOLASETRON

Brand Name: Anzemet®

Methods Administered: I.V., P.O.

Side Effects: Diarrhea; abdominal or stomach pain; headache; dizziness; light-headedness; fever or chills; fatigue

Notify Physician of These Side Effects: High or low blood pressure; blood in urine; painful urination; chest pain; fast heartbeat; severe stomach pain; rash, hives or itching; swelling of face, feet or lower legs; trouble breathing

DRONABINOL

Brand Name: Marinol®

Method Administered: P.O.

Side Effects: Dizziness; drowsiness; nausea or vomiting; false sense of well-being; trouble thinking

Notify Physician of These Side Effects (may be signs of an overdose): Amnesia; memory loss; confusion; hallucinations; delusions; anxiety; mental depression; fast heartbeat; severe drowsiness; false sense of well-being; decrease in motor coordination; slurred speech; constipation; problems urinating

Precautions: Avoid alcohol and central nervous system depressants (alcohol, pain medications, tranquilizers or sleeping medication) while taking dronabinol.

EPOETIN

Brand Names: Epogen®, Procrit®, Eprex®

Method Administered: S.Q. Injection

Side Effects: Tiredness and weakness; tingling, burning or prickling sensation; loss of strength or energy; muscle pain

Notify Physician of These Side Effects: Chest pain; shortness of breath; seizures; coughing; sneezing; sore throat; fever; weight gain; swelling of legs, arms, feet or hands

Precautions: Epoetin may cause seizures, especially during the first 90 days of treatment. Avoid driving, operating heavy machinery and any other activities that may pose danger if a seizure occurred while you performed them.

FILGRASTIM

Brand Names: Neupogen®, Leukine®

Method Administered: S.Q. Injection

Side Effects: Rash or itching; headache; pain in arms, legs, joints, muscles, lower back or pelvis

Notify Physician of These Side Effects: Redness or pain at injection site; fever; rapid or irregular heartbeat; sores on skin; wheezing

GRANISETRON

Brand Name: Kytril®

Methods Administered: I.V., P.O.

Side Effects: Abdominal pain; constipation; diarrhea; headache; agitation; dizziness; drowsiness; heartburn; indigestion; trouble sleeping

Notify Physician of These Side Effects: Fever; severe nausea or vomiting; chest pain; fainting; irregular heartbeat; shortness of breath; rash, hives or itching

ONDANSETRON

Brand Names: Zofran®, Zofran ODT®

Methods Administered: I.V., P.O.

Side Effects: Constipation; diarrhea; fever; headache; abdominal pain; burning, prickling or tingling sensation; drowsiness; dry mouth; feeling cold; itching

Notify Physician of These Side Effects: Chest pain; burning, pain or redness at injection site; shortness of breath; rash, hives or itching; trouble breathing; wheezing

OPRELVEKIN

Brand Name: Neumega®

Method Administered: S.Q. Injection

Side Effects: Red eyes; weakness; numbness or tingling of hands or feet; skin discoloration; rash at injection site

Notify Physician of These Side Effects: Fast or irregular heartbeat; sore mouth or tongue; white patches on mouth or tongue; shortness of breath; swelling of feet or lower legs; bloody eye; blurred vision; severe redness or peeling of skin

PALONOSETRON

Brand Name: Aloxi®

Methods Administered: I.V., P.O.

Side Effects: Headache; constipation; diarrhea

Notify Physician of These Side Effects: Headache not relieved with prescribed pain medication;

diarrhea not controlled within 24 hours with medications; constipation not relieved with medication

PAMIDRONATE

Brand Name: Aredia®

Method Administered: I.V.

Side Effects: Abdominal pain; body aches or pain; bone pain; constipation; diarrhea; joint pain; kidney problems

Notify Physician of These Side Effects: Decrease in amount of urine; headache; muscle pain or cramps; pain in jaw; nausea

PREDNISONE

Brand Names: Deltasone®, Liquid Pred®, Meticorten®, Orasone®, Panasol® and Prednicen-M®.

Method Administered: P.O.

Side Effects: Increase in appetite; indigestion; nervousness; restlessness; trouble sleeping; sense of well-being; nausea; vomiting; fluid retention

Notify Physician of These Side Effects: Blurred vision; frequent urination; hallucinations; hives or skin rash; abdominal pain or burning; black tarry stools; irregular heart beat; unusual bruising; wounds that do not heal; nausea or vomiting over 24 hours in duration

Precautions: Take medication at same time of day starting early in morning. Do not take at night or late in afternoon. Do not increase or decrease dose without physician's consent. Do not stop taking medication without notifying your physician.

ZOLEDRONIC ACID

Brand Name: Zometa®

Method Administered: I.V.

Side Effects: Fatigue; nausea; vomiting; bone pain; pain in the jaw; headache; decreased appetite

Notify Physician of These Side Effects: Nausea or vomiting not relieved within 24 hours with medications; headache or body pain not relieved with prescribed pain medication

Precautions: Take a daily multivitamin that contains 400 IU of Vitamin D and at least 500 mg. of calcium daily. Drink lots of fluids.

APPENDIX C

Resources

"Knowledge is of two kinds. We know a subject ourselves, or we know where we can find information on it."

—*Samuel Johnson*

One of the most important ways to gain control over your disease and reduce your anxiety is to get answers to your questions. Because you are an individual, your questions and needs may be different from other women's and may not be addressed by your healthcare team. This is when you can reach out to support resources and find out what you need to know. The good news is that most resources are available free of charge.

Tips for Getting Organized:
- Start a notebook for keeping information about your disease, treatment and recovery.
- Remove the tear-out pages in the back of this book and place them in your notebook.
- Write down your questions and then read through the following list of resources for breast cancer patients.
- Call or email the resource. In your notebook record your questions, the telephone number, when you called and whom you talked to.
- Print out information that you want to keep.
- Ask your healthcare team for the names of local sources of support or call your local hospital's library.

Finding Information on the Internet
The Internet is a valuable resource, but be sure that the sites you visit are recognized as having sound clinical information. Most national cancer organizations have sites, as do many medical schools and universities. Internet access is available at most public and hospital libraries if you do not have a home computer with access.

Suggestions for the Wisest Use of the Internet:
- Never substitute information found on the Internet for seeing or asking your healthcare provider about your concerns.
- Always seek information from reliable organizations and make sure that the information is dedicated to cancer education.
- Make sure the information is current. Look for the last update of the information on the site.

GENERAL RESOURCES

AMC Cancer Research Center's Cancer Information Line
1-800-525-3777
www.amc.org
Professional cancer counselors provide answers to questions about cancer, support and information on free publications. Equipped for deaf and hearing-impaired callers.

American Cancer Society (ACS)
1-800-ACS-2345 (1-800-227-2345)

www.cancer.org

Provides free, written information on breast cancer, support group information and referrals to Reach to Recovery program for peer interaction.

Association of Cancer Online Resources
1-212-226-5525

www.acor.org

Online cancer information system that archives online support groups, information on treatments and clinical trials, links to other cancer education, advocacy groups on the Internet and much more.

BreastCancer.net
www.breastcancer.net

Archives the latest news on breast cancer and allows quick and specific searches.

BreastCancer.org
www.breastcancer.org

Breast cancer education site including articles, news, newsletters and chats.

CancerIndex.org
www.cancerindex.org

Online index of cancer resources and Web sites providing information and support. Provides a collection of media clips on various breast cancers. To access media clips, choose "Breast Cancer" from the list on the main screen and then click on "Multimedia Breast Cancer Resources."

Cancerlinks.org
www.cancerlinks.org

A directory of other sites and resources on specific cancers.

Chemocare.com
www.chemocare.com

Web site designed to provide the latest information about chemotherapy side effects and self-care for patients, families and caregivers. Regularly updated by Cleveland Clinics.

Merck Manual Online Medical Library
www.merck.com/mmhe/index.html

Explains disorders, their symptoms, how they are diagnosed and how they can be treated. Based on the world's most widely used textbook of medicine, *The Merck Manual*, but written in everyday language for patients. Provided free of charge on the Internet by Merck & Co., Inc., as a public service.

National Cancer Institute (NCI)
1-800-4-CANCER (1-800-422-6237)

www.cancer.gov

The NCI Web site provides comprehensive information on breast cancer diagnosis, treatment, statistics, research, clinical trials and breast cancer news.

ADVOCACY GROUPS / ORGANIZATIONS

Avon Breast Crusade
www.avoncrusade.com

A fundraising effort that has raised over $585 million for breast cancer education and research in countries around the world.

National Breast Cancer Coalition
1-202-296-7477

www.natlbcc.org

Grassroots advocacy group of hundreds of member organizations and tens of thousands of individuals fighting breast cancer though action, advocacy and public education.

National Coalition for Cancer Survivorship
1-877-622-7937

www.canceradvocacy.org

Advocates for quality cancer care for all Americans and the empowerment of cancer survivors through federal policy initiatives.

Patient Advocate Foundation
(Employment Issues)

1-800-532-5274

www.patientadvocate.org

The Patient Advocate Foundation is a national nonprofit organization that serves as an active liaison between the patient and her insurer, employer and/or debt holders in matters relative to a diagnosis through case managers, doctors and attorneys. Patient Advocate Foundation seeks to safeguard patients through effective mediation, ensuring access to care, maintenance of employment and preservation of financial stability.

Susan G. Komen for the Cure
1-877-GO-KOMEN (1-877-465-6636)
www.komen.org
Offers information on all areas of breast cancer treatment and support.

BREAST RECONSTRUCTION

American Cancer Society
www.cancer.org
Search: breast reconstruction
Breast reconstruction after mastectomy information.

BreastCancer.org
www.breastcancer.org/pictures/treatment/
Pictures of breast cancer patients with different types of breast reconstruction.

Breast Implants
1-888-463-6332
www.fda.gov
Search: breast implants
Information on choosing an implant, the associated risks, FDA regulations and manufacturers of implants.

Center for Microsurgical Breast Reconstruction
www.diepflap.com
Explanations of DIEP and SGAP reconstruction procedures, timelines and before-and-after photos.

Medline Plus
www.nlm.nih.gov/medlineplus/breastreconstruction.html
Complete guide to different types of breast reconstruction.

COMPLEMENTARY AND ALTERNATIVE MEDICINE (CAM)

Glycemic Index
www.southbeach-diet-plan.com/glycemicfoodchart.htm
List of foods sorted by category shown on a scale from 0 to 100 based on the extent to which they raise blood sugar levels.

Office of Dietary Supplements (ODS), NIH
www.ods.od.nih.gov
Site offering research resources, frequently asked questions and fact sheets about supplements, all geared toward helping the public make informed decisions.

National Council Against Health Fraud
www.ncahf.org
Provides links to position papers and information about alternative and unproven treatments.

U.S. Food and Drug Administration (FDA)
www.fda.gov/Food/default.htm
Site for the Center for Food Safety and Applied Nutrition provides links to information on food safety, labeling, nutrition and cosmetics.

CANCER TREATMENTS CLINICAL ASPECTS

Cancer.gov: Breast Cancer Clinical Trials
www.cancer.gov/clinicaltrials
Information on choosing and participating in clinical trials, results of recent trials and resources for finding a trial.

Inflammatory Breast Cancer (IBC) Research Foundation
www.ibcresearch.org
General information, research, articles, news articles, discussion and commentary on inflammatory breast cancer.

National Cancer Institute

www.cancer.gov

The National Cancer Institute maintains a cancer treatment database providing prognostic, stage and treatment information on more than 1,000 protocol (treatment) summaries.

National Comprehensive Cancer Network: Breast Cancer Treatment Guidelines for Patients

www.nccn.org

Decision trees included on this site aid patients in choosing treatment and follow-up options. Also available in Spanish.

CHILDREN AND FAMILIES

Caring Bridge

www.caringbridge.org

Non-profit Web service that provides a free Web site to anyone going through a health crisis, treatment or recovery.

Kids Konnected

1-800-899-2866

www.kidskonnected.org

Kids Konnected is a non-profit organization that provides for the needs of the children of cancer patients. They offer a kid-friendly and informative Web site, a 24-hour hotline, leadership training, support groups, online forums, a teddy bear outreach program and other support tools for children and families.

EMPLOYMENT CONCERNS

American Cancer Society — Americans With Disabilities Act

http://www.cancer.org/docroot/MIT/mit_3_1_2.asp

Provides basic information about the Americans with Disabilities Act.

Family and Medical Leave Act

1-866-4 US WAGE (1-866-487-9243)

http://www.dol.gov

Search: FMLA

Web site includes a fact sheet about FMLA. The toll-free number reaches the Wage and Hour Division at the Department of Labor. They can tell you how to reach the division office nearest you.

National Coalition for Cancer Survivorship (NCCS) Employment

http://www.canceradvocacy.org/resources/employment.html

NCCS offers valuable information on your employment rights as a cancer survivor, including a free download of their publication *Working It Out.*

The US Equal Employment Opportunity Commission

http://www.eeoc.gov/facts/cancer.html

Includes frequently asked questions about cancer in the workplace and patients' and survivors' rights under the Americans with Disabilities Act.

HAIR CARE AND MAKE-UP

Look Good ... Feel Better

1-800-395-LOOK (5665)

www.lookgoodfeelbetter.org

A comprehensive online guide to caring for your hair and skin during cancer treatment. Contact your local American Cancer Society for free classes and instructions on make-up application and hair care during treatment.

INSURANCE AND FINANCES

Cancer.Net
http://www.cancer.net/patient/Library/
Financial+Resources
List of financial resources available through local and national service organizations for travel and housing assistance, medication and treatment cost assistance and general financial information.

Georgetown University Health Policy Institute
http://www.healthinsuranceinfo.net
The Health Policy Institute has prepared a consumer guide for getting and keeping health insurance for each state and the District of Columbia. The guides are accessible for printing or viewing online.

National Coalition for Cancer Survivorship (NCCS) Insurance
http://www.canceradvocacy.org/resources/insurance.html
NCCS offers tips about getting, keeping and affording health insurance, including a free download of their publication *What Cancer Survivors Need to Know About Health Insurance.*

LYMPHEDEMA

National Lymphedema Network
1-800-541-3259
www.lymphnet.org
Provides education and guidance to lymphedema patients, health care professionals and the general public.

MALE BREAST CANCER

ACS: Male Breast Cancer Resource Center
www.cancer.org
Search: male breast cancer
Information and links to other Web sites on male breast cancer.

MedicineNet.com
www.medicinenet.com/male_breast_cancer/article.htm
Provides online education about diagnosis and treatment of male breast cancer.

YourShoes® at Network of Strength
1-800-221-2141
www. networkofstrength.org
The 24-hour YourShoes Support Center can provide you with information about male breast cancer and help address your concerns. Through the Match Program you can be put in touch with a man who has survived male breast cancer.

PREGNANCY AND BREAST CANCER

Breast Cancer.org
www.breastcancer.org/tips/fert_preg_adopt/bc_pregnancy
Discussion of decisions about treatment during pregnancy.

Fertile Hope
www.fertilehope.org
Fertile Hope is a national non-profit organization dedicated to providing reproductive information, support and hope to cancer patients whose medical treatments present the risk of infertility.

Hope for Two: Pregnant With Cancer Network
1-800-743-4471
www.pregnantwithcancer.org
Connects pregnant women diagnosed with cancer to women who have lived through the experience.

PROSTHESIS

Check in the yellow pages of your telephone book, call your local unit of the American Cancer Society or ask your surgeon or nurse for references.

Network of Strength (Formerly Y-Me)
1-800-221-2141 (24-hour English hotline)
1-800-986-9505 (24-hour Spanish hotline)
www.networkofstrength.org
A wig and prosthesis program is available free to women who cannot afford to purchase these items.

ReForma
http://myreforma.com
Reusable, hypoallergenic and self-adhering prosthetic nipples available in two sizes and three colors.

Softee
1-866-605-8585
www.softeeusa.com
Site offering a wide selection of post-surgical products for recovery including reconstruction camisoles.

SEXUALITY

International Academy of Compounding Pharmacies
1-800-927-4227
www.iacprx.org
Allows patients to search for a local compounding pharmacist.

Pure Romance
1-866-ROMANCE
www.pureromance.com
Offers a range of intimate products, in-home parties and the Sensuality, Sexuality, Survival (SSS) program, which serves as a resource for women surviving cancer who have questions about renewing their intimacy.

SUPPORT GROUPS / ORGANIZATIONS

African-American Breast Cancer Alliance (AABCA)
1-800-ACS-2345
www.geocities.com/aabcainc
This organization provides education to African-American women on breast health, early detection and breast cancer support groups. For more information and to see if there is an alliance in your area, call the American Cancer Society at 1-800-ACS-2345.

Breast Cancer Network of Strength
1-800-221-2141 (24 Hour Hotline-English)
1-800-986-9505 (24 Hour Hotline-Spanish)
www.networkofstrength.org
Provides support and counseling through their 24-hour hotline YourShoes®. Trained volunteers, all of whom have had breast cancer, are matched by background and experience to callers whenever possible. Interpreters are available in 150 languages. Referrals for major cancer treatment centers are also available.

Cancer Care, Inc.
1-800-813-HOPE (1-800-813-4673)
www.cancercare.org
Offers free assistance to cancer patients through counseling, education, referral and direct financial assistance.

Living Beyond Breast Cancer
1-888-753-5222
www.lbbc.org
Provides interactive conferences, teleconferences, a toll-free information and support line, free newsletters and publications, low-cost informational recordings and a networking program.

Local Support Groups
Call your local American Cancer Society office for local support group meetings. Local numbers may be acquired by calling the national office at 1-800-ACS-2345. Or call your local cancer treatment center for support group information.

National Asian Women's Heath Organization (NAWHO)

www.nawho.org

The site explains the organization's program, Communicating Across Boundaries: The Asian American Woman's Breast and Cervical Cancer Program, and offers a free download on related cultural competency training.

National Coalition for Cancer Survivorship (NCCS)

1-877-NCCS-YES (1-877-622-7937)

www.canceradvocacy.org

Survivorship information and support. The Cancer Survival Toolbox, a CD of survival skills, is provided free (also available in Spanish).

Pink-Link

www.pink-link.org

A free online breast cancer support network with access to a member forum, online journals and breast cancer resources.

SHARE: Self Help for Women With Breast or Ovarian Cancer

1-866-891-2392

www.sharecancersupport.org

Offers survivor-led support to women with breast or ovarian cancer, their families and friends. Services include hotlines, survivor-led support groups, wellness programs, educational forums and advocacy activities.

Sharsheret (Jewish Women)

1-866-474-2774

www.sharsheret.org

Provides support and resources for young Jewish women facing breast cancer. Offers a peer support network connecting young women with others who share similar diagnoses and experiences, as well as education and outreach programs.

Sisters Network Inc. (African-American Women)

1-866-781-1808

www.sistersnetworkinc.org

African-American breast cancer survivorship organization. Promotes the importance of breast health through empowerment, support, breast education programs, resources, information and research.

The Wellness Community

Phone: 1-202-659-9709 Fax: 1-202-659-9301

www.thewellnesscommunity.org

The Wellness Community is a national non-profit organization dedicated to providing free emotional support, education and hope for people with cancer. There are 20 facilities nationwide. The Web site offers online support groups and an online newsletter for cancer patients.

Yes, I Can Action Now

www.yesicannow.org

"Yes, I Can Now" is a program created by Aventis Oncology for women with breast cancer. It is a Web and mail-based program providing patients with survivor stories, diet and exercise tips, medical information, treatment organizers and other valuable information. Patients can go online to sign up.

The Young Survival Coalition (Young Women)

1-877-972-1011

www.youngsurvival.org

An advocacy and awareness organization for young women who are diagnosed with breast cancer. The group offers support, information and education.

SURGERY

Breast Cancer Network of Strength
1-800-221-2141 (24 Hour Hotline-English)
1-800-986-9505 (24 Hour Hotline-Spanish)
www.networkofstrength.org
Gives referrals to major cancer treatment centers for second opinions or treatments not offered in some localities.

Caring Connections
www.caringinfo.org/stateaddownload
Caring Connections provides free advance directives and instructions for each state that can be opened as a PDF (Portable Document Format) file.

SURVIVORSHIP MAGAZINES

Breast Cancer Wellness Magazine
www.breastcancerwellness.org
Mission of magazine is to empower mind, body and spirit of women diagnosed with breast cancer. Go online for a free subscription.

Coping With Cancer
1-615-790-2400
www.copingmag.com
Coping with Cancer is America's consumer magazine for people whose lives have been touched by cancer. For a subscription go online or call.

CURE
1-800-210-CURE (2873)
www.curetoday.com
CURE is a magazine for cancer patients and their families, providing information on recent advancements in diagnosis, treatment and prevention of cancer. Healthcare providers and patients can go online to sign up for a free subscription.

MAMM
1-646-365-1350
www.mamm.com
MAMM is a magazine devoted to women diagnosed with breast and reproductive cancer. For a subscription go online or call.

SURVIVORSHIP RESOURCES

Imaginis
www.imaginis.com
Web site providing education and the latest news in breast cancer for professionals and patients. Sign up for the online newsletter to receive concise summaries on the latest news and information on breast cancer.

Reach To Recovery
National ACS Office 1-800-ACS-2345
www.cancer.org
This program of the American Cancer Society offers in-home visits from volunteers. Call your local ACS unit for an appointment. Volunteers will share helpful information for recovery, including range of motion exercises for the surgical arm.

Survivorship A-Z: Practical Information for Living Successfully After a Diagnosis
http://www.survivorshipatoz.org
Survivorship A-Z provides practical information survivors need to thrive in the "new normal" that exists after a life-changing diagnosis.

APPENDIX D

Recommended Reading

BREAST CANCER EDUCATION

Breast Cancer Support Partner Handbook
Judy C. Kneece, RN, OCN
Publisher: EduCare Publishing Inc.; 2009
ISBN: 1886665117
(Available at www.educareinc.com)

Breast Cancer Survival Manual:
A Step-by-Step Guide for the Woman
With Newly Diagnosed Breast Cancer
John Link, M.D., Carey Cullinane, M.D., M.P.H.,
Jane Kakkis, M.D., M.P.H., James Waisman, M.D.
Publisher: Holt Paperbacks; 2007
ISBN: 0805082344 (Available on Amazon)

Sexuality and Fertility After Cancer
Leslie R. Schover, Ph.D.
Publisher: Wiley; 09/97
ISBN: 0471181943 (Available on Amazon)

Timeless Healing
Herbert Benson, M.D., Marg Stark
Publisher: Scribner; 03/97
ISBN: 0684831465 (Available on Amazon)

COPING SKILLS

Coping With Life's Stressors
Susanna McMahon, Ph.D.
Publisher: Dell; 07/96
ISBN: 0440507359 (Available on Amazon)

The Feeling Good Handbook
David D. Burns
Publisher: Plume; 05/99
ISBN: 0452281326 (Available on Amazon)

The Human Side of Cancer: Living With
Hope, Coping With Uncertainty
Jimmie C. Holland, M.D., Sheldon Lewis
Publisher: Harper Paperbacks; 10/01
ISBN: 006093042X (Available on Amazon)

I Am Not My Breast Cancer: Women Talk
Openly About Love and Sex, Hair Loss and
Weight Gain, Mothers and Daughters, and
Being a Woman With Breast Cancer
Ruth Peltason
Publisher: Harper Paperbacks; 09/08
ISBN: 0061174076 (Available on Amazon)

Life Strategies: Doing What Works, Doing What Matters
Phillip C. McGraw, Ph.D.
Publisher: Hyperion; 01/06
ISBN: 0786890983 (Available on Amazon)

The Portable Therapist: Wise and Inspiring Answers to the Questions People in Therapy Ask the Most...
Susanna McMahon, Ph.D.
Publisher: Dell; 07/94
ISBN: 0440506034 (Available on Amazon)

DIET AND EXERCISE

The Breast Cancer Survivor's Fitness Plan (Harvard Medical School Guides)
Carolyn M. Kaelin, M.D., M.P.H.,
Francesca Coltrera, Josie Gardiner, Joy Prouty
Publisher: McGraw-Hill; 08/06
ISBN: 0071465782 (Available on Amazon)

Dr. Ann's 10-Step Diet: A Simple Plan for Permanent Weight Loss and Lifelong Vitality
Ann Kulze, M.D.
Publisher: Top Ten Wellness & Fitness; 09/08
ISBN: 0974832812 (Available on Amazon)

Eating Well, Staying Well During and After Cancer
Abby Bloch, Ph.D., R.D.,
Barrie R. Cassileth, Ph.D.,
Michelle D. Holmes, M.D., Dr. P.H.,
Cynthia A. Thomson, Ph.D., R.D.
Publisher: American Cancer Society; 10/03
ISBN: 0944235514 (Available on Amazon)

Eating Well Through Cancer: Easy Recipes & Recommendations During & After Treatment
Holly Clegg, Gerald Miletello, M.D.
Publisher: Self Published; 04/01
ISBN: 0961088877 (Available on Amazon)

INSPIRATIONAL

Cancer: 50 Essential Things to Do; Third Edition
Greg Anderson
Publisher: Plume; 02/09
ISBN: 0452290104 (Available on Amazon)

Chicken Soup for the Breast Cancer Survivor's Soul: Stories to Inspire, Support and Heal
Jack Canfield, Mark Victor Hansen, Mary Olsen Kelly
Publisher: Health Communications; 10/06
ISBN: 0757305210 (Available on Amazon)

Finding the "CAN" in Cancer
Terri Schinazi, Nancy Emerson, Susan Moonan
Publisher: Lulu.com; 04/07
ISBN: 143031365X (Available on Amazon)

Spinning Straw Into Gold: Your Emotional Recovery From Breast Cancer
Ronnie Kaye
Publisher: Fireside; 02/91
ISBN: 0671701649 (Available on Amazon)

The Triumphant Patient: Become an Exceptional Patient in the Face of Life-Threatening Illness
Greg Anderson
Publisher: iUniverse, Inc.; 10/00
ISBN: 0595131050 (Available on Amazon)

Uplift : Secrets from the Sisterhood of Breast Cancer Survivors
Barbara Delinsky
Publisher: Washington Square Press; 05/03
ISBN: 0743431375 (Available on Amazon)

References

American Cancer Society Consumer's Guide to Cancer Drugs
Wilkes, G., R.N., M.S., A.O.C.N., and Ades, T., R.N., M.S., A.O.C.N.,
Sudbury, Massachusetts: Jones and Bartlett Publishers, 2000.

The Breast: Comprehensive Management of Benign and Malignant Disorders, Third Edition
Bland, K., M.D., and Copeland, E., III, M.D., St. Louis: Elsevier Science, 2003.

Clinical Practice Guidelines in Oncology: Breast Cancer, Volume 1
National Comprehensive Cancer Network, 2009.
http://www.nccn.org/professionals/physician_gls/f_guidelines.asp.

Core Curriculum for Oncology Nursing
Itano, J., and Taoka, K., St. Louis: Saunders Company, 2005.

Diseases of the Breast, Third Edition
Harris, J., Lippman, M., Morrow, M., and Osborne, C.K.,
Philadelphia: Lippincott Williams & Wilkins, 2004.

Ferri's Clinical Advisor 2008: Instant Diagnosis and Treatment
Ferri, F., M.D., F.A.C.P., St. Louis: Mosby, 2008.

Guidelines for Detection, Prevention and Risk Reduction: Breast Cancer Risk Reduction, Volume 1
National Comprehensive Cancer Network, 2009.
http://www.nccn.org/professionals/physician_gls/f_guidelines.asp.

Guidelines for Detection, Prevention, and Risk Reduction: Genetic/Familial High Risk Assessment Breast and Ovarian Cancer, Volume 1
National Comprehensive Cancer Network, 2009.
http://www.nccn.org/professionals/physician_gls/f_guidelines.asp.

PDxMD: Hematology and Oncology
Ferrari, M., Britain: Elsevier Science, 2003.

Pocket Radiologist: Breast
Birdwell, R., M.D., Philadelphia: Saunders, 2003.

Psycho-oncology
Holland, J., M.D., New York: Oxford University Press, 1998.

Survivorship

The caterpillar views the cocoon as life threatening …
The butterfly views the cocoon as life-giving.

A cancer diagnosis is similar to the transformation of a caterpillar into a butterfly. At diagnosis, as a little caterpillar crawling along in life, you find yourself physically coming to a stopping place during treatment where you spin a cocoon around your body. Inside this safe web, you hibernate physically and emotionally. However, during this time, a strange phenomenon is occurring—strangely enough, you are changing your very essence.

Just like the caterpillar, after a period of dormancy, your treatments end—the cocoon breaks open. You emerge, a new and beautiful person—just like the butterfly. To your amazement, you can now fly! Time spent in the cocoon has transformed you.

No longer do you crawl, but now you can fly in a newfound freedom. You may not even recognize your former self. From your vantage point, you enjoy life from a new perspective. Your freedom brings joy into others' lives as they view your brilliance and brings you confidence as you spread your new wings. They are attracted by and amazed at the change they see in you. Peers look to you as a role model. You have emerged as a new creature, my dear one.

Cancer, though one of the scariest words you will ever hear, is surprisingly preparing you for an even better life. So use your time in the cocoon of treatment as a time to redefine yourself and your life. Your challenge is to live each day to its fullest. You are being set free to fly!

Glossary

It is important to understand the medical terminology related to your diagnosis and treatments. The following is a list of the most common medical terms used in breast cancer. If you do not understand the technical language used by your doctors or nurses, ask them to explain what they mean. Understanding the terms will enable you to make intelligent decisions.

A

ABSCESS — A collection of pus from an infection.

ABSOLUTE RISK REDUCTION — Absolute number of patients who will benefit from a treatment.

ACINI — The parts of the breast gland where fluid or milk is produced (singular: acinus).

ACUTE — Occurring suddenly or over a short period of time.

ADENOCARCINOMA — A form of cancer that involves cells from the lining of the walls of many different organs of the body. Breast cancer is a type of adenocarcinoma.

ADJUVANT TREATMENT — Treatment that is added to increase the effectiveness of a primary treatment. In cancer, adjuvant treatment usually refers to chemotherapy, hormonal therapy or radiation therapy after surgery to increase the likelihood of killing all cancer cells.

ALKYLATING AGENT — Type of chemotherapy drug used in cancer treatment.

ALLERGIC REACTION — Various physical symptoms that may include rash, hives, itching, nasal congestion, watery and red eyes, swelling of the throat or difficulty breathing that occur when the body reacts to a substance that it is exposed to or that is ingested.

Ask QUESTIONS.

BE INFORMED.

LIVE ONE DAY AT A TIME.

—JUDY M. SHEEKS, Survivor

*ABSOLUTELY
NOTHING IN MY LIFE
PREPARED ME
FOR CANCER—
EXCEPT GOD.*

*—KAY C. HARVEY
Survivor*

*AFTER CANCER,
LIFE MAY GET BACK TO
NORMAL, BUT IT WILL
NEVER BE THE SAME.
YOU WILL ALWAYS SEE
LIFE FROM A DIFFERENT
VANTAGE POINT.*

ALOPECIA — Refers to hair loss as a result of chemotherapy or radiation therapy administered to the head. Hair loss from chemotherapy is temporary. Hair loss from radiation may be permanent.

ALTERNATIVE MEDICINE — Treatment used instead of standard treatments. They generally are not recognized by the medical community as standard or conventional medical approaches.

AMENORRHEA — Absence or discontinuation of menstrual periods.

ANALGESIC — Medicine given to control pain; for example: Aspirin or Tylenol®.

ANEMIA — Condition marked by a decrease in the blood component hemoglobin that causes symptoms of fatigue, weakness, dizziness, inability to concentrate and shortness of breath. Many chemotherapy drugs cause a reduction in hemoglobin levels.

ANESTHESIA — Medication that causes entire or partial loss of feeling or sensation.

ANESTHESIOLOGIST — A doctor who specializes in giving drugs to prevent or relieve pain during surgery or other procedures being done in the hospital.

ANDROGEN — A male sex hormone. Androgens may be used in patients with breast cancer to treat recurrence of the disease.

ANEUPLOID — The characteristic of having either fewer or more than the normal number of chromosomes in a cell. This is an abnormal cell.

ANOREXIA — Severe, uncontrolled loss of appetite.

ANTIEMETIC — A medicine that prevents or relieves nausea and vomiting; used during, and sometimes after, chemotherapy.

ANTIMETABOLITES — Anticancer drugs that interfere with the process of DNA production, thus preventing cell division.

AREOLA — The circular field of dark-colored skin surrounding the nipple.

ASPIRATION — Removal of fluid or cells from tissue by inserting a needle into an area and drawing the fluid into the syringe.

ASYMPTOMATIC — Without obvious signs or symptoms of disease. While cancer may cause symptoms and warning signs, it may develop and grow without producing any symptoms, especially in its early stages.

ATYPICAL CELLS — Not usual; abnormal. Cancer is the result of atypical cell division.

AUTOLOGOUS — Tissue from your own body.

AXILLA — The armpit.

AXILLARY DISSECTION — Surgical removal of lymph nodes from the armpit. The tissue removed is sent to the pathologist to determine if the breast cancer has spread outside of the breast. The number of nodes dissected varies during surgery. Your physician can tell you how many nodes were removed.

AXILLARY NODES — Lymph nodes in the axilla (underarm). These nodes may be cut out and examined during surgery to see if the cancer has spread past the breast. The number of nodes in this area varies.

AXILLARY SAMPLING — Procedure where lymph nodes are removed from under the arm during breast cancer surgery to evaluate if cancer is present.

BENIGN TUMOR — An abnormal growth that is not cancer and does not spread to other parts of the body.

BILATERAL — Pertains to both sides of the body. For example, bilateral breast cancer would be on both sides of the body or in two breasts.

BIOLOGICAL RESPONSE MODIFIER — Treatment used that alters the body's natural response to stimulate bone marrow to make specific blood cells. Referred to as a colony stimulating factor.

BIOPSY — The surgical removal of a small piece of tissue or a small tumor for microscopic examination to determine if cancer cells are present. A biopsy is the most important procedure in diagnosing cancer.

BIOTHERAPY — Treatments used to stimulate the body's immune system.

BLOOD COUNT — A test to measure the number of red blood cells (RBCs), white blood cells (WBCs) and platelets in a blood sample.

BONE MARROW — The soft, fatty substance filling the cavities of the bones. Blood cells are manufactured in the bone marrow. Chemotherapy affects the bone marrow, resulting in a temporary decrease in the number of cells in the blood.

BONE MARROW BIOPSY AND ASPIRATION — A procedure in which a needle is inserted into the center of a bone, usually the hip, to remove a small amount of bone marrow for microscopic examination.

BONE SCAN — A procedure in which a trace amount of radioactive substance is injected into the bloodstream to illuminate the bones under a special camera to see if the cancer has spread to the bones.

BRCA 1 AND BRCA 2 — Genes identified to increase risk of hereditary

Anxiety is treated by doing something. If it is on your mind, do something about it.

Breast cancer prompts a desire to take action.

—JUDY E. WINDSOR
Survivor

BECAUSE A WISE PATIENT KNOWS HER ENERGY IS LIMITED, SHE ALLOTS HER TIME TO THINGS SHE ENJOYS MOST AND SAYS "NO" TO THE OTHERS.

breast cancer.

BREAST CANCER — A potentially fatal tumor, because of its ability to leave the breast and go to other vital organs and continue to grow if it is not removed from the body. These are breast cells that are abnormal with uncontrolled growth.

BREAST IMPLANT — A round or teardrop-shaped sac inserted into the body to restore the shape of the breast. May be filled with saline water or synthetic material.

BREAST-CONSERVING SURGERY — Surgery that removes cancer while saving the basic cosmetic appearance of the breast including the nipple and areola.

BREAST SELF-EXAM (BSE) — A procedure to examine the breasts thoroughly once a month to detect any changes or suspicious lumps. Exams should be practiced at the end of the menstrual period or seven days after the start of the period and should be performed monthly at the same time.

CALCIFICATIONS — Small calcium deposits in breast tissue seen on mammography. They are the smallest object detected on a mammogram. Deposits are the result of cell death. Occurs with benign and malignant changes.

CAM — Stands for <u>C</u>omplementary, <u>A</u>lternative <u>M</u>edicine.

CANCER — A general term used to describe more than 100 different uncontrolled growths of abnormal cells in the body. Cancer cells have the ability to continue to grow, invade and destroy surrounding tissue, leave the original site and travel via lymph or blood systems to other parts of the body where they can set up new cancerous tumors.

CANCER HAS GIVEN ME A PURPOSE. IT HAS MOST ASSUREDLY OPENED BOTH MY EYES AND MY HEART.

—*ROSE-MARIE BOWMAN GANN*
Survivor

CANCER CELL — A cell that divides and reproduces abnormally with uncontrolled growth. This cell can break away and travel to other parts of the body and set up another site; this is referred to as metastasis.

CAPSULAR CONTRACTURE — Fibrous tissues that form around an implant and cause changes in the shape of the implant and potential pain.

CARDIOLOGIST — Physician specializing in heart disease.

CLAVICLE — The collarbone.

CARCINOEMBRYONIC ANTIGEN (CEA) — A blood test used to monitor women with metastatic breast cancer to help determine if the treatment is working. This is not a test specific for cancer.

218

CARCINOGEN — Any substance that initiates or promotes the development of cancer. For example, asbestos is a proven carcinogen.

CARCINOMA — A form of cancer that develops in tissues covering or lining organs of the body, such as the skin, the uterus, the lung or the breast.

CARCINOMA IN SITU — An early stage of development, when the cancer is still confined to the tissues of origin and has not spread outside the area. In situ carcinomas are highly curable.

CAT SCAN OR CT SCAN — An imaging exam that uses X-rays to create cross-sectional pictures of the body.

CELL — The basic structural unit of all life. All living matter is composed of cells.

CELLULITIS — Infection occurring in soft tissues. Your surgical arm has an increased risk for cellulitis because of the removal of lymph nodes. Pain, swelling and warmth occur in the area.

CHEMOTHERAPY — Treatment of cancer by use of chemicals. Usually refers to drugs used to treat cancer.

CLINICAL TRIAL — A scientific study, generally involving a large number of test subjects (or patients), that is conducted to prove or determine the effectiveness of a drug or treatment program. Limited experimental evidence and preliminary studies prior to the clinical trial has shown or suggested the potential effectiveness and usefulness of the drug or treatment.

COBRA — Consolidated Omnibus Budget Reconciliation Act of 1985. A health insurance available if you are terminated or laid off from your job. This health insurance would remain in effect for a period of 18 months after the job is terminated.

COMBINATION CHEMOTHERAPY — Treatment consisting of the use of two or more chemicals to achieve maximum kill of tumor cells.

COMBINED MODALITY THERAPY — Two or more types of treatments used to supplement each other. For instance, surgery, radiation, chemotherapy, hormonal or immunotherapy may be used separately or together for maximum effectiveness.

COMPLEMENTARY MEDICINE — Treatment often used to enhance or complement standard treatments. For example, massage therapy.

COMPLETE BLOOD COUNT (CBC) — A laboratory test to determine the number of red blood cells, white blood cells, platelets, hemoglobin and other components of a blood sample.

COMPUTERIZED TOMOGRAPHY SCANS — Commonly called CT or CAT scans. These specialized X-ray studies detect cancer or metastasis.

CANCER REMINDS YOU OF A VALUABLE LESSON—DON'T WASTE A HAPPINESS OPPORTUNITY.

CRY WHEN YOU MUST. REMEMBER, IT COULD BE WORSE. JUST DO YOUR BEST. CRY AND YOU'LL FEEL BETTER. DANCE ALSO IF POSSIBLE.

—AUDREY E. MITCHELL
Survivor

CANCER ATTACKS
THE BODY FIRST AND
THEN IT INVADES THE
SPIRIT. SOMETIMES
THE BODY IMPROVES
MORE QUICKLY THAN
THE SPIRIT.

CONTRAST AGENT — Compounds used to improve the visibility of internal bodily structures during an X-ray image or an MRI.

COOPER'S LIGAMENTS — Flexible fibrous elastic bands of tissue passing from the chest muscle into the breast tissues between the lobes of the breasts, providing shape and support for the breasts.

CORE BIOPSY — Removal (with a large needle) of a section (core) of a lump. The core is sent to the lab to see if the lump is benign or malignant.

CYST — An abnormal sac-like structure that contains liquid or semi-solid material; is usually benign. Lumps in the breast are often found to be harmless cysts.

CYTOLOGY — The study of cells that have been sloughed off, cut out or scraped off organs; cells are microscopically examined for signs of cancer.

CYTOTOXIC — Drugs that can cause the death of cancer cells. Usually refers to drugs used in chemotherapy treatments.

DELAYED RECONSTRUCTION — Reconstruction performed at any time after breast cancer surgery.

DEPRESSION — A mental condition marked by ongoing feelings of sadness, despair, loss of energy, difficulty dealing with normal daily life, feelings of worthlessness and hopelessness, loss of pleasure in activities, changes in eating or sleeping habits, and thoughts of death or suicide.

DETECTION — The discovery of an abnormality in an asymptomatic or symptomatic person.

DEXA SCAN — Dual Energy X-ray Absorptiometric scan. An imaging test that measures bone density to diagnose osteoporosis.

DIAGNOSIS — The process of identifying a disease by its characteristic signs, symptoms and laboratory findings. With cancer, the earlier the diagnosis is made, the better the chance for a cure.

DIAPHANOGRAPHY (DPG) — A non-invasive procedure (no cutting) that uses ordinary light as an investigative tool to detect breast masses. Also called transillumination.

DIEP RECONSTRUCTION — A type of breast reconstruction in which blood vessels called Deep Inferior Epigastric Perforators (DIEP) are removed along with the skin and fat connected to them from the lower abdomen. Muscle is not used.

DON'T WITHDRAW
OR ISOLATE YOURSELF.
REACH OUT AND TALK.
SPILL YOUR EMOTIONS.

—KATHY MANOS
Survivor

DIFFERENTIATED — The similarity between a normal cell and the cancer cell; defines what degree of change has occurred. Cancer cells that are well differentiated are close to the original cell and are usually less aggressive. Poorly differentiated cells have changed more and are more aggressive.

DIPLOID — The characteristic of having two sets of chromosomes in a cell. This is normal for a breast cell.

DNA — One of two nucleic acids (the other is RNA) found in the nucleus of all cells. DNA contains genetic information on cell growth, division and cell function.

DOSE-DENSE CHEMOTHERAPY — Same amount (dose) of chemotherapy drugs given in a shorter period of time. Usually every two weeks rather than every three weeks.

DOUBLING TIME — The time required for a cell to double in number. Breast cancer has been shown to double in size every 23 to 209 days. It would take one cell, doubling every 100 days, eight to ten years to reach one centimeter (⅜ inch, or the size of the tip of your small finger).

DUCTAL CARCINOMA IN SITU — A cancer inside the ducts of the breast that has not grown through the wall of the duct into the surrounding tissues. Sometimes referred to as a precancer. Good prognosis is involved with in situ cancers.

DUCTAL PAPILLOMAS — Small, noncancerous, finger-like growths in the mammary ducts that may cause a bloody nipple discharge. Commonly found in women 45 to 50 years of age.

EDEMA — Excess fluid in the body or a body part that is described as swollen or puffy.

ENDOCRINE MANIPULATION — Treating breast cancer by changing the hormonal balance of the body to prevent hormone-dependent cancer cells from multiplying.

ESTROGEN — A female hormone, secreted by the ovaries, that is essential for menstruation, reproduction and the development of secondary sex characteristics, such as breasts. Some patients with breast cancer are given drugs to suppress the production of estrogen in their bodies.

ESTROGEN RECEPTOR ASSAY (ERA) — A test that is done on cancerous tissue to see if a breast cancer is hormone-dependent and may be treated with

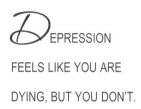

DEPRESSION FEELS LIKE YOU ARE DYING, BUT YOU DON'T.

EVEN THOUGH BREAST CANCER TOTALLY DISRUPTS YOUR LIFE, IT IS ONLY A TEMPORARY DETOUR.

—SHELLY BELKA
Survivor

hormonal therapy. The test will reveal if your cancer is estrogen receptor positive or negative.

ESTROGEN RECEPTORS (ER) — Describes cells that have a protein to which the hormone estrogen will bind. Cancer cells that are estrogen receptor positive need estrogen to grow. Tumor is tested by the pathologist after surgery to determine if cells are estrogen positive or estrogen negative.

EXCISIONAL BIOPSY — Surgical removal of a lump or suspicious tissue by cutting the skin and removing the tissue.

EXTERNAL BEAM RADIATION — High dose of X-ray beams delivered to the site of cancer by a machine called a linear accelerator.

FAMILIAL CANCER — Cancer occurring in families more frequently than would be expected by chance.

FAMILY AND MEDICAL LEAVE ACT (FMLA) — Law that allows eligible employees to take up to 12 work weeks in any 12-month period off from work for personal illness.

FATIGUE — A condition marked by extreme tiredness and inability to function due to lack of energy.

FAT NECROSIS TUMOR — A hard, noncancerous lump caused by the destruction of fat cells in the breast due to trauma or injury.

FERTILITY — The ability to have children.

FIBROADENOMA — A noncancerous, solid tumor most commonly found in younger women.

FIBROCYSTIC BREAST CHANGES OR CONDITION — A noncancerous breast condition in which multiple cysts or lumpy areas develop in one or both breasts. It can be accompanied by discomfort or pain that fluctuates with the menstrual cycle. Large cysts can be treated by aspiration of the fluid they contain.

FINE NEEDLE ASPIRATION — A procedure to remove cells or fluid from tissues using a needle with an empty syringe. Cells or breast fluid, extracted by pulling back on the plunger, are analyzed by a physician.

FLAP NECROSIS — Cell death of flap tissues transplanted from another area of the body during reconstruction; caused by lack of blood supply to the tissues.

EVERY TIME YOU REFUSE TO ASK QUESTIONS, YOU HAMPER YOUR OWN ABILITY TO COPE.

FINDING THE HUMOR IN BREAST CANCER HAS BROUGHT ME TREMENDOUS PHYSICAL AND PSYCHOLOGICAL HEALING.

—*JANE HILL*
Survivor

FLOW CYTOMETRY — A test done on cancerous tissues that shows the aggressiveness of the tumor. It shows how many cells are in the dividing stage at one time, commonly referred to as the "S" phase, and the DNA content of the cancer, referred to as the ploidy. This reveals how rapidly the tumor is growing.

FREE FLAP — Tissues (skin and fat with or without muscle) removed from an area of the body that are cut free from their original blood supply and reattached at the new reconstruction site.

FROZEN SECTION — A technique in which a part of the biopsy tissue is frozen immediately, and a thin slice of frozen tissue is mounted on a microscope slide for a diagnostic examination by a pathologist.

FROZEN SHOULDER — Surgical shoulder which has a severely restricted range of motion and is painful.

G

GALACTOCELE — A clogged milk duct often associated with childbirth.

GAMMA-DETECTION PROBE — Instrument used during sentinel node biopsy to identify radiation uptake of first nodes that drain a tumor.

GENES — Segments of DNA that contain hereditary information that is transferred from cell to cell; genes are located in the nucleus of the cell.

GENETIC — Refers to the inherited pattern located in genes for certain characteristics.

GLUTEUS (GLUTEAL) FLAP — Tissues composed of muscle, fat and blood vessels removed from the buttocks and used to reconstruct the breast.

GLYCEMIC INDEX — Measure of the increase in the level of blood glucose (a type of sugar) caused by eating a specific carbohydrate.

H

HEALTHCARE DIRECTIVES — A written document that instructs others about your healthcare wishes, including appointing a healthcare agent and specific healthcare instructions, should you be unable to make decisions on your own.

HEMATOMA — A collection of blood that can form in a wound after surgery, an aspiration or an injury.

FOR A PERSON TO LEARN TO LIVE AT PEACE WITH UNCERTAINTY AND YET NOT BE PARALYZED BY IT IS A MASTERFUL SIGN OF MATURITY.

GET THE FACTS ABOUT YOUR CANCER. IT IS THE ONLY WAY YOU CAN MAKE AN INFORMED DECISION.
—*Survivor*

HUMOR HELPS. GO OUT EACH DAY WITH JOY.
—*MILDRED HYDRICK*
Survivor

HIDING BEHIND PRETENSE IS DRAINING. IT ROBS YOU OF THE LOVE AND CARING YOU NEED. OPEN UP. TALK. LET PRETENSE BE A THING OF THE PAST.

HEMOGLOBIN — A component inside red blood cells that binds to oxygen in the lungs and carries it to all the tissues in the body.

HER2/NEU — Human epidermal growth factor receptor 2 is a protein identified in breast cancer indicating increased aggressiveness.

HORMONAL THERAPY — Treatment of cancer by alteration of the hormonal balance. Some cancers will only grow in the presence of certain hormones.

HORMONES — Chemicals secreted by various organs in the body that help regulate growth, metabolism and reproduction. Some hormones are used as treatment following surgery for breast, ovarian and prostate cancers.

HORMONE RECEPTOR ASSAY — A diagnostic test to determine whether a breast cancer's growth is influenced by hormones or if it can be treated with hormones.

HOT FLASHES — A sensation of heat and flushing that occurs suddenly. May be associated with menopause or some chemotherapy medications.

HYPERPLASIA — An abnormal, excessive growth of cells that is benign.

IMMEDIATE RECONSTRUCTION — Breast reconstruction performed immediately after breast cancer surgery.

IMMUNE SYSTEM — A complex system by which the body protects itself from outside invaders that are harmful to the body.

IMMUNOLOGY — The study of the body's mechanisms of resistance against disease and invasion by foreign substances—the body's ability to fight a disease.

IMMUNOTHERAPY — A treatment that stimulates the body's own defense mechanisms to combat diseases such as cancer.

IMMUNOSUPPRESSED — Condition of having a lowered resistance to disease. May be a temporary result of lowered white blood cells from chemotherapy administration.

INCISIONAL BIOPSY — A surgical incision made through the skin to remove a portion of a suspected lump or tissue.

INFILTRATING CANCER — Cancer that has grown through the cell wall of the breast area in which it originated, and into the surrounding tissues.

INFILTRATING DUCTAL CARCINOMA — A cancer that begins in the mammary duct and has spread to areas outside the duct.

INFORMATION ABOUT MY CANCER WAS NECESSARY FOR ME TO ONCE AGAIN FEEL IN CONTROL OF MY LIFE.

—ANN PARKER
Survivor

INFLAMMATION — Reaction of tissue to various conditions that may result in pain, redness or warmth of tissues in the area.

INFLAMMATORY CARCINOMA — Very aggressive cancer in the lymphatics of the breast; requires immediate treatment with chemotherapy for disease control.

INFORMED CONSENT — Process of explaining to the patient the risks and complications of a procedure or treatment before it is done. Most informed consents are written and signed by the patient or a legal representative.

IN SITU — In place, localized and confined to one area. A very early stage of cancer.

INTEGRATIVE MEDICINE — Combination of both evidence-based or mainstream medicine and complementary therapies such as massage, yoga, etc.

INTERNAL BREAST RADIATION — Radiation therapy that places the radiation source inside of the breast for short periods of time; given after breast cancer surgery.

INTERNAL MAMMARY NODES — Lymph nodes located in the area near the breastbone.

INTRADUCTAL — Residing within the duct of the breast. Intraductal disease may be benign or malignant.

INTRAMUSCULAR (I.M.) — To receive a medication by needle injection into the muscle of the body.

INTRAVENOUS (I.V.) — Entering the body through a vein.

INVASIVE CANCER — Cancer that has spread outside its site of origin and is growing into the surrounding tissues.

INVERTED NIPPLE — The turning inward of the nipple. Usually a congenital condition; but, if it occurs where it has not previously existed, it can be a sign of breast cancer.

LACTATION — Process of being able to produce milk from the breasts.

LATISSIMUS DORSI — Muscle tissue from the back used for breast reconstruction.

LESION — An area of tissue that is diseased.

LEUKOCYTE — A white blood cell or corpuscle.

ILLNESS IS THE OPPORTUNITY TO THINK ABOUT HOW YOU WANT TO SPEND YOUR LIFE. YOU DONT WANT TO WASTE IT WORKING TO ACQUIRE WHAT YOU DON'T NEED, SEEING THOSE YOU DON'T WANT TO SEE AND DOING WHAT YOU DON'T WANT TO DO.

IF YOU ASK FOR WHAT YOU NEED, YOU MAY NOT GET IT. BUT THE ODDS ARE FAR WORSE IF YOU DON'T ASK.

LETTING GO OF ALL THE "YOU SHOULDS" IN YOUR LIFE AND REPLACING THEM WITH "I WANT" BRINGS AN ENORMOUS SENSE OF FREEDOM TO LIVE LIFE WITH RENEWED ENERGY.

LEUKOPENIA — A decrease in the number of white blood cells (where the count is less than 5000); increases a person's susceptibility to infection.

LINEAR ACCELERATOR — A machine that produces high-energy X-ray beams to destroy cancer cells.

LIVER SCAN — A way of visualizing the liver by injecting into the bloodstream a trace dose of a radioactive substance which helps visualize the organ during X-ray.

LIVING WILL — Document signed by an individual stating her wishes in medical care issues if she is unable to properly communicate or make decisions.

LOBULAR — Pertaining to the part of the breast that is furthest from the nipple, the lobes.

LOCALIZED CANCER — A cancer still confined to its site of origin.

LOCAL RECURRENCE — Cancer that recurs in the area of the primary tumor after a period of time when cancer was non-detectable but has not spread to distant organs.

LUMP — Any kind of abnormal mass in the breast or elsewhere in the body.

LUMPECTOMY — A surgical procedure in which only the cancerous tumor and an area of surrounding tissue is removed. Usually the surgeon will remove some of the underarm lymph nodes at the same time. This procedure is also referred to as a tylectomy.

LYMPH — A clear fluid circulating throughout the body in the lymphatic system that contains white blood cells and antibodies.

LYMPH NODES — Also called lymph glands. These are rounded body tissues in the lymphatic system that vary in size from a pinhead to an olive and may appear in groups or one at a time. The principal ones are in the neck, underarm and groin. These glands produce lymphocytes and monocytes (white blood cells which fight foreign substances) and serve as filters to prevent bacteria from entering the bloodstream. They will filter out cancer cells but will also serve as a site for metastatic disease. The major ones serving the breast are in the armpit. Some are located above and below the collarbone and some in between the ribs near the breast-bone. There are three levels of lymph nodes in the underarm area of the breast and another around the breastbone. The number of nodes varies from person to person. Lymph nodes are usually sampled during surgery to determine if the cancer has spread outside of the breast area.

LYMPHATIC VESSELS — Vessels that remove cellular waste from the body by filtering through lymph nodes and eventually emptying into the vascular (blood) system.

LIVE LIFE ONE DAY AT A TIME. YOU CAN'T CHANGE YESTERDAY. FORGET THOSE "IF ONLY" THOUGHTS. WORRYING ABOUT TOMORROW ONLY MAKES THINGS WORSE.

—HARRIETT BARRINEAU
Survivor

LIFE AFTER A CANCER DIAGNOSIS CAN BE VIEWED AS A CHALLENGE OR AS A PREDICAMENT TO BE ENDURED. HOW YOU DETERMINE TO EXPERIENCE YOUR OWN JOURNEY IS UP TO YOU.

LYMPHEDEMA — A swelling in the arm (or extremities) caused by excess fluid that collects after the lymph nodes have been removed by surgery or affected by radiation treatments.

M

MACROCYST — A cyst that is large enough to be felt with the fingers.

MAGNETIC RESONANCE IMAGING (MRI) — A magnetic scan; a form of X-ray using magnets instead of radiation. MRI gives a more clearly defined picture of fatty tissue than X-ray.

MAGNIFICATION VIEW — Special enlarged views to magnify an area for greater detail of suspicious finding. Used in mammography.

MALIGNANT TUMOR — A mass of cancer cells. These cells have uncontrolled growth and will invade surrounding tissues and spread to distant sites of the body, setting up new cancer sites; this process is called metastasis.

MAMMARY DUCT ECTASIA — A noncancerous breast disease most often found in women during menopause. The ducts in or beneath the nipple become clogged with cellular and fatty debris. The duct may have gray to greenish discharge, a lump you can feel, and can become inflamed, causing pain.

MAMMARY GLANDS — The breast glands that produce and carry milk by way of the mammary ducts to the nipples during pregnancy and breastfeeding.

MAMMOGRAM — An X-ray of the breast that can detect tumors before they can be felt. A baseline mammogram is performed on healthy breasts usually at the age of 35 – 40 to establish a basis for later comparison.

MARGINS — The area of tissue surrounding a tumor when it is removed by surgery.

MASTALGIA — Pain occurring in the breast.

MASTECTOMY — Surgical removal of the entire breast, including nipple, areola, lymph nodes and some of the surrounding tissue.

- **MODIFIED RADICAL MASTECTOMY** — The most common type of mastectomy. Breast skin, nipple, areola and underarm lymph nodes are removed. The chest muscles are saved.

- **PROPHYLACTIC MASTECTOMY** — A preventative procedure sometimes recommended for patients at a very high risk for developing cancer in one or both breasts.

LEARNING TO "LET GO" OF THINGS WE CAN'T CHANGE IS ONE OF THE MOST IMPORTANT STEPS TO EASING OUR SUFFERING.

MUSIC HAS ALWAYS BEEN AN IMPORTANT PART OF MY LIFE. WHENEVER I FELT THE NEED FOR A BOOST, I'D START SINGING.

—LOUISE K. EDWARDS
Survivor

*M*EDICAL BILLS

HAVE BEEN

OVERWHELMING.

BUT, BY THE GRACE OF

GOD, I'M TRYING.

—*Survivor*

- **RADICAL MASTECTOMY (HALSTED RADICAL)** — The surgical removal of the breast, breast skin, nipple, areola, chest muscles and underarm lymph nodes.

- **SEGMENTAL MASTECTOMY (PARTIAL MASTECTOMY/LUMPECTOMY)** A surgical procedure in which only a portion of the breast is removed, including the cancer and the surrounding margin of healthy breast tissue.

- **SUBCUTANEOUS MASTECTOMY** — Performed before cancer is detected. A procedure that removes the breast tissue but leaves the outer skin, areola and nipple intact. (This is not suitable with a diagnosis of cancer.)

MASTITIS — An infection occurring in the breast. Pain, tenderness, swelling, redness and warmth may be observed. Usually responds to antibiotic treatment.

MENOPAUSE — The time in a woman's life when the menstrual cycle ends and the ovaries produce lower levels of hormones; usually occurs between the ages of 45 and 55.

METASTASIS — The spread of cancer from one part of the body to another through the lymphatic system or the bloodstream. The cells in the new cancer location are the same type as those in the original site.

MICROCALCIFICATIONS — Particles observed on a mammogram that are found in the breast tissue, appearing as small spots on the picture. Usually occur from calcium deposits caused by death of breast cells that may be benign or malignant. When clustered in one area, may need to be checked more closely for a malignant change in the breast.

MICROCYST — A cyst that is too small to be felt but may be observed on mammography or ultrasound screening.

MICROMETASTASIS — The undetectable spread of cancer outside of the breast that is not seen on routine screening tests. Metastasis is too limited to have created enough mass to be observed.

MITOTIC RATE — Rate of cell division and growth of a cancerous tumor.

*M*ANY TIMES,

A GOOD DOSE OF

ASSERTIVENESS—

ASKING FOR WHAT YOU

NEED—CAN BE AS

THERAPEUTIC AS A

GOOD DOSE

OF MEDICINE.

MULTICENTRIC — Describes cancers or suspicious microcalcifications located over more than one quarter of the breast.

MULTIFOCAL — Describes cancers or suspicious microcalcifications located within one quarter of the breast.

MYELOSUPPRESSION — A decrease in the ability of the bone marrow cells to produce blood cells, including red blood cells, white blood cells and platelets. This condition increases susceptibility to infection, increases risk of bleeding and produces fatigue.

NADIR — The time after chemotherapy when blood cell counts reach their lowest levels. According to the type of blood cells affected by different drugs, an increase in infection, fatigue and bleeding occur.

NECROSIS — Death of a tissue.

NEEDLE BIOPSY — Removal of a sample of tissue from the breast using a wide-core needle.

NEEDLE LOCALIZATION — Procedure to mark an area of suspicion in the breast for the surgeon by inserting a needle before surgery.

NEGATIVE NODES — Lymph nodes that do not have evidence of cancer after surgical removal and pathological evaluation.

NEO-ADJUVANT CHEMOTHERAPY — Chemotherapy given before surgery to treat breast cancer.

NEOPLASM — Any abnormal growth. Neoplasms may be benign or malignant, but the term usually is used to describe a cancer.

NEUTROPENIA – Low blood count values of neutrophil cells (type of white blood cells that fight infection); increases potential for infections.

NODULARITY — Increased density of breast tissue, most often due to hormonal changes, which cause the breast to feel lumpy in texture. This finding is called normal nodularity, and it usually occurs in both breasts.

NODULE — A small, solid mass.

NUCLEAR GRADE — An evaluation of the size and shape of the nucleus in tumor cells and the percentage of tumor cells that are in the process of dividing or growing.

ONCOGENE — Certain stretches of cellular DNA. Genes that, when inappropriately activated, contribute to the malignant transformation of a cell.

ONCOLOGIST — A physician who specializes in cancer treatment.

ONCOLOGY — The science dealing with the physical, chemical and biological properties and features of cancer, including causes, the disease process, and therapies.

NOTHING IS MORE FRIGHTENING THAN THE WORD, "CANCER."

NO MATTER HOW DISAPPOINTING, THE TRUTH IS A LOT BETTER THAN A LURKING FEAR.

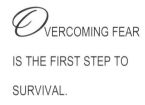

OVERCOMING FEAR IS THE FIRST STEP TO SURVIVAL.

—LISA BOCCARD
Survivor

229

ONLY YOUR FAITH CAN HELP YOU TO ACCEPT AND MOVE ON, NOT WITHOUT REGRETS AND SADNESS ABOUT YOUR LOSS, BUT WITH HOPE AND COURAGE TO FACE THE FUTURE IN SPITE OF YOUR LOSS.

PEOPLE HURT. THE HUMAN SPIRIT IS SENSITIVE TO LOSS. THIS IS NORMAL. EMOTIONAL HEALING MAY TAKE LONGER THAN YOUR PHYSICAL HEALING.

—Survivor

ONCOTYPE DX® — Test performed by evaluating 21 known genes in tumor cells of women with early stage breast cancer to evaluate the potential for breast cancer recurrence and need for chemotherapy.

ONE-STEP PROCEDURE — A procedure in which a surgical biopsy is performed under general anesthesia and if cancer is found, a mastectomy or lumpectomy is done immediately as part of the same operation.

OOPHORECTOMY — The surgical removal of the ovaries, sometimes performed as a part of therapy for breast cancer to reduce hormonal stimulation.

ORGASM — A state of physical and emotional excitement that occurs at the climax of sexual intercourse.

OSTEOPOROSIS — Softening of bones that occurs with age, calcium loss and hormone depletion increasing risk of fracture.

PALLIATIVE TREATMENT — Therapy that relieves symptoms, such as pain or pressure, but does not alter the development of the disease. Its primary purpose is to improve the quality of life.

PALPATION — A procedure using the hands to examine organs such as the breast. A palpable mass is one you can feel with your hands.

PATHOLOGIST — A physician with special training in diagnosing diseases from samples of tissue under a microscope.

PATHOLOGY — The study of disease through the microscopic examination of body tissues and organs. Any tumor suspected of being cancerous must be diagnosed by pathological examination.

PECTORALIS MUSCLES — Muscular tissues attached to the front of the chest wall and extending to the upper arms. These are under the breast and are divided into the pectoralis major and the pectoralis minor muscles.

PEDICLE FLAP – Tissues to reconstruct the breast that are taken from another area of the body, such as the stomach, buttocks or back, and remain attached to their original blood supply.

PER ORALLY (P.O.) — To take a medication by mouth.

PERMANENT SECTION — A technique in which a thin slice of biopsy tissue is mounted on a slide to be examined under a microscope by a pathologist in order to establish a diagnosis.

PHLEBITIS — Inflammation in a vein or veins.

PHYTOCHEMICALS — Chemical components found in plants (vegetables, fruits and nuts) that have a beneficial effect on health.

PLATELET — A cell formed by the bone marrow and circulating in the blood that is necessary for blood clotting. Platelet transfusions are used in cancer patients to prevent or control bleeding when the number of platelets has decreased.

PLOIDY — The number of chromosome sets in a cell.

PORT, LIFE PORT, PORT-A-CATH — A device surgically implanted under the skin, usually on the chest, that enters a large blood vessel and is used to deliver medication, chemotherapy, blood products and also is used to obtain blood samples. A port is usually inserted if a person has veins in the arm that are difficult to use for treatment or if certain types of chemotherapy drugs are to be given.

POSITIVE NODES — Lymph nodes removed during surgery that have cancer cells present after being studied by a pathologist.

PRECANCEROUS — Abnormal cellular changes that are potentially capable of becoming cancer. These early lesions are very amenable to treatment and cure. Also called pre-malignant.

PRETREATMENT MULTIDISCIPLINARY CONFERENCE — Meeting and discussion attended by different types of physicians involved in the treatment of breast cancer. Usually attended by a radiologist, surgeon, oncologist, radiation oncologist, reconstructive surgeon, genetic counselor, nurse navigator and other healthcare providers. Individual case is presented to the group after a positive biopsy and before any surgical intervention or treatment is started. Group discussion allows all physicians to offer their best clinical advice on the particular case under review before any final treatment decision is made.

PRIMARY TUMOR — First or original site of a cancer.

PROGESTERONE — Female hormone produced by the ovaries during a specific time in the menstrual cycle. Causes the uterus to prepare for pregnancy and the breasts to get ready to produce milk.

PROGESTERONE RECEPTOR ASSAY (PRA) — A test that is done on cancerous tissue to see if a breast cancer is progesterone hormone dependent and can be treated by hormonal therapy.

PROGESTERONE RECEPTORS (PR) — A receptor protein in breast cells to which progesterone will attach. Breast cancer cells that are PR+ depend on the hormone progesterone to grow and usually respond to hormonal therapy.

PROGNOSIS — A prediction of the course of the disease—the future prospect for the patient. For example, most breast cancer patients who receive treatment early have a good prognosis.

Pursue happiness, joy and peace for the same reason you take chemotherapy or radiation—it is part of your battle plan against cancer.

Plan to simplify your life. Use your time and energy to do important things. Instead of polishing silver, polish your emotional reserves with things that make you smile, whatever they are.

PUT YOUR EMPHASIS
ON CONTROLLING YOUR
LIFE AND TREATMENTS,
NOT CONTROLLING
YOUR CANCER. YOUR
EMPHASIS SHOULD BE
ON HOW TO LIVE BETTER.

QUIET YOUR
ANXIETY BY BREATHING
DEEPLY AND FOCUSING
ON A REPETITIVE
POSITIVE WORD.

REALIZE THAT
SELF-CARE MEANS
AVOIDING RELATION-
SHIPS THAT ARE
EMOTIONALLY DRAINING.
CANCER IS ENOUGH TO
DEAL WITH. AVOID TOXIC
PEOPLE AND SITUATIONS
WHEN POSSIBLE.

PROLACTIN — A female hormone that stimulates the development of the breasts and later is essential for starting and continuing milk production.

PROPHYLACTIC MASTECTOMY — Removal of high-risk breast tissue to prevent future development of cancer.

PROSTHESIS — An artificial form. In the case of post-mastectomy breast cancer patients, a breast form that can be worn inside a bra.

PROTOCOL — A schedule of selected drugs and treatment time intervals known to be effective against a certain cancer.

PTOSIS — The natural drooping of an organ, such as the breast, caused by aging.

QUACKERY — Treatments, drugs or devices that claim to prevent, diagnose or cure diseases or health conditions, including cancer, that are known to be false or have no proven scientific evidence on which to base their claims.

RADIATION ONCOLOGIST — A physician specifically trained in the use of high energy X-rays to treat cancer.

RADIATION THERAPY — Treatment with high energy X-rays to destroy cancer cells.

RADIOLOGIST — A physician who specializes in diagnoses of diseases by the use of X-rays.

RADIOTHERAPY — Treatment of cancer with high-energy radiation. Radiation therapy may be used to reduce the size of a cancer before surgery or to destroy any remaining cancer cells after surgery. Radiotherapy can be helpful in shrinking recurrent cancer to relieve symptoms such as pain and pressure.

RANGE OF MOTION — The normal movement capability of a limb that is measured in degrees of a circle.

RECONSTRUCTION — The rebuilding of the breast mound after surgical removal. Surgery performed by a reconstructive surgeon using implants or body tissues.

RECURRENCE — Reappearance of cancer after a period of remission.

REGIONAL INVOLVEMENT — The spread of cancer from its original site to nearby surrounding areas. Regional cancers are confined to one location of the body. Regional involvement in breast cancer could include the spread to the lymph nodes or to the chest wall.

REHABILITATION — Programs that help patients adjust and return to full, productive lives. May involve physical therapy, the use of a prosthesis, counseling and emotional support.

RELAPSE — The reappearance of cancer after a disease-free period.

RELATIVE RISK REDUCTION — Figures derived by taking the absolute number of women benefiting from a therapy and translating it into a percentage of increase or decrease.

REMISSION — Complete or partial disappearance of the signs and symptoms of disease in response to treatment. The period during which a disease is under control. A remission, however, is not necessarily a cure.

RETRACTION — The process of skin pulling in toward breast tissue, often referred to as dimpling.

RISK FACTORS — Anything that increases an individual's chance of getting a disease such as cancer. The risk factors for breast disease include having a first degree relative with breast cancer, early menstruation, late menopause, first child after 30 or no children.

RISK REDUCTION — Techniques used to reduce your chances of getting a certain cancer. For example, reducing your dietary fat may help prevent breast cancer.

S

S PHASE — A test that is performed to determine how many cells within the tumor are in a stage of division.

SALINE — Substance that contains salt.

SARCOMA — A form of cancer that arises in the supportive tissues such as bone, cartilage, fat or muscle.

SECONDARY SITE — A second site in which cancer is found. Example: cancer in the lymph nodes near the breast is a secondary site.

SECONDARY TUMOR — A tumor that develops as a result of metastasis or spreads beyond the original cancer.

RECOVERY PRESCRIPTION: DO SOMETHING NEW OR GOOD FOR YOURSELF EVERY DAY.

RIGHT NOW, I'M MORE ASSERTIVE. I FIGURED ONE OF THE WORST THINGS POSSIBLE HAS ALREADY HAPPENED TO ME, SO WHAT HAVE I GOT TO FEAR?

—MARYANN EUBANKS
Survivor

SAYING "NO" TO SOMETHING YOU DON'T WANT TO DO IS SAYING "YES" TO YOURSELF.

*S*TRESSED SPELLED

BACKWARDS IS

DESSERTS. TURN

YOUR STRESS INTO

SOMETHING GOOD.

SENTINEL LYMPH NODE MAPPING — A procedure used to identify the first nodes draining a cancerous tumor by injecting a dye or radioactive contrast agent.

SENTINEL NODE(S) — First identified node or nodes that drain lymphatic fluid from a cancerous tumor.

SERMs (SELECTIVE ESTROGEN RECEPTOR MODULATORS) — Antihormonal drugs that can slow down or stop the growth of cancers that need estrogen to grow. Drugs in this group include tamoxifen, toremifene and raloxifene.

SEROMA — Collection of fluid (noncancerous) under the skin that feels soft and spongy.

SIDE EFFECTS — Usually describes situations that occur after treatments. For example, hair loss may be a side effect of chemotherapy; fatigue may be a side effect of radiation therapy.

SPICULATED — Describes shape of tumor margin that has long needle-like protrusions into surrounding tissues.

SSRIs — Selective Serotonin Reuptake Inhibitors are a class of drugs that increase serotonin in the brain. Used in the treatment of depression.

STAGING — An evaluation of the extent of the disease, such as breast cancer. A classification based on stage at diagnosis which helps determine the appropriate treatment and prognosis. In breast cancer, the classification is determined by whether the lymph nodes are involved; whether the cancer has spread to other parts of the body (through the lymphatic system or bloodstream) and set up distant metastasis; and the size of the tumor. Five different stages (0 – 4) are used in breast cancer with levels in each stage. Stage IV is the most serious.

STELLATE — Appearing on mammography as a star-shape because of the irregular growth of cells into surrounding tissue. May be associated with a malignancy or some benign conditions.

STEREOTACTIC NEEDLE BIOPSY — A biopsy done while the breast is compressed under mammography. A series of pictures locate the lesion, and a radiologist enters information into a computer. The computer calculates information and positions a needle to remove the finding. A needle is inserted into the lump, and a piece of tissue is removed and sent to the lab for analysis. May be referred to as a stereotactic core biopsy.

STOMATITIS — Inflammation of the gastrointestinal tract creating discomfort and a potential for infection. May be caused by chemotherapy drugs.

SUBCUTANEOUS (S.Q. OR S.C.) — To receive a medication by needle injection into the fatty tissues of the body.

*S*HARING WITH

OTHER BREAST

CANCER PATIENTS IS

VERY IMPORTANT.

YOU CANNOT,

MUST NOT, NEED NOT

DO IT ALONE!

—*FELICIA SMITH*
Survivor

SUPRACLAVICULAR NODES — The nodes located above the collarbone in the area of the neck.

SYMPTOMS — Changes you can feel that may or may not be visible to others.

SYSTEMIC — Pertaining to the whole body.

T

TAMOXIFEN — Anti-estrogen drug that may be given to women with estrogen receptive tumors to block estrogen from entering the breast tissues. May produce menopause-like symptoms, including hot flashes and vaginal dryness. Currently being used with high risk women in clinical trials to prevent breast cancer and with women who have had breast cancer to prevent recurrence.

TESTOSTERONE — Major male hormones found in lower amounts in females. Testosterone in females impacts and increases the sex drive and the ability to experience orgasm.

THROMBOCYTOPENIA — A decrease in the number of platelets in the blood, resulting in the potential for increased bleeding and decreased ability for clotting.

TISSUE — A collection of similar cells. There are four basic types of tissues in the body: epithelial, connective, muscle and nerve.

TRAM — Stands for transverse rectus abdominis muscle, the tissue that is used to reconstruct a breast using the major stomach muscle attached to its original blood supply.

TRANSILLUMINATION — The inspection of an organ by passing a light through the tissues. Transmission of the light varies with different densities.

TREATMENT MODALITIES — Different types of treatment. For example: surgery, chemotherapy, radiation therapy and hormonal therapy.

TRIPLE NEGATIVE BREAST CANCER — Breast cancer that shows after testing that the tumor is receptor negative for estrogen (ER), progesterone (PR) and HER2 receptors (human epidermal growth factor receptor 2).

TUMOR — An abnormal tissue, swelling or mass, may be either benign or malignant.

TUMOR GROWTH RATE — Time required for a specific tumor to double in size. Same type of tumor varies in time from person to person.

STRESS IS BETTER MANAGED WHEN IT IS ANTICIPATED. KNOWING WHAT'S AHEAD ALLOWS YOU TO PREPARE TO BUFFER YOUR OWN STRESS. ASK QUESTIONS SO YOU CAN BE PREPARED.

THE REALITY OF NO BREASTS MADE ME FEEL LIKE AN "IT." IT WAS TRULY SILENT SUFFERING. YET, NOW, I CAN TALK ABOUT IT, WHEN BEFORE, I WAS MORTIFIED.

—*Survivor*

TWO-STEP PROCEDURE — When surgical biopsy and breast surgery are performed in two separate surgeries.

U

ULTRASOUND EXAMINATION — The use of high frequency sound waves to locate a tumor inside the body. Helps determine if a breast lump is solid tissue or filled with fluids.

ULTRASOUND GUIDED BIOPSY — The use of ultrasound to guide a biopsy needle to obtain a sample of tissue for analysis by a pathologist.

V

VACUUM-ASSISTED BIOPSY — Biopsy procedure in which an instrument cuts tissues and uses a vacuum to withdraw them into a container.

W

WET/MOIST DESQUAMATION — Condition where the top layers of the skin peel or slough off, exposing red, tender skin that oozes fluid. Condition may occur in late stages of radiation therapy.

WHITE BLOOD CELLS — Components of the blood, also known as leukocytes, that are able to kill bacteria and other invaders in the body. Low white blood cells—identified after a complete blood count is performed—causes one to be more susceptible to infections.

USE YOUR CANCER DIAGNOSIS AS THE EXCUSE TO DO WHAT YOU HAVE ALWAYS WANTED TO DO. PEOPLE WON'T CHALLENGE YOU NOW WITH QUESTIONS LIKE "ARE YOU SURE?"

WE MUST FIGHT WORRY LIKE WE DO CANCER. WE MUST TAKE EVERY EFFORT KNOWN TO GET RID OF IT.

Index

T

U

V

W

Y

Survivorship

Most think that a diagnosis of cancer will end their life, when in reality it changes their life.

Life after cancer may get back to normal, but it will never be the same. You will always see life from a different vantage point.

After cancer treatment the battle to heal your body may be over, but the battle to get on with life and your happiness has just begun.

It is easy to delay gratification or happiness—waiting until the perfect time in the future. You have to retrain yourself to grasp the happiness each day brings and not feel guilty. This is the power of living in the present. Cancer has taught you a powerful lesson—don't waste a happiness opportunity.

—*Judy Kneece*

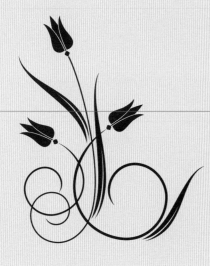

Tear-Out Worksheets

The following tear-out worksheets are designed to help you custom manage your cancer experience. Tear out the worksheets and place them in a notebook.

Topics Include:

- Managing My Fears
- Surgery Questions
- Tumor Location and Size / Appearance after Surgery
- Surgical Decision Evaluation / Reconstructive Decision Evaluation
- Reconstructive Surgery Questions / Reconstructive Surgery Options
- Surgical Discharge Questions / Surgical Discharge Notes
- Drain Bulb Record
- Medical Oncologist Questions / Medical Oncology Consultation Notes
- Radiation Oncologist Questions / Radiation Oncology Consultation Notes
- Personal Healthcare Provider Record
- Personal Treatment Record
- Patient Appointment Reminder
- Personal Plan for Recovery
- Healthcare Symptoms Record
- Personal Treatment Barriers Assessment
- Survivorship Surveillance Guidelines
- Inspirational

Cancer Can't Rob Me

Today is another new day and I can choose to use it in many ways. I did not choose to have cancer, but I can choose how I am going to respond and what I plan to do with today. Today is mine to make choices. This day can be a new beginning for me, if I so choose.

Today can be the day that I decide to exchange those things which weigh my spirit down for a lighter load of faith and trust. I can change my perception of cancer as a "robber" of my health and my future and change it into a vehicle to transport me into a life rich in understanding. This understanding will strengthen me and make me valuable to others who will walk the same path after me.

I can choose:

- To see cancer as a "challenge" instead of as a defeat.
- To demystify cancer by learning about my disease rather than cowering in fear of the unknown.
- To give up concentrating on the "things I can't control" and replace them with thoughts of "what I can control."
- To respond with a spirit of "I can" instead of "I can't."
- To ask for help and not try to face the challenge alone.
- To face my fears with a plan for steps of action against them.
- To look for the blessings in the events of today instead of focusing on losses.
- To add to my life the things I have always wanted to do but postponed until the right time.

Today is the time:

- To use my spiritual faith as a vehicle to understand why and to give me hope.
- To let go of anger, bitterness and resentments, which only slow down my recovery.
- To see my cancer experience as a new tool for personal growth.
- To offer my support and share what I'm learning with others who may need my help.

Therefore, I choose for today:

Peace and not anxiety,

Good and not evil,

Love and not hate,

Gain and not loss.

When today becomes tomorrow, this day will

be gone forever, leaving in its place what I choose today.

I, alone, can choose to use today wisely—

Cancer Can't Rob Me Of This Day!

—Judy Kneece, RN, OCN

MANAGING MY FEARS

In the first column, list all of the fears and worries you are presently facing. In the second column, list the name of the most appropriate person with whom to verbalize these fears. In the third column, think about and list things you can do to change or reduce these fears.

Fears	Person(s) Involved	Things I Can Do

"You can gain strength, courage, and confidence by every experience in which you really stop to look fear in the face.
The danger lies in refusing to face the fear, in not daring to come to grips with it. You must do something you think you cannot do."

—Eleanor Roosevelt

MANAGING MY FEARS

"To fight fear—ACT.
To increase fear—wait,
put off, postpone."

—David Joseph Schwartz

Fears	Person(s) Involved	Things I Can Do

SURGERY QUESTIONS WORKSHEET

Check the questions you would like to have answered.
Tear out this sheet and take it to your surgical consultation.

Surgeon's Name: _____ Date: _____

General Questions

- ☐ What is the name of the type of breast cancer I have?
- ☐ How large is the tumor?
- ☐ Is the tumor in situ (inside ducts or lobules) or invasive (grown through walls of ducts or lobules)?
- ☐ Do you expect cancer cells to be found in my lymph nodes?
- ☐ Do you expect that the cancer has invaded anything else (skin, muscle, bones, other organs)?
- ☐ Is there any evidence from my mammogram that there might be cancer anywhere else in this breast or in the opposite breast?
- ☐ Does my type of cancer have an increased risk of being found in the same breast or occurring, at a future time, in the opposite breast?

Additional Questions _____
_____
_____

Lumpectomy Questions

- ☐ Am I a candidate for a lumpectomy?
  If so, how do you expect my breast to appear after surgery, considering the size of the lump and tissue you need to remove compared to the size of my breast, or the position of the lump in the breast?
- ☐ Do you think the cosmetic results will be acceptable?
- ☐ Which of the lumpectomy procedures do you plan to use (lumpectomy or wide excision)?
- ☐ Am I a candidate for sentinel lymph node biopsy?
  If so, do you evaluate the removed sentinel lymph node(s) during surgery or after surgery?
- ☐ Will you remove lymph nodes by a separate incision under my arm?
- ☐ What do you consider the advantages and disadvantages of a lumpectomy for my case?
- ☐ Will a lumpectomy give me the same chance for control of my cancer as a mastectomy?
- ☐ Will I need to have radiation therapy after a lumpectomy?
- ☐ How long will I be in the hospital?
- ☐ Will I have drains in the incision after surgery?
- ☐ Will I go home with drains?
- ☐ When do you expect the drains to be removed?
- ☐ How long will I need to be away from my job?

Additional Questions _____
_____

W • 5

SURGERY QUESTIONS

Mastectomy Questions

- ☐ Which type of mastectomy do you plan to perform? (Refer to pages 34 – 35)
- ☐ What do you think are the advantages and disadvantages of having a mastectomy?
- ☐ In my particular case, does mastectomy offer a better chance of control of my cancer?
- ☐ Am I a candidate for sentinel lymph node biopsy?

    If so, do you evaluate the removed sentinel lymph node(s) for cancer during surgery or after surgery?
- ☐ How many lymph nodes do you plan to remove?
- ☐ Will I have drain bulbs in my incision after surgery? If so, how many?
- ☐ Will I go home with drains in place?
- ☐ When are drains usually removed?
- ☐ Will I have to have stitches/sutures removed? When and where will this be done?
- ☐ How long will I be in the hospital?
- ☐ When should I be able to resume my normal activities?
- ☐ Are there any types of limitations that I should expect in my surgical arm in the future?
- ☐ When can I plan to return to work?

Additional Questions _____

_____

Reconstruction Questions

- ☐ Am I a candidate for immediate reconstruction?
- ☐ Can you provide me with information about immediate reconstruction?
- ☐ Tell me the advantages and disadvantages of immediate reconstruction.
- ☐ Could you provide me with information on the use of implants and the potential use of my body tissues for reconstruction?
- ☐ Do you foresee anything in my present health status which could prevent me from having either type of reconstruction?

Additional Questions _____

_____

Final Questions

- ☐ Is there anything else you need to tell me about my cancer or surgery?
- ☐ Do you have any written information on my cancer or surgery?
- ☐ Do you recommend any books or DVDs?
- ☐ Do you recommend any support groups or a professional counselor?
- ☐ If I have additional questions, whom should I call and whom should I speak with (nurse/physician)?

Additional Questions _____

_____

TUMOR LOCATION & SIZE

Tumor Location

Ask your physician to draw where your tumor is located in your breast and the estimated amount of tissue that will be removed during surgery.

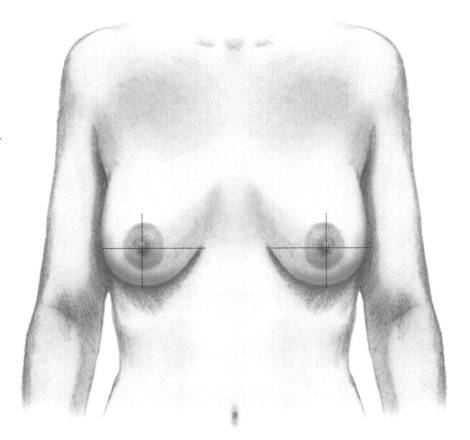

Tumor Size

Ask your physician to draw the estimated size of your tumor on this chart.

Tumor size is the largest dimension of the tumor. Results are reported in centimeters (cm) or millimeters (mm).

- 10 mm equals 1 cm
- 1 cm equals ⅜ inch
- 1 inch equals 2.5 cm

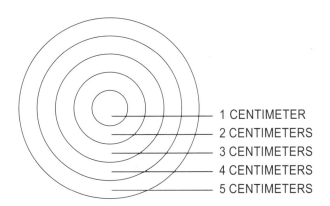

- 1 CENTIMETER
- 2 CENTIMETERS
- 3 CENTIMETERS
- 4 CENTIMETERS
- 5 CENTIMETERS

APPEARANCE AFTER SURGERY

Ask your surgeon to draw your planned incision.

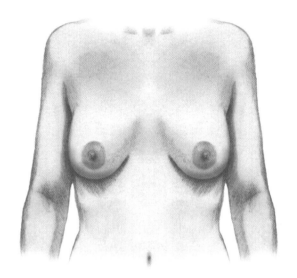

Lumpectomy Scar

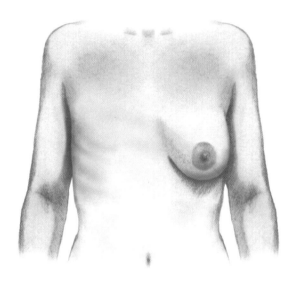

Right Mastectomy Scar

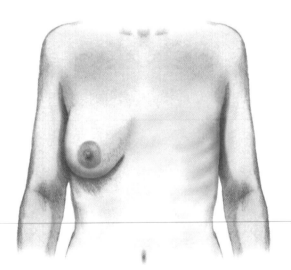

Left Mastectomy Scar

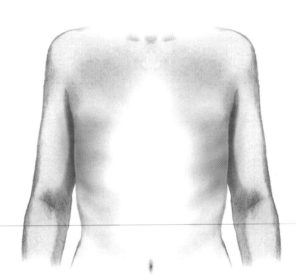

Bilateral Mastectomy Scars

SURGICAL DECISION EVALUATION

If you have been told that you are a candidate for a lumpectomy or a mastectomy, making the decision is often difficult. This self-questionnaire is designed to help you explore your innermost thoughts and desires about outcomes of the surgical options by choosing between two probing questions that only you can answer. Take this short assessment to help make a decision that agrees with your desired outcomes.

Answer the following questions to help uncover your true feelings. The statements are in pairs. Read both statements before you answer. **Choose only one answer between the two statements that best states how you feel at this time.** You will circle either A or B in the column on the right for each section.

A I would **resent** losing my breast. B. I would **accept** losing my breast.	A B
A. My breasts are **very important** to how I feel about my self-image. B. My breasts are **not that important** to how I feel about my self-image.	A B
A. My goal is to **preserve** my body image (breast), if possible. B. My goal is to **reduce my chances of local recurrence** (in breast) to the lowest level possible.	A B
A. **I don't want to lose my breast** and be required to wear a prosthesis or have reconstructive surgery. B. **I would rather lose my breast** to reduce the chance of recurrence to the lowest level.	A B
A. I would, **without increased anxiety,** perform breast self-exam or go for clinical exams on the lumpectomy breast. B. I would **worry** about recurrence in the remaining breast tissues after lumpectomy.	A B
A. **I'm not a worrier;** I would see my doctor as needed. B. **I would worry** about the cancer coming back in my remaining breast tissues.	A B
A. I would **agree** to go to radiation therapy five days a week for six to seven weeks to save my breast. B. I would **rather not** have to travel back to the hospital for six to seven weeks for radiation therapy.	A B
A. **I don't mind going to radiation** for six to seven weeks to keep my breast. B. I don't have time to keep going back to the hospital. **I want to get this over.**	A B
A. To keep my breast, I could **accept changes** after radiation therapy such as increased lumpiness and a decrease in size. B. I would **be anxious** about monitoring a breast that had lumpy changes after radiation.	A B
A. These changes (lumpiness, change in size) are **minor** compared to not having my breast. B. It would **overwhelm** me to feel my breast after having had cancer in it.	A B
A. I feel that my breast is **important** to my sexuality and self-esteem; without a breast I would feel less sexually attractive to my partner. B. My partner does **not care** if I have a breast or not; our relationship would not change if I lost my breast.	A B
A. **I do not think** I would ever feel sexy again without my breast. B. **I do think** I could feel sexy again without my breast.	A B

Add the number of A's and B's you selected. Total A's _____   Total B's _____

The highest number shows your inclination to prefer this type of surgical procedure:

A = Lumpectomy   B = Mastectomy

This is a guide, not the answer, as to your inclination toward surgical options.

If your initial choice is mastectomy, continue with questions about reconstruction on the next page.

RECONSTRUCTIVE DECISION EVALUATION

If your total for mastectomy had the higher number, or if you simply prefer mastectomy, you now need to consider your options for reconstructive surgery. Continue to choose between the two statements in the same manner.

A. I **would dislike** wearing an external prosthesis (breast form) daily. B. I **would rather** wear an external prosthesis than to have additional surgery.	A B
A. I **don't** want to have to wear a **prosthesis** because it would be a daily reminder of having lost my breast to cancer. I want my body image to be back to normal as soon as possible. B. I would **do anything to avoid** additional surgery.	A B
A. I **do** want to be able to wear low-cut clothing or go braless. B. I **don't** want to wear low-cut clothing or go braless.	A B
A. I **don't** want to have to wear a prosthesis to maintain my body image. B. I **would rather** wear a prothesis than have more surgery.	A B

Add the number of A's and B's you selected. Total A's _____ Total B's _____

Your inclination to prefer reconstruction or no reconstruction procedure: **A = Reconstruction B = Prosthesis**

Delayed or Immediate Reconstruction

A. I **would rather have time to recover** from my mastectomy and treatments before I have reconstructive surgery. B. I would **rather have all of my surgeries** performed at the time of my breast cancer surgery than to have to return after chemotherapy or radiation therapy.	A B
A. **Additional surgery is too much** to undergo when my anxiety is so high about my cancer. B. **Let's do it all now** and get it over with; I don't like putting things off that I need to do.	A B
A. I want to **take my time** finding a reconstructive surgeon and studying the different types of reconstructive surgery before I make a decision. B. I **understand** my reconstructive options and feel comfortable with the recommended reconstructive surgeon.	A B
A. Reconstructive surgery is too important to **make a fast decision** when I am overwhelmed about my cancer. B. Why should I have to **wait** to have my body image restored?	A B

Add the number of A's and B's you selected. Total A's _____ Total B's _____

Your inclination to prefer delayed or immediate reconstruction: **A = Delayed B = Immediate Reconstruction**

Remember, your decisions need to be made according to how **you feel** about the changes your surgical choice would have on you. Each option has advantages and disadvantages to consider. **Survival rates are equal.** Talk to a variety of healthcare professionals (surgeon, medical oncologist, radiation oncologist, plastic surgeon, nurse) and women about the types of surgeries to arrive at your final conclusion.

RECONSTRUCTIVE SURGERY QUESTIONS WORKSHEET

Check the questions you would like to have answered.
Tear out this sheet and take it to your reconstructive consultation.

Surgeon's Name _____ **Date** _____

- ☐ What type of reconstructive surgery do you recommend for me (autologous or implant)?

- ☐ If autologous (my own body tissues), which type of surgery do you recommend? (See reverse side of this sheet for descriptions of surgery types.)

- ☐ If an implant, what kind of implant do you recommend? Will the implant be placed under the muscle?

- ☐ What are the advantages and disadvantages of the recommended surgery?

- ☐ May I see photographs and talk to some of your patients?

- ☐ What can I expect to look like after surgery?

- ☐ Will you reconstruct my nipple and areola?

- ☐ How much feeling (sensation) will I have in my reconstructed breast?

- ☐ How will my breast feel when touched (soft, firm)?

- ☐ Will this surgery cause me to have additional scars?

- ☐ Will my surgery cause any restrictions on future physical activities (employment, sports or ability to exercise)?

- ☐ How many surgical procedures will my reconstruction require?

- ☐ How long will I be in surgery for each of these procedures?

- ☐ How long will I be in the hospital for each procedure?

- ☐ How often will I need a return appointment with you?

- ☐ How long will it take to complete the reconstruction process?

- ☐ How long before I can return to work or normal activities after each procedure?

- ☐ How much will it cost and how much should my insurance cover?

- ☐ In the future, what problems could potentially occur after reconstructive surgery?

Additional Questions _____

_____

_____

_____

_____

RECONSTRUCTIVE SURGERY OPTIONS

Comparison of Breast Reconstruction Procedures

TYPE	ADVANTAGES	DISADVANTAGES	RECOMMENDED FOR	NOT RECOMMENDED FOR
Tissue Expander and Implant	▪ Short surgical time ▪ Low initial cost	▪ Multiple fillings of expander with saline ▪ 2nd surgery for implant ▪ Capsular contracture ▪ Leakage or rupture	▪ Medium size breast (400 – 800 cc) ▪ Lumpectomy defect ▪ Tight skin from radiation therapy	▪ Previous radiation therapy may limit size
Fixed-Volume Implant Only (Saline or Silicone)	▪ Short surgical time ▪ One-step procedure ▪ Lower initial cost	▪ Capsular contracture ▪ Leakage or rupture	▪ Small breast (200 – 400 cc)	▪ Thin skin flaps ▪ Radiation therapy
Latissimus Dorsi Flap **(Pedicle Flap) Muscle and Tissue**	▪ Autologous tissues: skin, fat and muscle transfer ▪ Small donor scar on back	▪ Muscle weakness ▪ Potential seroma ▪ Flap necrosis risk (1%)	▪ Small to medium size breast (200 – 600 cc) ▪ Lumpectomy defect ▪ Tight skin from radiation therapy	
TAP Thoracodorsal Artery Perforator (Free Flap) Tissues Only	▪ Autologous tissues: skin and fat only ▪ No muscle removed ▪ Small donor scar	▪ Potential seroma ▪ Flap necrosis risk	▪ Small to medium sized breast (200 – 600 cc) ▪ Lumpectomy defect ▪ Tight skin from radiation therapy	▪ Extremely thin women
TRAM Flap Transverse Rectus Abdominis Myocutaneous (Pedicle Flap)	▪ Autologous tissues: skin, fat and muscle ▪ Pedicle flap ▪ Tummy tuck	▪ Scar on abdomen ▪ Muscle weakness ▪ Extended operative time ▪ 6 – 12 wks. recovery ▪ Abdominal wall hernia ▪ Flap necrosis risk	▪ Mastectomy	▪ Previous abdominal surgery or liposuction ▪ Certain physical conditions ▪ Cigarette smokers (some physicians)
DIEP Deep Interior Epigastric Perforator (Free Flap)	▪ Abdominal tissues: skin and fat only ▪ No muscle removed ▪ Potential return of nerve sensations in area	▪ Additional scar on abdomen ▪ Extended operative time from microscopic reattachment ▪ Flap necrosis risk	▪ Mastectomy	▪ Previous abdominal surgery or liposuction ▪ Certain physical conditions ▪ Cigarette smokers (some physicians) ▪ Extremely thin women
Inferior Gluteus Flap (Free Flap)	▪ Autologous tissues: muscle, fat and blood vessels removed from lower buttocks	▪ Scar at donor site ▪ 6 – 12 weeks recovery ▪ Extended surgical reattachment time ▪ Flap necrosis risk	▪ Mastectomy	▪ Cigarette smokers (some physicians) ▪ Extremely thin women
S-GAP Superior Gluteal Artery Perforator (Free Flap)	▪ Autologous tissues: skin and fat only ▪ No muscle removed ▪ Potential return of nerve sensations in area	▪ Scar at donor site ▪ Shorter recovery ▪ Extended surgical reattachment time ▪ Flap necrosis risk	▪ Mastectomy	▪ Cigarette smokers (some physicians) ▪ Extremely thin women ▪ Excessively heavy women

SURGICAL DISCHARGE QUESTIONS   WORKSHEET

Prior to leaving the hospital, your nurse will provide you with verbal and written instructions concerning your care. You will also receive a list of symptoms that might occur and need to be reported to the doctor. During your hospitalization, it may be helpful to write down any questions as they occur. When your doctor makes the final hospital visit, you may want to be prepared to clarify the following. Check the questions you wish to have answered.

- ☐ If you do not remember what your doctor said about your surgery or diagnosis the day you had surgery, ask for clarification.

- ☐ What activities should I avoid until my next appointment?

- ☐ Are there any special exercises or recommendations regarding the use of my arm?

- ☐ Will the numbness, tingling or sensations experienced be temporary or permanent?

- ☐ What type of pain is normal after my type of surgery?

- ☐ What medications will I take for pain?

- ☐ Will I be given any prescriptions for medication to take home?

- ☐ Do I resume previous medications (especially estrogen-type medications)?

- ☐ When can I shampoo my hair?

- ☐ When can I shower or take a tub bath?

- ☐ How do I care for my surgical dressing?

- ☐ When can I remove my surgical dressing?

- ☐ When can I drive?

- ☐ When do I need to make my next appointment?

- ☐ When will my drains (if present) be removed?

- ☐ When will I have sutures or stitches removed?

- ☐ Will I be referred to any other doctors or have any other treatments?

    If so, when will I see these doctors? Who will make the appointments?

- ☐ When will my pathology report be available?

- ☐ Is there anything that I can do to ensure a speedy recovery?

Ask your nurse to write down any appointment dates or names of doctors that you will be referred to for further evaluation concerning treatment.

Additional Questions _____

_____

_____

_____

SURGICAL DISCHARGE NOTES

DRAIN BULB RECORD

Measure and record drainage of bulb(s) each time you empty a drain.

Take this record to your physician.

Date	Time	Drain 1	Drain 2	Total

DRAIN BULB RECORD

Measure and record drainage of bulb(s) each time you empty a drain.
Take this record to your physician.

Date	Time	Drain 1	Drain 2	Total

MEDICAL ONCOLOGIST QUESTIONS

Your Medical Oncologist specializes in treatment of cancer using chemotherapy, hormonal and immunotherapy. Check the questions you would like to have answered.
Tear out this sheet and take it to your appointment with the oncologist.

Oncologist's Name: _____ **Date:** _____

My Treatment:

☐ What kind of treatment will I receive (chemotherapy, hormonal, immunotherapy)?

☐ On what schedule will I receive these treatments?

☐ How long will I receive treatments?

☐ How long will each treatment take?

☐ Where will I receive my treatments (office, clinic, hospital)?

☐ Can someone come with me when I receive my treatments?

☐ Will I feel like driving myself home after my treatment, or do I need a driver?

☐ Will any other tests be given before or while I receive my chemotherapy?

☐ Will I need radiation therapy?

☐ Do you have written information on my cancer or treatment plans?

Preparing for My Treatments:

☐ Should I eat before I come for my treatments?

☐ Can I take vitamins or herbs if I so choose?

During My Treatments:

☐ What side effects will I experience from the treatments (nausea, hair loss, changes in blood cell counts, etc.)?

☐ Will I be given medications to treat the side effects?

☐ What kind of protection precautions to my skin should I take during chemotherapy (exposure to sunlight)?

☐ When I complete my treatments, how often will I return for checkups?

☐ How will you evaluate the effectiveness of the treatments?

My Medications:

☐ What are the names of the drugs?

☐ Are the drugs given by mouth or into a vein?

☐ Will I need a port (device implanted under the skin) to receive any I.V. medications or will you use a vein in my arm?

Changes in My Body and Life:

☐ Will I continue to have menstrual periods? If not, when will they return?

☐ Should I use birth control? What type do you recommend?

☐ Will I be able to conceive and bear a child after treatment?

☐ What physical changes should I report to you or to your nurse during treatment?

☐ Can I continue my usual work or exercise schedules, or will I need to modify them during treatments?

☐ Are there any precautions my family should take to limit exposure to the chemotherapy during my treatments (shared eating utensils, bathroom facilities)?

Additional Questions _____

_____

MEDICAL ONCOLOGY CONSULTATION NOTES

RADIATION ONCOLOGIST QUESTIONS

WORKSHEET

A Radiation Oncologist treats cancer with radiation therapy.
Check the questions you would like to have answered.
Tear out this sheet and take it to your radiation consultation.

Physician's Name: _____ **Date:** _____

☐ How many radiation treatments will I receive?

☐ How long will my first visit take to mark the area?

☐ How do you mark the area that will be radiated?

☐ What kind of soap and bath do you recommend during my treatments?

☐ Is there anything that I can not use during my treatment (deodorant, perfume, lotions to the chest or back, etc.)?

☐ Can I wear a bra or my prosthesis during radiation treatments?

☐ Do you have written information on radiation therapy for the breast area?

☐ What side effects are considered normal during radiation therapy?

☐ What side effects, if they occur, should I report immediately?

☐ In the future, what changes could potentially occur in the radiated breast?

Additional Questions _____

_____

_____

_____

_____

_____

_____

W • 19

RADIATION ONCOLOGY CONSULTATION NOTES

PERSONAL HEALTHCARE PROVIDER RECORD

Primary Physician

Name

Telephone

Address

Nurse

Surgeon

Name

Telephone

Address

Nurse

Reconstructive Surgeon

Name

Telephone

Address

Nurse

Oncologist

Name

Telephone

Address

Nurse

Radiation Oncologist

Name

Telephone

Address

Nurse

Breast Health Navigator

Name

Telephone

Address

WORKSHEET

Personal Healthcare Provider Record

Breast Health Center

Name

Telephone

Address

Hospital

Name

Telephone

Address

Pharmacy

Name

Telephone

Address

Social Worker

Name

Telephone

Address

Support Group

Name

Telephone

Address

Other

Name

Telephone

Address

PERSONAL TREATMENT RECORD

Name _____ Diagnosis Date _____

Cancer Type _____ Tumor Size _____ Node Status _____

ER/PR Status _____ HER2_____ Oncotype DX® Score _____

Baseline Vital Signs: Blood Pressure _____ Pulse _____ Respirations _____ Weight _____

Allergies _____ Routine Medications _____

Surgery

Surgery Date: _____ Type: _____

Reconstructive Surgery Date: _____ Type: _____

Chemotherapy Treatments

Start Date: _____ End Date: _____

Name of Chemotherapy Drugs: Chemotherapy Treatment Dates:

_____   _____ _____ _____

_____   _____ _____ _____

_____   _____ _____ _____

_____   _____ _____ _____

_____   _____ _____ _____

_____   _____ _____ _____

Radiation Therapy

Start Date: _____ End Date: _____ Type: _____

Hormonal Therapy

Drug Name: _____ Start Date: _____ End Date: _____

Drug Name: _____ Start Date: _____ End Date: _____

Physical Therapy

Range of Motion: _____ Start Date: _____ End Date: _____

Lymphedema Treatment: _____ Start Date: _____ End Date: _____

PERSONAL TREATMENT RECORD

Chemotherapy Treatment Notes

_____
_____
_____
_____
_____
_____
_____
_____
_____
_____
_____
_____

Dates of Treatment

_____
_____
_____
_____
_____
_____
_____
_____
_____
_____
_____
_____

PATIENT APPOINTMENT REMINDER   WORKSHEET

Tear this worksheet out and place it where you can easily write down questions between visits.

Next Scheduled Appointment

Physician _____ **Date** _____ **Time** _____

It is helpful to write down questions for your nurse or physician prior to your visit.
It is also helpful to keep a list of thoughts which need to be communicated to your healthcare team.

Questions to ask physician _____

_____
_____
_____
_____
_____
_____
_____
_____

Questions to ask nurse _____

_____
_____
_____
_____
_____
_____
_____
_____

Remember to tell physician/nurse _____

_____
_____
_____
_____
_____
_____
_____

PATIENT APPOINTMENT REMINDER

Next Scheduled Appointment

Physician _____ **Date** _____ **Time** _____

It is helpful to write down questions for your nurse or physician prior to your visit.
It is also helpful to keep a list of thoughts which need to be communicated to your healthcare team.

Questions to ask physician _____

_____

_____

_____

_____

_____

_____

_____

_____

Questions to ask nurse _____

_____

_____

_____

_____

_____

_____

_____

_____

Remember to tell physician/nurse _____

_____

_____

_____

_____

_____

PERSONAL PLAN FOR RECOVERY

Take the time to plan steps of action in every area of your life for maximum recovery. Inventory your life and make the adjustments you feel will restore a sense of control.

Support System

Personal: Identify at least two people you can talk to openly.

I can talk to: _____ and _____

Information: Identify sources of correct information on breast cancer.
Check the resource section of this book.

Physician: _____ Phone: _____

Physician: _____ Phone: _____

Nurse: _____ Phone: _____

Organization: _____ Phone: _____

Organization: _____ Phone: _____

Organization: _____ Phone: _____

Organization: _____ Phone: _____

Support: Identify your local support groups by calling the American Cancer Society.

Breast Cancer Patients: _____ Phone: _____

Support Partner Groups: _____ Phone: _____

Children's Classes: _____ Phone: _____

Spiritual: Identify people who can help you deal with the spiritual aspects of your illness.

_____ Phone: _____

_____ Phone: _____

_____ Phone: _____

"Planning is like a road map.

It can show us the way and head us in the right direction and keep us on course.

Planning means mapping out how to get from here to where we want to be.

Planning is the power tool for achievement, the magic bridge to our goals and our success."

—Wynn Davis

PERSONAL PLAN FOR RECOVERY

☐ **Fears:** Name your fears and plan steps of action to address them. Complete the Fear Management worksheet on page W • 3.

☐ **Diet:** Evaluate your diet.

I plan to make the following changes: _____

☐ **Exercise:** Plan a program of exercise to restore and maintain your physical condition.

I plan to: _____

I will check with my doctor about starting my exercise program: (date) _____

I am starting an exercise program: (date) _____

I am going to ask (person) to join me: _____

☐ **Personal Appearance:** Make plans to enhance your self-esteem and personal appearance during treatment. If taking chemotherapy, check out a "Look Good...Feel Better" class, sponsored by the American Cancer Society.

I plan to: _____

☐ **Time Management:** Plan to make lifestyle changes: (Employment, Social, Civic duties)

I plan to start: _____

I plan to stop: _____

☐ **Family Management:** Make changes in your household.

I need to delegate chores for: _____

I need to hire help for: _____

I need to stop doing: _____

☐ **Personal Fulfillment:** Think of things you want to do more of or things you want to begin to do. Think selfishly. You deserve it!

I want to add the following goals, hobbies or pleasurable events to my life.

I plan to: _____

_____

☐ **Reaching Out:** A spirit of gratefulness and an effort on your part to help others is very rewarding. Plan to say "thank-you" to those who play an important part in your life and recovery. Plan to give back to others who are in need.

People to write or thank: _____

Things I would like to do to help others: _____

Congratulations!
You have just taken steps to plan your psychological and social recovery.
Refer to this sheet when in doubt of what you can do to speed your recovery.

HEALTHCARE SYMPTOMS RECORD

WORKSHEET

Your physician needs to know about changes in your health. Use this chart to record any symptoms you have experienced since your last visit. Take the chart with you to your checkup to help you remember which symptoms to report.

General Symptoms	Date	Date	Date	Date
Fever or chills				
Fatigue				
Dizzy/Fainting				
Headaches				
Vision Change				
Weight loss				
Weight gain				
Numb hands/feet				
Hot flashes				
Night sweats				
Nervousness				
Depression				
Forgetfulness				
Vaginal dryness				
Sexual changes				
Can't sleep				
Poor appetite				
Pain (# and location)				
Gastrointestinal				
Nausea				
Vomiting				
Indigestion				
Constipation				
Diarrhea				
Stomach pain				
Stomach swelling				
Blood in stool				
Problems swallowing				
Urinary				
Painful/frequent urination				
Inability to control urine				
Blood in urine				
Respiratory				
Shortness of breath				
Chest pain				
Cough				
Breast/Chest Wall				
Lump, discharge, rash				
Pain				

HEALTHCARE SYMPTOMS RECORD

Your physician needs to know about changes in your health. Use this chart to record any symptoms you have experienced since your last visit. Take the chart with you to your checkup to help you remember which symptoms to report.

General Symptoms	Date	Date	Date	Date
Fever or chills				
Fatigue				
Dizzy/Fainting				
Headaches				
Vision Change				
Weight loss				
Weight gain				
Numb hands/feet				
Hot flashes				
Night sweats				
Nervousness				
Depression				
Forgetfulness				
Vaginal dryness				
Sexual changes				
Can't sleep				
Poor appetite				
Pain (# and location)				
Gastrointestinal				
Nausea				
Vomiting				
Indigestion				
Constipation				
Diarrhea				
Stomach pain				
Stomach swelling				
Blood in stool				
Problems swallowing				
Urinary				
Painful/frequent urination				
Inability to control urine				
Blood in urine				
Respiratory				
Shortness of breath				
Chest pain				
Cough				
Breast/Chest Wall				
Lump, discharge, rash				
Pain				

PATIENT TREATMENT BARRIERS ASSESSMENT   WORKSHEET

Patient Name: _____ **Date:** _____

Listed below are obstacles (barriers) that may prevent you from getting the healthcare you need during your cancer treatment. It is essential that your healthcare team understand your needs. This sheet has been designed to help you identify your current situation. Please read the following list and mark the items that identify your present situation. Return this sheet to the physician or nurse in charge of your care.

Communication

☐ Primary language other than English   Language: _____

☐ Cannot read or write

☐ Hearing Obstacle: ○ Hard of Hearing   ○ Hearing Aid   ○ Deaf

☐ Vision Obstacle: ○ Vision impairment   ○ Blind

☐ Problems understanding medical language

☐ Problems filling out medical forms

☐ No telephone

☐ No permanent address

☐ Other:_____

Financial

☐ Insurance: ○ No Insurance ○ Underinsured

☐ Pre-existing financial debts or obligations impacting decisions

☐ No funds for food

☐ No paid leave from work for illness

☐ Prescription medication assistance needed

☐ Medical equipment or supplies assistance needed

☐ Other: _____

Transportation

☐ No transportation available

☐ Public transportation needed

☐ No funds for public transportation

☐ Other: _____

Family Care

☐ Child care during treatment needed

☐ Responsible for older adults living in my home

☐ Housing

☐ Other: _____

PATIENT TREATMENT BARRIERS ASSESSMENT

Personal Care

☐ Need home care assistance for eating, bathing, dressing, toileting and/or walking

☐ Need prosthesis

☐ Need wig

☐ Need medical equipment

☐ Need help with nutrition

☐ Need help learning new job skills

☐ Other: _____

Coping

☐ I have a history of coping difficulties (depression or anxiety).

☐ I am presently under the care of a: ○ Counselor ○ Psychologist ○ Psychiatrist

☐ I have no personal support system at home.

☐ I would like to speak with a spiritual leader. My faith: _____

☐ I am concerned about the impact of my diagnosis on my present career or occupation.

☐ Other: _____

Treatment

☐ I would like a second opinion.

☐ I do not understand how treatment decisions will be made.

☐ I do not understand my treatment plan recommendation.

☐ I have religious beliefs that need to be considered by my healthcare team during treatment:

  ○ Blood transfusions   ○ Narcotics for pain control   ○ Other: _____
  ○ Medications containing alcohol   ○ Abortion

☐ I have questions that I need answered by a: ○ Doctor ○ Nurse

☐ Other: _____

Cultural

☐ I have citizenship problems.

☐ Other:_____

SURVIVORSHIP SURVEILLANCE GUIDELINES — WORKSHEET

You have completed your treatment for breast cancer. To monitor your future health, your healthcare team will recommend a follow-up schedule for physician visits and screening tests. It is important to understand when you are to return to your physician for your healthcare check-ups. The American Society of Clinical Oncology (ASCO) recommends surveillance guidelines for breast cancer patients after completion of treatment. Your surveillance may be conducted by your oncologist or a primary care physician.

Physician Surveillance Visits

Physician who will provide follow-up surveillance after cancer treatment:

☐ **Medical Oncologist**   Name:_____   Telephone:_____

☐ **Primary Physician**   Name:_____   Telephone:_____

☐ **Other:**_____

Recommended Physician Visit Schedule:
(Ask someone on your healthcare team to mark the appropriate surveillance recommendations.)

1 – 3 years past treatment   ☐ every 3 months   ☐ every 4 months   ☐ every 6 months   ☐ other:_____

4 – 5 years past treatment   ☐ every 3 months   ☐ every 4 months   ☐ every 6 months   ☐ yearly

6 years or more past treatment ☐ every year   ☐ other:_____

Returning to your physician for a physical exam and update of your history is the most important thing you can do to protect your future health. It has been proven that a physician's exam and review of your recent physical changes is the number one way that most recurrences are detected. Make the most of this opportunity by preparing to report any changes you have experienced since your last exam. Write down any changes you experience so that you don't forget. Report these changes early in the visit so your physician will have time to further evaluate the change.

During your physical exam, your doctor will look for any physical changes that relate to your general health and/or any symptoms that may suggest your cancer has recurred locally or spread to another part of your body (systemic disease). In addition to performing a careful breast exam, your doctor will closely examine your entire chest wall and check for lymph node enlargement in other areas of your body. Your heart and lungs will be listed to, and your abdomen, liver, spleen, neck and other areas will be checked for swelling or tenderness. Your neurological (nerve) functioning will also be checked by the physician for signs associated with recurrence.

Surveillance Recommendations

Breast Self-Exam   (Ask for written instructions if you do not know how to perform.)

Mammography   ☐ every 6 months   ☐ yearly   ☐ not needed   ☐ other:_____

Pelvic Examination   ☐ yearly   ☐ every 2 years   ☐ every 3 - 5 years   ☐ other:_____

Bone Density Scan   ☐ yearly   ☐ every 2 years   ☐ every 3 - 5 years   ☐ other:_____

Diagnostic Testing   (MRI, PET, CAT Scan, Chest X-ray, Bone Scan, Ultrasound, etc.)
Tests are now recommended for surveillance testing **only** when you have symptoms that indicate a need. Your physician will order test when needed.

SURVIVORSHIP SURVEILLANCE GUIDELINES

Symptoms to Report to Physician: Breast or Chest Wall Changes

- Change in size, shape or contour of the lumpectomy breast or non-surgical breast

- Nipple discharge that is clear or bloody from the lumpectomy breast or non-surgical breast

- Nipple inversion on lumpectomy breast or non-surgical breast

- A new lump that may feel like a small pea in lumpectomy breast, non-surgical breast or on chest wall

- Thickening in breast tissues or on the chest wall after mastectomy

- Changes in the skin: dimpling (pulling in of skin), scaly appearance, orange peel appearance, rash, redness or discoloration on lumpectomy breast, non-surgical breast or chest wall

- A lump in the underarm area

Symptoms to Report to Physician: Body or General Health Changes

- New lump or thickening in area above the collarbone

- Chronic bone pain or tenderness in an area

- Chest pain with shortness of breath

- Chronic cough

- Persistent abdominal pain or abdominal swelling

- Headaches, dizziness, fainting or rapid changes in vision

- Increasing fatigue unrelated to treatments

- Inability to control urine or bowels

- Persistent nausea or loss of appetite

- Changes in weight, especially weight loss

Do not hesitate to report any other changes you observe to your physician. The most common way recurrence is discovered is when a patient reports symptoms or changes she has experienced. Don't ignore any change as being unimportant. Instead, let your physician or nurse make the decision. What may seem unimportant to you may be important to your healthcare team.

Thankfulness In My Circumstances

Today is another new day. I can choose to reflect on the things that I have lost, or I can choose to reflect on the reasons I still have to be thankful.

I am thankful for:

- The diagnosis of cancer instead of a fatal heart attack, because I prefer to live.
- The alarm clock that jolts me awake in the morning, because it means I am still alive.
- The cold floor under my feet, because I can still get out of bed on my own.
- The dirty dishes after breakfast, because my family and I have food to eat.
- The mounds of dirty laundry in the basket, because I am surrounded by people I love.
- The telephone that doesn't stop ringing, because I have friends who care about how I am doing.
- The covering of dust on my furniture, because I can still see.
- The lawn that needs mowing and the house that needs painting, because I have a home.
- The bills that I drop in the mailbox almost daily, because I still have an income.
- The doctor's appointment I have to make this afternoon, because I live in a country where I can receive medical care.
- The prosthesis that hugs my chest, because it reminds me that I am a survivor and not a statistic of breast cancer.
- The too-thin hair on my head, because there are treatments for my disease.
- The clothes that clinch my thighs and hug my waist after my weight gain, because I can still eat.
- The parking place finally located at the top of the medical parking garage, because I can still walk.
- The shadow that trails behind me as I walk to the office, because I can be out in the sunshine.
- The long wait in the doctor's office, because I am not a hospitalized or homebound patient.
- The waiting room conversation complaining about high medical costs, because I live in a country with free speech.
- The repetitive blood draws I face, because I am still a candidate for treatment.
- The nurse's questions about my health over the past weeks, because I can still remember.
- The doctor's cold stethoscope on my chest, because I can still feel.
- The news about my blood work, because I can still experience hope.
- The insurance paperwork, because I have financial help with my medical bills.
- The overwhelming exhaustion I feel as I fall into bed at the end of the day, because it means I have been alive and productive for another day.
- The nighttime prayer I whisper, because I have a God who still cares about me.

My blessings may come in disguise, but I cherish every one of them.

—Judy Kneece, RN, OCN

Becoming a Cancer Survivalist

American Heritage Dictionary defines a **Survivalist** as: *"One who has personal survival as a primary goal in the face of difficulty, opposition and especially the threat of a natural catastrophe (death)."* Survivalists take a difficult situation and somehow manage to turn it into a challenge instead of a defeat. Survivalists learn to maximize the positives in their lives and deal with the negatives.

Survivalists are realistic. They accept their cancer diagnosis but refuse to accept it as an automatic death sentence. Rather, they view it as a caution light, warning them to take actions to better manage their health and build an even better quality of life.

Survivalists refuse to adopt the helpless, hopeless victim cliché. They are determined to influence their illness and consequently, their future. They know that what they do can make a difference.

Survivalists know that coping and emerging from this disease means admitting their physical, mental and spiritual needs. Recovery means more than drugs and surgery. It also means facing the toughest demons—fear, anxiety and depression—and latching onto help when needed.

Survivalists feel responsible for their health. They depend on their physician, not as a dictator, but as a partner in recovery.

Survivalists reach out for valuable support—with partners, family, friends, support groups and healthcare professionals. They seek help without feelings of guilt, shame or inadequacy. They know that this is one of the most precious parts of being human—people helping people.

Survivalists take care of their bodies. They eat what is healthy, exercise regularly, get adequate rest, eliminate smoking, monitor alcohol intake and smile often.

Survivalists pay attention to the mental pollutants that seep into their lives. They identify their sources of stress. They learn how to modify the things they can and accept the things they cannot change.

Survivalists indulge themselves by saying "no" to those things that feel uncomfortable and "yes" to those things that feel good and right. They liberate themselves from stressful or unproductive situations and work to create pleasurable ones.

Survivalists apply their spiritual faith to make sense of suffering and find meaning and purpose to their situation.

Survivalists are grateful. They invest time identifying their blessings. They share their love and appreciation generously and often with those who have blessed their lives.

Survivalists refuse to carry around the emotional baggage of resentment, anger, bitterness, envy or jealousy. They know that these things can only drag them down as they struggle to recover. Therefore, they abandon the things that make them powerless. They release others from the bondage of their expectations.

Survivalists know that life and death are inevitable and that both are business issues, so they take action. That includes preparing a will, a medical power of attorney, instructions for personal property, end of life directives (living will), and having frank discussions with family members about these decisions.

Survivalists give back to others who are struggling with the same challenges. They encourage, they teach, they support, they provide hope and they share what they have learned. They volunteer to make life better for others. They believe that a shared trial is half a trial and that a shared joy is a double joy.

Survivalists do not postpone happiness. They know that only this minute is guaranteed to anyone. They know that joy is not dependent on circumstances, but on how they view them. Joy is a product of the mind and not circumstances.

—Judy Kneece, RN, OCN